Speaking of
How to Prevent Common Diseases

Dr. Ajit S. Puri did his MBBS, MD (in Clinical Medicine) from the Government Medical College at Amritsar and Patiala — He received training in various specializations of cardiology, allergy and applied immunology, diabetes, and also neurology in the UK. He was awarded fellowships from the Indian College of Allergy and Applied Immunology, the Indian College of Physicians, the International College of Angiology in the USA; life membership of the Association of Physicians of India, Cardiological Society of India, and founder membership of the Geriatric Society of India. He has worked in several recognized positions both in India and abroad. Presently he is working as Senior Consultant, Department of Medicine, Mohan Dai Oswal Cancer Treatment and Research Foundation, Ludhiana in India. Dr. Puri has presented papers at important medical conferences and published articles in medical journals both in India and abroad. He has also contributed monographs on diabetes, hypertension, emergency medical treatment, warning signals of diseases, heart diseases (in vernacular), urinary tract infection, high blood uric acid, and has given radio/TV talks on some of these problems here and in other countries.

Dr. Puri has visited the UK, the USA, Switzerland, Canada, Sri Lanka, Nepal, Holland, Austria, West Germany, Belgium, Italy, France, Luxembourg, many a time, in pursuit of his mission for creating mass realization and to widen his horizons in the areas of his specialization. He was also invited to Japan in connection with his mission. He has participated in important meetings, seminars, clinical meetings of the General Medical Council, London; the Jephcott Lecture and Reception of the Royal Society of Medicine in London; the Autumn Scientific Meeting of the North of England Neurological Association, and has worked as a visiting member of faculty at the Newcastle General Hospital in UK. Dr. Puri has also visited various foreign universities, hospitals — the George Washington University Hospital (USA), University of Newcastle upon Tyne, the Charing Cross Hospital London, the University of Sheffield (UK), the University of Colombo (Sri Lanka), the Toronto General Hospital (Canada), and has interacted with noted medical specialists on important medical topics.

The author has a wide experience of over a span of three decades in the early detection, prevention and treatment of common serious diseases. He has worked assiduously in various fields of medicine in India and abroad. The significance of his pioneering work lies in creating mass consciousness regarding some of the fatal diseases which afflict mankind.

"... admirable press releases ... congratulations on this excellent publication."

Lord Walton of Detchant
(UK)

"We are recommending your book to several American institutions ..."

R. R. Dash
Counsellor (Health)
Embassy of India
Washington, USA

"... written in simple, clear language ... will be a great help to people in the health fields."

Sr. M. Nirmala
Missionaries of Charity
Calcutta, India

"If prevention of illness is indeed better than cure, then this book is certainly an excellent guide to good living for the common man."

The Observer

"... first ever book on preventive medicine based on clinical approach ... renewed international action about disease prevention, especially stresses the urgent need for global awareness programme for halting the spread of common but fatal diseases-many of which kill human beings silently, and the book has been acclaimed world wide for enlightening world citizens to lead a reasonable disease-free life."

The Indian Express

Your Health Guide

speaking of
How to Prevent Common Diseases

AJIT S. PURI
MD, DSc. (Honoris Causa), **FICP, FCAI, FICA**

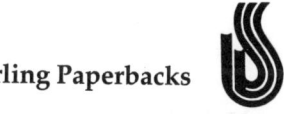

Sterling Paperbacks

STERLING PAPERBACKS
An imprint of
Sterling Publishers (P) Ltd.
A-59, Okhla Industrial Area, Phase-II,
New Delhi-110020.
Tel: 26387070, 26386209; Fax: 91-11-26383788
E-mail: sterlingpublishers@airtelbroadband.in
ghai@nde.vsnl.net.in
www.sterlingpublishers.com

Speaking of
How to Prevent Common Diseases

©2007, Ajit S. Puri

ISBN 978 81 207 3466 1

First Edition 2000

Second Revised Edition 2001

Third Revised Edition 2007

All rights are reserved. No part of this publication may be reproduced, stored in a retrieval system or transmitted, in any form or by any means, mechanical, photocopying, recording or otherwise, without prior written permission of the original publisher.

Published by Sterling Publishers Pvt. Ltd., New Delhi-110020.

*Dedicated to the memory of Mother Teresa
for her love of the poor and the sick*

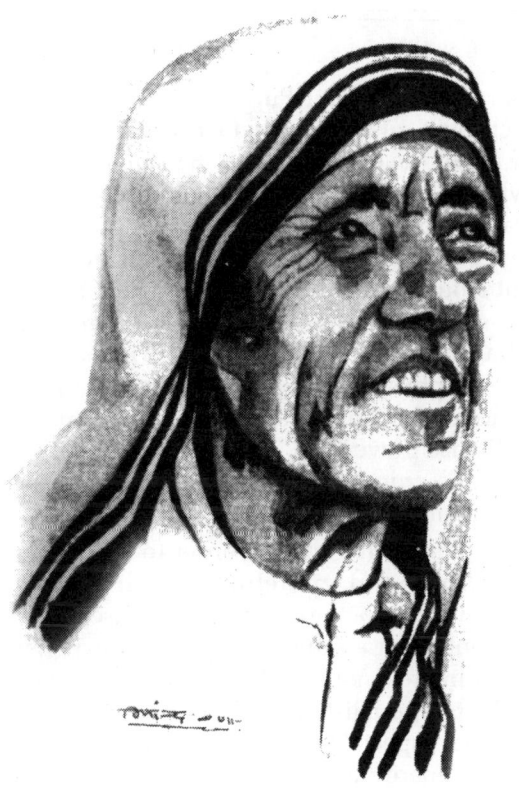

This book is a humble tribute to the apostle of love and peace, **Mother Teresa**, who devoted her life to redirect the destiny of those suffering and struck by terminal illnesses. It seeks to enhance the level of mass awareness, irrespective of age, religion, country, economic status, in relation to the early detection, prevention and treatment of common but lethal diseases.

FOREWORD

It is many years since Dr. Ajit Puri first wrote to me, having consulted a neurological textbook which I had written, asking for my advice about the diagnosis and management of some of his patients who had presented to him with difficult diagnostic problems. I was happy to respond as best as I could at a distance, and later enjoyed meeting with him, first at his brother's home in Government House, Bombay, in 1971, and then later on more than one occasion when he visited London. From all my talks with him, I have recognised that Dr. Puri is a dedicated, enthusiastic, caring physician. He believes, properly, that clinical medicine is concerned not just with diagnosis and management but also with disease prevention, and he also emphasises in the following pages the crucial importance of activities concerned primarily with community health.

Dr. Puri has written this book in order to draw attention to important principles and guidelines relating to the early diagnosis and prevention of the commoner diseases which afflict mankind. The book is based upon his personal experience and will plainly be of interest not only to family physicians but also to medical students, specialist physicians and others working in the healthcare field, especially in the community. I congratulate Dr. Puri upon his energy and initiative and am glad to know that he has dedicated the book to the late Mother Teresa, who did so much throughout her life for the under-privileged.

Oxford   Lord Walton of Detchant
                                                    TD, MA, MD, DSc, FRCP

Former Professor of Neurology and Dean of Medicine, University of Newcastle upon Tyne; former President, British Medical Association, Royal Society of Medicine and General Medical Council; former Warden, Green College, Oxford; former President, World Federation of Neurology.

PREFACE TO THE THIRD EDITION

The book has been primarily written for early diagnosis, prevention and treatment of common but fatal diseases so that such diseases could be diagnosed and/or prevented in infancy and the individual is saved from its serious and fatal complications.

The book proved enlightening and useful. Its first two editions have been acclaimed worldwide in 36 countries.

For this edition I have rethought the whole text to update its contents. Each chapter has been revised, some sections have been rewritten and there have been numerous additions and alterations.

There has been a constant exchange of views with world acclaimed medical authorities of different countries. Besides mentioning the discussions on varied topics in different chapters of the book in previous editions, one discussion has been added to the chapter on kidney under the sub-head urinary tract infection- benign enlargement of the prostate.

Likewise, another unusual manifestation of hypothyroidism, a rare case, earlier reported from Ukraine has been included in the chapter on the thyroid gland.

The last chapter on exercise has been revised and expanded.

The book has been appreciated by the World Health Organization (WHO). Dr. B.P. Kean, Director, External Cooperation and Partnerships, WHO, Geneva, Switzerland conveyed the collective comments that have been printed on the back of the jacket. The WHO team has placed the book at the international level.

For constant encouragement, I owe my gratitude to Lord Walton, former President of the British Medical Association and Royal Society of Medicine who also wrote the foreword to this book. I am glad to mention that in his letter of November 21, 2006 he wrote: "I was happy to write a foreword for your original book on *How to Prevent Common Serious Diseases*".

Presentation of the book to the noted personalities of India and abroad continued with press coverage that helped in propagating the aim of the book. After presentation to the Vice-President of India, Ms. Maneka Gandhi, a noted human and animal rights activist, and to some governors of the Indian states, the book was presented to the present Prime Minister of India, Dr. Manmohan Singh. The event was highlighted through the Press Information Bureau, Government of India on the internet.

The book was presented to the Chief Minister of Delhi Ms. Sheila Dixit, the Prince of Wales and the Duchess of Cornwall during their visit to Patiala, and also to Chaudhary Pervaiz Elahi, Pakistan Chief Minister of Punjab, on his visit to Patiala. I am grateful to Capt. Amrinder Singh, Indian Chief Minister of Punjab, for his presence during various presentations. I am equally grateful to S. Tejveer Singh, IAS, Deputy Commissioner of Patiala and journalist Jaswant Singh Puri for their active participation in various book presentations.

As mentioned in the earlier editions, I am highly thankful to my various friends both in India and abroad for their continued help for the completion of this book. My thanks are also due to Sterling Publishers for their cooperation.

Patiala   AJIT S. PURI
India

PREFACE TO THE FIRST EDITION

Health is the soul that animates
all the enjoyments of life
which fade and are tasteless without it.

Sir W. Temple

It is important to prevent, diagnose and treat, at the earliest, various serious disorders, especially the occult/hidden diseases, which are likely to go unnoticed in the beginning for various reasons, and which may surface when they have already reached an advanced stage. At such a stage, the treatment of such diseases can be costly or prohibitive anywhere, and at that point the disease may yet be fatal. Some of such diseases may be listed as: cancers, heart/lung diseases, diabetes, high blood pressure, high blood cholesterol/uric acid, neurological/abdominal/thyroid gland disorders, diseases of the kidneys, etc.

It may be emphasized that for an early diagnosis of such diseases, it is always important to carry out various tests and examinations of both adults and children at regular intervals. For this purpose medical camps need to be organized. It comes under the head, 'Clinical Epidemiology', i.e. the science dealing with the prevalence of diseases in a defined population through population surveys. It is a handy tool for the prevention of various serious diseases, especially the occult ones.

In a clinical epidemiology session of the Joint Annual Conference of the Association of Physicians of India, held at Guwahati, January 1994 and at New Delhi, January 2001, I had the privilege to participate and elaborate my views. It was stressed that there was no way out except for an epidemiological study of various diseases to prevent the spread among the masses. Some of the medical camps that were organized by me, yielded fruitful results in this regard.

In this book, important guidelines for early and effective control of some of the fatal diseases are given. I feel that it is important that such vital information reaches all concerned, and that people take appropriate timely steps to prevent the occurrence of serious diseases.

It hardly needs stressing that one should not be afraid of the knowledge of the early warning signals/symptoms of various deadly diseases. As has been aptly remarked, "The real tragedy of life is when men are afraid of the Light". Hence, the significance of urgent understanding and attention in respect of various lethal diseases, that are a potential threat to human life and happiness, cannot be ignored.

It may be averred that the prevention and cure of fatal diseases is essentially a corporate endeavour involving both the patient and the physician.

I am grateful to the distinguished medical personalities of the various countries, mentioned in the text, with whom I had discussions on varied topics which indeed proved valuable in preparing this book. Still more, I am indebted to Lord Walton (U.K.) for kindly writing the foreword of this book, and who has been a guiding spirit for more than three decades in my mission.

I also owe thanks to various outstanding bodies/personalities like the WHO, the UN, the President of the Swiss Confederation, the Counsellor of the Government of Romania etc. for showing a keen interest in disseminating information regarding this book.

I am equally grateful to my various friends both in India and abroad who have helped me in this task at its various stages.

Patiala   AJIT S. PURI
India

What we know here is very little;
But what we are ignorant of is immense.
                                                    -de Laplace

CONTENTS

Foreword	vi
Preface to the Third Edition	vii
Preface to the First Edition	ix

1.	Cancers and Their Prevention	1
2.	Diseases of the Heart	21
3.	Diabetes	60
4.	High Blood Pressure (Hypertension)	74
5.	High Blood Cholesterol	79
6.	High Blood Uric Acid	84
7.	Stroke, Epilepsy, Poliomyelitis (Diseases of the Nervous System)	90
8.	Tuberculosis	125
9.	Allergy and Bronchial Asthma	151
10.	Diseases of the Abdomen and Ultrasonography	164
11.	Diseases of the Kidneys	169
12.	Diseases of the Thyroid Gland	219
13.	Tropical Diseases	235
14.	Leprosy	272
15.	AIDS and Other Sexually - Transmitted Diseases	273
16.	Diseases of Old Age	277

Appendices

I.	Smoking and Tobacco Chewing-Related Diseases	287
II.	Alcohol and Diseases	289
III.	Obesity and Diseases	292
IV.	Sudden Cardiac Death (SCD)	294
V.	Urgent Tests for the Detection of Various Common Serious Diseases	296
VI.	Urgent Tips: First Aid for Prevention / Immediate Control of Some Common Serious Diseases	300
VII.	Urgent Dietary Measures for the Prevention of Common Serious Diseases	310
VIII.	Exercise — for the Prevention/Treatment of Common Serious Diseases	314
	Index	317

1
CANCERS AND THEIR PREVENTION

Cancers are growths which may develop in any part of the body. Their exact cause is still unknown. The growth spreads locally and soon to distant organs, either by blood or lymphatics.

An early diagnosis is of paramount necessity in the treatment of such malignant disorders. Cancerous growth is usually painless in the beginning. By the time the patient seeks medical advice, the disease might have reached an advanced stage. Hence, it is highly desirable to detect the early growth of cancerous origin before it is too late. It is axiomatic then that an early detection is of the utmost importance to ensure recovery. Broadly speaking, the following are the major warning signals:

1. Persistently troublesome cough; blood in sputum; unusually hoarse voice.
2. Persistent indigestion, difficulty in swallowing.
3. Continuous pain in abdomen — gastric/duodenal peptic ulcer; inflamed gallbladder (cholecystitis) /gallstones (cholelithiasis).
4. Change in bowel habits (i.e. alternating constipation and diarrhoea); blood in stool.
5. Thickening/lump in breast or anywhere else; bleeding or discharging from nipple.
6. Nodule/lump or change in the size of testis; swelling or feeling of heaviness/discomfort in testis.
7. Swelling/nodule in connection with thyroid/parotid gland.
8. Blood in urine; change in bladder habits (see later at page 5).

9. Unusual vaginal bleeding or discharge; contact bleeding after intercourse.
10. Severe recurrent headaches with or without vomiting, particularly worsening while coughing or bending forward and downward; epileptic fits; neurological deficits or unexplained psychological symptoms as detailed on page 7, under the head 'brain tumours'.
11. A skin/mouth sore/ulcer that does not heal; old scar that repeatedly heals and breaks down.
12. Obvious change in wart, mole, birthmark or any other spot on the skin.
13. Glandular swelling/s in the neck, armpit or groin, etc.
14. Persistent pallor of eyes (jaundice).
15. Unexpected bleeding anywhere in the body.
16. Loss of weight without any obvious cause.
17. Unexplained low grade fever, or loss of appetite.

The above signals may be elaborated further so that they become clear to the masses:

1. Persistent cough, blood in sputum

For persistent cough, blood in sputum of recent origin in a middle-aged person, suspect cancer of the lungs (bronchogenic carcinoma). Another equally important cause is lung tuberculosis which should be suspected irrespective of age.

2. Unusual hoarseness

Unusually hoarse voice that does not completely respond to usual medical treatment may be a signal of some growth in the larynx which may be either benign (papilloma) or malignant. However, tuberculosis of the larynx is another important cause of hoarseness and it is usually secondary to pulmonary tuberculosis which may remain unrecognized, i.e., the symptoms of laryngeal tuberculosis may precede the symptoms of lung tuberculosis. Under any circumstances, immediate services of an ENT specialist must be availed of for laryngoscopy/precise diagnosis since laryngeal tuberculosis and carcinoma may stimulate each other, both in signs and symptoms, and a delay in diagnosis may prove distressing.

3. Persistent indigestion

For persistent indigestion (dyspepsia) of a vague type (i.e. when the pain in abdomen has no relation to meals as in peptic ulcer discussed at serial 5), loss of appetite, loss of weight in a middle-aged person, suspect carcinoma of the stomach. It is generally between 3-6 months after the onset of symptoms that the patient seeks medical advice.

4. Difficulty in swallowing

For progressive difficulty in swallowing (dysphagia) in a middle-aged person, suspect carcinoma of the oesophagus (food-pipe). Or, there could be cancer of the pharynx. Some usual notable causes of dysphagia are anaemia, foreign body, inflammatory stricture, hysteria, especially in women. Medical students need to understand that cancer predisposing condition like Barrett's oesophagus resulting from recurrent oesophagitis (inflammation of oesophagus) ought to be prevented. Selected cases should undergo oesophgoscopy test once or more times as the case may be so that early appropriate steps could be taken well in time. Neglected cases may develop adenocarcinoma of the oesophagus.

5. Gastric/duodenal peptic ulcer

For pain in the upper part of the abdomen, half an hour to an hour after meals, suspect gastric peptic ulcer. If there is pain in the same region, 1.5-3 hours after meals, and it is relieved only when the patient eats something (said to be hunger pain), suspect duodenal peptic ulcer. Although malignancy in duodenal ulcer (DU) is not common but gastric ulcer (GU) can silently develop a gastric carcinoma. Urgent treatment of GU must be carried out and the offending organism H. pylori eradicated with suitable antibiotics. One needs to live in good sanitary conditions, avoid infected food/water for the prevention of H. pylori infection. Better socioeconomic status helps. Non-steroidal anti-inflammatory drugs (NSAIDS) may cause peptic ulcer disease (PUD) and should be avoided especially in cases that have previous history of PUD, are smokers and/or alcoholics. The drugs are so notorious that they may cause serious complications of PUD including bleeding / perforation of gut and many a time without any preceding symptoms.

6. Inflamed gallbladder/gallstones

People who get an attack of acute cholecystitis (inflamed gallbladder) in which there is an acute pain in the right upper part of the abdomen should not delay surgical intervention for removing the gallbladder after the medicinal treatment is over, as such a gallbladder is always prone to malignant change. The prevention of the cancer of the gallbladder lies in the removal of the inflamed gallbladder after the acute episode is over.

In the same way, the gallbladder of patients who are suffering from chronic cholecystitis, i.e., long-standing inflammation of the gallbladder, should also be removed without delay. Similarly, in gallstones, the gallbladder should be removed as there is always associated chronic inflammation of the gallbladder.

7. Change in bowel habits

For recent/sudden change in bowel habits, i.e., alternating constipation and diarrhoea with the formation of a ball of wind or of a lump in the abdomen, passing of blood through the rectum or blood in stool, loss of appetite and weight, in a middle-aged person, suspect cancer of the colon or of the rectum. Sometimes, bleeding piles may alone be a signal of a malignant growth in a middle-aged person.

8. Lump/thickening in the breast or anywhere

A lump/thickening in the breast and/or bleeding or discharge from the nipple of a middle-aged female should immediately be got diagnosed and treated as it is always prone to malignant change (breast cancer). In general, the appearance of a painless swelling anywhere in the body, suspect malignancy (see page 13 — self-examination of the breasts).

9. Testes

For nodule/lump or change in the size, or swelling or heaviness in respect of a testis, in a middle-aged person, cancer of the testis should be suspected. People with an undescended testes should keep in mind the possibility of malignancy in such a testis, in middle or late life. Hence, it is advisable to lower it to its proper place by an operation (page 13 — self-examination of the testes).

10. Thyroid gland

For swelling or palpable nodule in connection with the thyroid gland, one should immediately report to the physician, lest it becomes malignant or toxic. A toxic thyroid swelling may lead to a thyroid crisis which is a case of emergency. Big thyroid swelling (goitre) may cause pressure symptoms like difficulty in swallowing, breathing or hoarseness of voice, etc. (One will find more details in the chapter on the 'diseases of the thyroid gland').

11. Parotid glands

These are situated on each side of the face below the ears. Any swelling in relation to these glands should be immediately got examined for early diagnosis of cancerous growth in relation to these glands.

The parotid glands are one of the three main pairs of salivary glands, the other two being the submaxillary and sublingual glands which are lying mostly in the floor of the mouth. Out of all these pairs of glands, the parotid glands are more prone to diseases like tumours, or inflammatory lesions.

12. Blood in urine

One should be cautious whenever there is blood in urine (haematuria). Medical people know that it could be a symptom of carcinoma of the kidney, the urinary bladder, the prostate, papilloma (benign) of the urinary bladder or of the pelvis of the kidney, or tuberculosis of the kidney. A middle-aged person has to be cautious on all these accounts. In a child the carcinoma of the kidney usually presents itself as a lump in the abdomen, and blood in the urine is a late feature. Tuberculosis of the kidney may be curable with medicinal treatment in early cases. Later, surgery may be required.

13. Change in bladder habits

In the case of urinary complaint which has been described at page 178 under the topic 'benign enlargement of the prostate (BEP)', and also passing of blood in the urine after the age of 40, one should suspect carcinoma of the prostate. In 75% cases, classical urinary symptoms are a late feature.

A digital-rectal examination (DRE) of the prostate by the concerned physician/surgeon is the best means for diagnosing early operable tumours of the prostate. Hence all men beyond 40 should take care to report to their doctors for DRE once they get any such urinary complaint.

Besides DRE, an ultrasonographic examination of the prostate, together with ultrasonographically guided needle biopsy of the affected/cancerous portion of the gland, for histopathological examination, will help in early diagnosing/detecting the condition. The blood test for prostate-specific antigen (PSA) should also be carried out although it has its own limitations. In some of the cases, increased serum level of prostatic acid phosphatase gives a clue in the diagnosis of occult cases of the prostate cancer. PSA and prostatic phosphatase are produced by prostate tissue. Those having a family history of prostate cancer should in no case delay these investigations.

Once a prostate cancer is diagnosed at an earlier or later stage, a bone scan, magnetic resonance imaging (MRI) of the abdomen, etc. are a must to exclude the spread of cancerous growth from the prostate to other parts of the body.

14. Female genitals

(i) Bleeding through vagina, in addition to her normal menstruation, or following intercourse (contact bleeding) in a 40-50 years old woman may be a signal of the cancer of the cervix. Other causes of contact bleeding are erosion of cervix, mucous polyp, etc. An immediate report to the gynaecologist is important for an early diagnosis of a cancerous lesion, if any.

(ii) Post-menopausal/intermenstrual bleeding through the vagina, may be a signal of the cancer of the body of the uterus. It usually occurs later in life, say, after menopause, but it can occur at a younger age as well.

(iii) Irregular bleeding through the vagina, around the age of 35-45, may be a signal indicating fibroid tumour of the uterus (benign). This will, in most of the cases, require surgical intervention. If neglected, though relatively infrequent, the possibility of a malignant change cannot be ruled out. However, even a benign growth is very troublesome to the woman as she feels markedly run down due to irregular and/or excessive bleeding from the vagina.

(iv) Irregular bleeding through the vagina, usually during early pregnancy may be a signal of hydatidiform mole. It is a benign tumour in which the placenta is transformed into a large number of cysts which look like a bunch of grapes. However, if spontaneous abortion occurs, profuse bleeding may follow which should give a clue of the condition.

If timely action is not taken, i.e., the disease remains undetected, a hydatidiform mole may follow chorionepithelioma which is one of the most malignant growths arising in the body of the uterus. It may follow an abortion, or, in neglected cases, it may progress till the end of pregnancy/labour. In late cases, there is always a risk of the growth spreading and the disease may even prove fatal.

Although the occurrence of a hydatidiform mole is not uncommon, one should not consider this condition straightway; other causes of bleeding through the vagina during the period of pregnancy must be given equal weightage to avoid unnecessary apprehension.

It is worthwhile to point out here that ultrasonography is important for early detection of various cancers, viz. of kidneys, urinary bladder, uterus (the most important being the cervix), testes, liver, gallbladder, prostate (as already mentioned) etc. Likewise upper gastrointestinal endoscopy is valuable for early diagnosis of various disorders of the oesophagus, stomach and duodenum. Similarly, colonoscopy and sigmoidoscopy are useful for locating early lesions of the colon or of the rectum. (More details in Chapter 10)

15. Brain tumours

It must be kept in mind that though headache is a presenting symptom of certain brain tumours, it is a fairly late feature of the disease. It may not be present in many of the early cases of brain tumour. Hence brain tumour should be diagnosed long before the headache appears, keeping in view the various symptoms with which a brain tumour presents initially, and for which the sufferer is expected to consult his physician for the early diagnosis or exclusion of a brain tumour. An urgent computed tomographic (CT) scanning or magnetic resonance imaging (MRI) is usually required for a precise diagnosis. However, severe recurrent headaches with or without vomiting, increasing by coughing/stooping, is an important warning signal of brain tumour. It may also be noted that vomiting as well as papilloedema (which the neurologist/ophthalmologist confirms after examining the fundi with the help of ophthalmoscope) are late manifestations of brain tumour. Besides headache, some of the other presenting symptoms of the brain tumour which must be kept in mind by the masses are given below:

(i) Epileptic attacks

If the epileptic attacks occur after the adult age and/or are not controlled or increase in frequency even with the administration of antiepileptic drugs, the possibility of a brain tumour must be suspected. A detailed account of epilepsy is given in Chapter 7.

(ii) Neurological deficits

Various neurological deficits like visual-field defects, or impaired vision in one or both the eyes, squint, diplopia (double vision); tinnitus (ringing in ears) particularly in one of the ears, unilateral deafness; loss of smell (anosmia), especially on one side; difficulty in swallowing (dysphagia), nasal regurgitation; weakness in one of the limbs or of the limbs of the same side; difficulty in speech, including reading and writing; unsteadiness in legs while walking, or in hands while doing some work; tremors, stiffness or involuntary movements, etc., should be kept in mind.

(iii) Unexplained psychological symptoms

Like depression, loss of memory, sudden change in personality/behaviour, etc. are also important to bear in mind.

16. Skin/oral cavity

For persistent and progressive ulceration of the skin / oral cavity, an old scar or ulcer that repeatedly heals and breaks down, suspect malignancy. Likewise, a painless nodule in any of these areas should arouse the suspicion of malignancy. Even a change in a wart/mole/birth mark, etc., malignancy of the skin should be suspected.

17. Glandular swellings

For glandular swelling/s in the neck, axillae, groin, etc., one should consult the physician for exclusion of cancerous growths like lymphosarcoma, etc. Another cause of glandular enlargement could be tuberculosis, which is curable in early cases with medicinal treatment. However, it must be borne in mind that enlargement of glands is a common occurrence as a result of inflammation called lymphadenitis. Hence a careful interpretation is needed.

18. Jaundice

There are several causes of jaundice (pallor of eyes). Yet the possibility of the malignancy of the bile duct, the gallbladder, the pancreas, the liver, etc. must be excluded before it is too late. Hepatitis is an equally serious cause of jaundice. It may be mentioned that normal serum bilirubin is 0.3-1.0 mg/dl and clinically jaundice is detectable when bilirubin levels are more than 2.5 mg/dl. Hence the need for suspecting the cases at the earliest possible. Jaundice is the most significant symptom of liver involvement. Hence whenever there is the slightest suspicion of jaundice, a thorough probe must be made for establishing the diagnosis.

19. Unexpected bleeding

For unexpected bleeding from any part of the body, in a child/adult, like oozing of blood from the gums, haemorrhagic spots/areas on the skin, or excessive bleeding from the nose, say, after a blow, or profuse bleeding following tooth extraction or minor injury, the possibility of early acute leukaemia must be considered for precise diagnosis.

It is important to point out that leukaemias should be given due consideration and all efforts must be made to treat and control the condition.

Chronic leukaemia: As compared to acute leukaemia, chronic leukaemia usually manifests itself at a later age, say at the age of 30-50 years, and has a different presentation from acute leukaemia. The disease remains hidden and the patient reports after months/years of the onset of the ailment, and in some cases it may be diagnosed accidentally during a routine medical check-up.

However, the disease can be diagnosed in infancy, and besides a clinical examination/suspicion by the physician who may happen to examine the case, we need the expertise of a clinical pathologist/laboratory technician competent to spot out such cases from the routine tests like total leucocyte count (TLC), differential leucocyte count (DLC) and, above all, from the examination of the peripheral blood film (PBF), especially for immature cells, etc.

Enlargement of the spleen and/or glands of the body (prominently cervical), tenderness on the sternum, i.e., the bone lying in front of the middle of the chest (so-called sternal tenderness), may be considered some of the relatively/moderately early symptoms/signs.

Both in acute and chronic cases of leukaemia, a bone marrow examination and some other special tests are 'a must' to confirm the diagnosis.

Recovery in the case of leukaemia, whether acute or chronic, depends on the age of the patient, and on the type/variety of the leukaemia diagnosed finally. There should be no unnecessary panic when the possibility of leukaemia is being considered. Many cases go well with their disease for several years before they begin to show. A middle-aged case of chronic leukaemia with some unusual complaints/symptoms detected for the first time by the author has still been continuing rather satisfactorily for the last seventeen years or so. He has retired from his job after completion of his tenure and has been living a fairly normal life. The idea of writing this is that the leukaemia patient or his family members should never go away with the idea that mortality is the rule in all such cases, as we see in some of the Indian movies.

However, it is very important to mention that a very scientific approach is required for the treatment of such cases. The patient needs the thorough guidance of the physician in respect of diet, exertion, stress, etc. He should undergo periodic check-ups, and blood-tests should be repeated, as advised. Above all, only the prescribed drugs should be taken by such patients. We lost one of our patients who on his own had shifted to other drugs, in spite of the fact that the prognosis of the case was rather good, and this fact was also confirmed by the late Dr. M.M. Wintrobe, a noted haematologist in the USA, who had also authored the book, *Clinical Hematology* (Lea & Febiger, Philadelphia), and to whom the detailed clinical data of the case were sent for a thorough probe/investigation. Later the peripheral blood films of this case were also taken to the USA for discussion by the author.

Interestingly, the patient mentioned earlier also got carried away when some unauthentic approach for his treatment was suggested to him, but it came to the notice of the author in time, and he, to substantiate his views/line of action, sent the case to the Tata Memorial Hospital, Mumbai, which probably saved the patient from the likely tragedy. The patient referred to above, is at present progressing satisfactorily with his disease by following instructions as well as the treatment religiously.

Finally, it may be stressed that a great realization is required among the masses regarding blood cancers, but somehow, leukaemias are lagging far behind in cancer awareness campaigns/programmes.

20. Other signals of cancer

Include unexplained loss of weight/low-grade fever and/or loss of appetite. A thorough/exhaustive investigation is required in such cases to detect the site of the cancer, especially when these symptoms cannot be explained properly.

While concluding the various signals of cancers, it is re-stressed that one must report to the concerned physician/surgeon/specialist whenever one experiences any of the above warning signals. It should be clearly indicated that any of these may not finally prove to be related to cancer. However, it is important that proper check-ups/tests are carried out to rule out the possibility of malignancy.

Besides the above-mentioned signals, some of the important topics (given-below) require the urgent attention of the reader.

Self-examination of the breasts and the testes

Everyone can examine herself/himself for the early detection of two important common cancers, viz., cancer of the breast in females, and cancer of the testes in males. The steps in this regard are as follows:

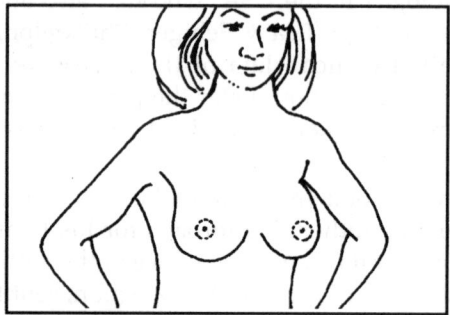

Look in a mirror for detecting any change
in the shape of either of your breasts.

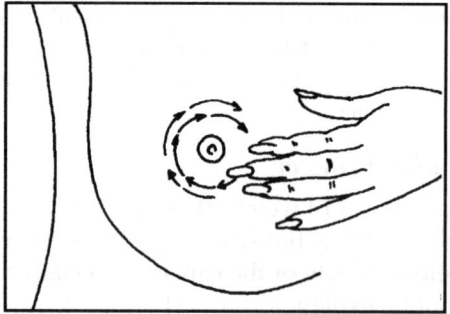

While standing or lying down, feel each breast with your fingers
to check for any thickening/lump in any of the breasts.

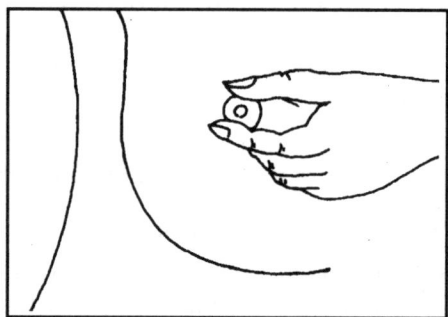

Squeeze the nipple to check for any bleeding or discharge.

Fig. 1. Steps for self-examination of the breasts.

1. Self-examination of the breasts

(i) See if there is any change in the shape of either of your breasts. You should stand in front of a long wall mirror for comparing the shape.

(ii) Feel your breast one by one with the help of your fingers for any thickening/lump in any of them.

(iii) Also squeeze the nipple of each of your breasts, and see if there is any bleeding or discharge (Fig. 1).

Self-examination of the breasts needs to be urgently popularized among women, since the incidence of breast cancer is on the rise. Particular attention is required to be paid in the rural areas where the level of awareness is low, and even *panchayats* or rural local bodies may be involved in such a campaign.

2. Self-examination of the testes

(i) Palpate each of your testes lightly with the help of your fingers and the thumb. The examination should not be done in a cold atmosphere as the skin of the testes constricts in the cold, and a proper examination may not be possible.

(ii) Look for any change in the size of the testes or a nodule/lump in any of them.

Regular check-up/urgent tests for prevention of cancer

1. Women should have a breast examination by a doctor every three years after the age of 20, and every year after the age of 40, and self-examination every month, as per the procedure mentioned above. Also, a woman after the age of 40 should undergo mammography every 1-2 years. It is an ideal tool for detecting breast cancer while a tumour is very small, less than 1.00 cm, before it can be felt. More frequent mammography is required in women who have a family history of breast cancer. It may be noted that with this procedure breast cancer can be detected almost three years earlier than it would otherwise be detected on physical/clinical examination. It involves a very low/limited as well as safe exposure to radiation. Mass realization in this respect is urgently required. Magnetic resonance imaging (MRI) is recommended in

women who are at a very high risk as this test is better than routine mammography.
2. Self-examination of the testes should be done by men every month after the age of 40.
3. A Papanicolaou's smear (commonly called Pap smear) is recommended, every year, after the age of 40, for the exclusion of the cancer of the cervix in females. This test plays an effective role in detecting precancerous and cancerous cervical lesions. It is valuable in a cervical cancer screening programme. Pap testing may be started at a younger age say after the age of 21 in case the individual is sexually active as the cancer of the cervix is most commonly caused by human papilloma virus (HPV) and there is a risk of sexual transmission of the virus. An ultrasound, preferably transvaginal sonography, should also be carried out to rule out the malignancy of the endometrium (i.e. inner linning of the uterus).
4. Both in men and women, digital-rectal examination (DRE) and proctoscopy examination, should be done every year after the age of 40, to exclude the possibility of cancer of the rectum and the anal canal. DRE will also be useful for diagnosing the cancer of the prostate (especially those with a family history of prostate cancer). Serum prostate specific antigen (PSA) is an important test for early detection of prostate cancer. This test should be carried out at least two days after DRE, since palpation of the prostate during this procedure is likely to cause more secretions of this enzyme in to the blood. Similar precautions are required following X-ray/s of the abdomen. If possible, even though it is a bit cumbersome, a colonoscopy/sigmoidoscopy examination should be carried out every 3-5 years, to exclude cancer of the colon and of the rectum. A simple test of stool for blood or RBC, and if need be occult blood, is also required, at least yearly.
5. Examination of the urine for blood/RBC, or occult blood should be done every year in both sexes after the age of 40, for an early detection of cancer of the urinary tract. In females, urine tests should not be done during menstruation period as the blood may then contaminate the urine. More precisely, ultrasonography of the urinary tract is required.

6. Ultrasonographic examination of the abdomen may be done every year, especially after the age of 40, to exclude malignancy of the various organs of the abdomen, including prostate. It is a safe test and has no radiation hazards, unlike X-ray/CT scan.
7. Chest X-rays may be carried out yearly after middle age, especially of those who are prone to the cancer of the lungs like chronic smokers, to exclude asymptomatic lesion of this disease. In selected cases, sputum for malignant cells, computed tomography (CT) of the lung may be done.

It is important to discuss here some of the related topics, and provide some relevant information about the female breast and the use of female hormones with special reference to malignancy. However, it is no less important to study some of the details about the male breast, including carcinoma of the male breast, which, if it develops, spreads much more rapidly than cancer of the female breast.

Female breasts

Breasts in a woman may be small. There is a misconception that unusually small breasts may not be normal, and it is seen that females, especially young unmarried girls, take hormonal treatment (oestrogens) unnecessarily which has severe adverse side-effects.

If a woman has normal menstruation and the secondary sex characters are normally developed, such small breasts should be taken within normal limits, and no treatment is required. However, the woman may also be checked up by a gynaecologist for any pathology in the uterus/ovaries, etc. A simple per vaginal (PV) examination, and transvaginal sonography is all that may be required. But in spite of this, the woman with small breasts usually feels perturbed, which may be due to cosmetic considerations.

The author happened to come across such a case of unusually small breasts, in a young girl, who felt constantly disturbed, and was taking hormones, of course, with no signs of improvement. She was asked to stop the hormones immediately, and was examined by a gynaecologist, who reported that she was perfectly all right, the only finding was that she had very small breasts. In spite of repeated assurances, the girl hardly felt satisfied, and was not convinced that her breasts were normal, though smaller in size. The details of the case were sent to USA for the views of Dr. Charles W. Lloyd who is a specialist on the subject, and has contributed a chapter in the *Text Book of Endocrinology* (W.B. Saunders Company, USA). Dr. Lloyd, while expressing his views on unusually small breasts in an otherwise normal female, wrote to the author ".... This is not unusual. It seems to be analogous to other conditions in which a normal person has an organ that does not develop quite as much as would be expected. In some men, the penis is smaller than usual, although they are perfectly normal. We have found that when a woman is endocrinologically normal, i.e., all other secondary sex structures are normally developed and ovulation and menstruation are normal, there isn't much that can be done about small breasts. The explanation seems to be that there is an individual variation in responsiveness of the tissues. The breasts simply do not respond in the usual amount to normal hormone values. It is generally found that they will not have significant growth of the breasts even though large amounts of oestrogen are given. Perhaps there is some difference in the levels of the other factors than oestrogen that are important for normal breast development. Some of these women have considerable growth of the breasts when they become pregnant and lactate. Probably this is due to the influence of pituitary or placental lactogenic substances ...".

Hence it is obvious that probably there is an individual variation that in some females breasts remain small, while in others they are normal and even large. However, such small breasts will not in any way affect the health or growth of the female concerned. Many of such cases which we could follow, showed that their breasts worked in a normal way i.e. for lactation following delivery, and the breasts also, to some extent, increased in size.

Malignancy and use of female hormones

There is a word of great caution that a female should not take hormones indiscriminately. These should only be taken with the advice of a specialist for the period specified. Even when the woman is on an oral contraceptive, a regular check-up of blood pressure is required, as all oral contraceptives cause a significant rise in blood pressure. Even a heart attack/stroke may be precipitated with the use of hormones. Also, the hormones may cause an increase in blood sugar levels, various blood lipids and body weight. Likewise, blood coagulability may also be increased with their continuous usage. Hence the need for precaution at every step.

In older women, while administering hormones, say to tide over the troublesome period of menopause, it must be ensured that she has no hidden malignancy. It is, therefore, advisable that the breasts are examined for any lump, and mammography of both the breasts is done. At the same time, a Pap smear and an ultrasonographic examination of the uterus must be carried out to exclude the malignancy of the uterus, especially of the cervix. It should be noted that hormones increase the risk of cancer of the uterus and breast. Hence awareness in this respect is an important step in the prevention of cancer of these parts of the body.

Male breasts

At birth, breasts (mammary glands) are similar in size in both sexes. The breasts remain rudimentary in males throughout life, while in females changes occur during puberty and pregnancy as a result of the influence of various female hormones in the body.

However, in males, the breasts may get abnormally enlarged. This condition is called gynecomastia.

Gynecomastia

Enlarged breasts in a male may be one of the developmental anomalies of the breast like polymastia, in which a man has more than two breasts, or amastia, where there is absolutely no breast or there has been no development of the breast at all, etc. However the condition of enlarged male breasts i.e. gynecomastia may be entirely familial i.e. the male breasts in all the members of a family may be enlarged.

A transient gynecomastia may occur in a newly-born male, and also in some elderly men, probably due to some hormonal imbalance.

A significant gynecomastia may be seen when the testes are destroyed either due to some infection or malignancy, or when the testes are absent since birth.

Gynecomastia also manifests in advanced liver diseases, as well as during long starvation, and again it occurs under the influence of hormones of the body.

Further, gynecomastia may be noted in cases of cancer of the lung (bronchogenic carcinoma) as a result of increased levels of oestrogen.

Hence gynecomastia is an important topic and the author also contributed a review article on the subject to one of the issues of the *Punjab Medical Journal*.

Gynecomastia may be unilateral or bilateral, i.e. either one or both the breasts may be enlarged. The cases of gynecomastia in which there is no underlying pathology, will have no symptoms except that the patient may feel slight discomfort or pain, and sometimes it may become a serious case of psychological upset, like the case of small breasts in a female, described earlier. However, if the patient feels markedly perturbed, enlarged breasts in males may be removed surgically (mastectomy).

In a case where the gynecomastia is as a result of some disease, the symptoms of the underlying pathology should be evident, and one has to pay attention to such a primary disease for the treatment of the patient as a whole. Even some drugs like digitalis, methyldopa, chlorpromazine may also cause gynecomastia. It is clear in such cases, gynecomastia is only due to the side-effect of these drugs, and may require reduction/ stoppage or the change of such drugs.

Carcinoma of male breast

One should not delay in detecting carcinoma of the male breast, and such cases should not be neglected saying that the patient is suffering from gynecomastia, especially in early cases. The disease usually occurs in one of the breasts, while gynecomastia may occur in both the breasts.

A cancer of the female breast is much more common than the cancer of the male breast. The possible cause could be some abnormality in oestrogen metabolism of the body. Furthermore, carcinoma of the male breast occurs at a later age than the carcinoma of the female breast. But the prognosis of male breast carcinoma is deadly; since the breast is much smaller than a female breast, the cancer will quickly spread locally into the chest wall as well as to the distant organs, and therefore, the urgent treatment should never be delayed. The signs to watch for are: any change in, around or beneath the nipple and areola either in size, shape or texture, particularly in men above 50 years of age. Any of these signs may develop singly or together and definitely require a specialist's opinion.

Hence, there should be urgent mass realization about male breast cancer as well, and all men especially above 40, should be vigilant on this account, even though, as mentioned above, it is less common than the carcinoma of the female breast. Approximately one case of carcinoma of the male breast occurs out of 100 cases of female breast cancer. But once it appears, it is likely to be fatal if timely/quick action is not taken.

Vaccination

It is important to introduce mass vaccination programme where vaccine can help in the goal of preventing cancer of any type. In this context Hepatitis B vaccine needs a special reference. This vaccine is advocated for the prevention of chronic hepatitis that may lead to liver cancer. On similar lines more vaccines are being developed e.g. HPV vaccine for the prevention of cancer of the cervix and Helicobacter pylori vaccine for the prevention of gastric cancer.

General measures for prevention of cancer

1. Avoid smoking and tobacco chewing. (See Appendix I also).
2. Alcoholic beverages should be generally avoided. However, if one drinks, one should consume it only in moderation. (Refer to Appendix II).
3. In women, oestrogen therapy should be taken for the duration prescribed by the specialist, as already explained earlier on page 16.
4. To avoid radiation, X-rays and CT scans should only be done when necessary. For those working at the site of radiation, the use of protective devices are mandatory for their safety.

5. It is recommended to take high fibre (green vegetables, fruits, whole wheat/cereals), and low-fat diet (less intake of saturated fats like ghee, butter, cream, egg-yolk, etc.) —refer to Appendix VII.
6. One should try to avoid living in highly-polluted areas.
7. Too much sunlight is also to be avoided.
8. One should take regular exercise as it significantly reduces the risk of cancers (see Appendix VIII).
9. One needs to be aware of early warning signals of cancers (see page 1)

National programme

A programme at the national level would go a long way for detecting and treating the cancer at an early stage, and its awareness among citizens.

2
DISEASES OF THE HEART

Under the occult diseases of the heart, one ought to know about:
Coronary artery disease (CAD),
Rheumatic heart disease (RHD) and
Congenital heart disease (CHD).

1. Coronary artery disease - CAD
(also called ischaemic heart disease - IHD)

Much is known about coronary artery disease (CAD), and therefore, only salient features of the disease shall be elaborated.

How is CAD an occult/asymptomatic/hidden disease?

CAD is indeed a silent human killer. Although the disease process starts in coronary arteries early in childhood, it continues progressing very gradually through years / decades, and becomes significant enough only later in life, say at the age of 40, or earlier. The reason is that no symptom of the disease occurs till more than 50-60% of the surface area of the coronary arteries is involved. Out of sudden deaths, as a result of CAD, 50% patients may not have any symptom earlier, and such may be the cases which have never gone through tests for detection of CAD.

Hence such a fatal disease remains masked for a long time, but if one knows about it, it can be checked/arrested, and mortality in the prime years of life, when one is at the height of one's career, can be prevented. The CAD in young people i.e. of less than 40 years of age has reached an epidemic proportion and the disease follows a malignant course. There is a rapid increase of IHD cases all over the globe and it is estimated that by the year 2020, IHD would be the most common cause of death. Hence the need for caution.

What are coronary arteries?

There are two coronary arteries, right and left, which supply oxygenated blood to muscular walls of the heart. The left coronary artery divides into two main branches. Both right and the main branches of the left coronary arteries divide further into several smaller branches supplying blood to their respective portion of the heart. The lesion of CAD may occur either in the main blood vessel/branch, or in any of the smaller branches of the coronary arteries. The disease process may occur either at one place, or even at several places of the coronary arteries or its branches, i.e. in a person either the main vessel or many of the branches may be involved at the same time.

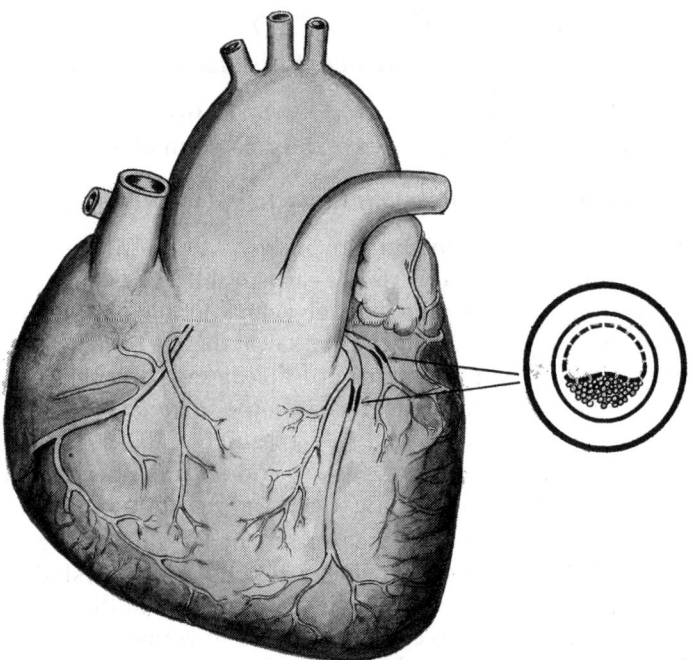

Fig. 2. Narrowing of the coronary arteries, and a sectional view showing deposition of fatty material (atherosclerosis).

Diseases of the Heart

The heart, which is egg-shaped, is a hollow muscular organ (consisting of four chambers) and is about the size of a fist. It supplies oxygenated blood to the whole body which is necessary for its proper functioning. Even for its own working, the muscular walls of the heart need oxygenated blood which is supplied by the coronary arteries. Hence if coronary arteries are diseased, called CAD, their calibre will become narrow, and so less blood will flow through them. Thus the supply of oxygenated blood to the walls of the heart will suffer.

What is the cause of CAD?

In the walls of the coronary arteries, a fatty material gets deposited called atherosclerosis. As mentioned earlier, it starts in early childhood, and as the years pass, this process of atherosclerosis continues, and ultimately the walls of the coronary arteries start thickening and their lumen starts narrowing (Fig. 2). The process is so slow that in about the third decade a partial blockage of the lumen of the coronary arteries/ its branches may manifest itself, and during the next 10 years i.e. in the fourth decade a complete blockage of the coronary arteries may occur. When the blockage is partial, less blood will flow in coronary arteries, and so less blood will be supplied to the muscular wall of the heart. And whenever there is less supply to the muscular wall of the heart, the patient experiences pain in the chest. The severity of pain has a direct relation to the blood supply to the wall of the heart. If the supply is adversely affected/suddenly cut off in the coronary arteries or one of its branches, the patient may get a severe pain in the chest called myocardial infarction or heart attack. In the beginning, the patient may get only temporary pain in the chest called angina pectoris.

Likewise atherosclerosis may affect blood vessels of central nervous system leading to stroke or earlier to it transient ischaemic episode (mentioned in the chapter of stroke), blood vessels of the lower limbs causing intermittent claudication and in late cases even gangrene may develop. Renal artery stenosis may occur as a result of atherosclerosis, and carotid arteries may be affected at their division in the neck.

What is angina pectoris?

As mentioned above, whenever the blood supply of the muscular wall of the heart starts suffering, clinical manifestations of CAD occur. Although there may be a mild blockage in a coronary artery, and thus a depletion in the supply of blood to the walls of the heart, yet this supply may be enough when the patient is at rest. But this supply may not remain adequate when the patient exerts, i.e. when he/she walks, or does some mechanical work. This leads to pain in the chest, and this is called angina pectoris. This pain is temporary, and when the patient stops walking or exerting, the pain diminishes. This pain will also stop when the patient takes some drugs which dilate the coronary arteries, like glyceryl trinitrate, which acts quickly when kept below the tongue or chewed. However, such a pain recurs when the patient resumes walking/exerting.

Besides exertion, in some other circumstances, the blood supply of the walls to the heart may suffer e.g. when the patient takes heavy meals, which put a stress on the heart, or when there is a mental/emotional strain caused by anxiety, worry or bad news. An attack of angina may also be precipitated on exposure to cold which may cause spasm/narrowing of coronary arteries.

In anginal pain, the patient feels as if the pain will take the life away. The pain occurs in the centre of the chest below the sternum, or on its left side. The patient may feel tightness or pressure/weight-like pain in the chest. True pain rarely occurs. The pain hardly lasts for 1-2 minutes, or at the most 10 minutes. As a general principle, pain anywhere in the chest either in front or back of the chest should be considered anginal if it occurs on exertion or during other conditions described, and relieved by rest in about 1-5 minutes and earlier if the patient takes glyceryl mitrate below the tongue. Such a patient should be investigated thoroughly. A detailed questioning is required by the physician while taking the history of the case. The patient often ignores such a pain, or starts doing less exertion so that the pain does not occur again. Hence, awareness/knowledge in this regard is highly needed, so that the patient reports in time and gets himself investigated before it is too late.

Diseases of the Heart

The above-said group of cases belongs to stable angina pectoris i.e. in which pain appears on exertion or during other circumstances mentioned above.

There is another group of anginal cases which is a step ahead of the above group and is called unstable angina pectoris. In this group pain occurs much more frequently with a little exertion. Even a small activity may cause pain in the chest, or at times it may occur even during the period of rest. It is obvious that in these cases the coronary arteries are involved much more than in a case of stable angina pectoris. However, there may not be a complete blockage of the flow of blood in coronary arteries/ branches as occurs in cases of a heart attack, in which a very severe pain stays for a long period, and is usually relieved by a pain-killer injection.

The cases of unstable angina should be treated/evaluated on the lines of heart attack. An emergency line of treatment is essentially required in such cases in a well-equipped hospital. If immediate steps are not taken, the patient may suffer from a heart attack, which must be prevented. In some of the cases when drug therapy is not working satisfactorily, even an urgent coronary angiography including angioplasty (ballooning) or surgery may have to be undertaken.

It may be said that a case of unstable angina is like a pendulum of a clock. With timely detection as well as treatment, the pendulum can be made to swing towards stable angina or complete relief, and if proper action is delayed, the pendulum may move to the worst side i.e. the patient may get a heart attack. Hence unstable angina is a danger signal of a heart attack, and it must alert the patient or his attendant to take immediate action, preferably in a hospital.

What is heart attack (also called myocardial infarction, coronary artery thrombosis or coronary occlusion)?

In case angina pectoris is ignored, and the disease is allowed to progress, the blockage in coronary arteries/or in its branches may go on increasing. The end-result of such a severe blockage in coronary arteries/branches would be that the blood supply of a part of heart muscle (supplied by the respective branch of coronary artery) may suddenly stop completely leading to severe damage/ injury/necrosis/death of the affected portion of the heart muscle.

However, the patient may directly go into the stage of heart attack without undergoing the stage of angina pectoris.

There may be only sudden spasm/narrowing/constriction of a coronary artery or its branches, either of a normal vessel or already involved coronary artery as a result of atherosclerosis. If the spasm is momentary, the patient may get only angina, but if it is a prolonged one, blood supply of a portion of heart muscle will suffer adversely, leading to a heart attack.

As regards clinical manifestations in a heart attack, the patient suddenly gets very severe pain in the centre of the chest (retrosternal) which may radiate to the left upper arm. In some cases, the pain may radiate to the back of the chest or towards the neck/lower jaw. In a typical case, the pain may only be present in any of these areas i.e. back of the chest or the neck, etc.

Unlike the pain in angina, the pain in a heart attack is not relieved by rest, or by the administration of quick-acting coronary dilator drugs like glyceryl trinitrate. It may last more than half an hour, and may be accompanied by profuse sweating. The pain, truly speaking, may be highly unbearable, the worst the patient has ever suffered/experienced and may be only relieved by a strong analgesic/pain-killer. The patient may even get breathlessness/syncope/vertigo. Some patients may quickly go into shock called cardiogenic shock which becomes a grave emergency, and the patient may die if proper aid is not given. However, a patient may die even instantaneously if the heart attack is very severe. Hence, after the immediate first aid (as detailed in Appendix VI) he should be shifted to the hospital. Such patients are treated in an intensive care unit (ICU) of the hospital. The sooner the patient is given aid, the lesser will be the damage to the heart. Emergency treatment of myocardial infarction should be immediately started as we have only first four hours to save the myocardium from damage. Early treatment prevents serious/fatal complications. For this reason, in some of the places, there are mobile cardiac care units. The van, duly-equipped, reaches the place of emergency in no time, and the patient receives proper treatment in the van itself on the way to hospital. If some fatal complications occur on the way, they are also tackled right in the van. Many lives can be saved with such timely treatment.

Hence, early diagnosis as well as treatment is important to save the life of a patient in a case of a heart attack. One must bear in mind the solitary important warning signal to detect cases of heart attack, in most of the cases, that whenever there is pain in chest/difficulty in breathing/syncope (transitory unconsciousness)/vertigo (dizziness), especially in middle age, the physician should be consulted for an immediate check-up. Further, cases of stable/unstable angina pectoris may precede a heart attack and thus should be considered a most important early warning signal.

Are there any risk factors responsible for CAD?

Yes, there are several factors which increase the process of atherosclerosis in the coronary arteries, and in a patient more than 1-2 factors may be operating at the same time. Awareness of all such factors is important so that the CAD could be prevented right from the beginning.

Some of the factors/diseases have been discussed in separate chapters like those on diabetes, high blood pressure, high blood cholesterol, high blood uric acid, etc. Also, there are appendices on smoking and tobacco chewing, obesity and diseases, and on diet, etc. An elevated plasma homocystein level is also an important risk factor in the causation of CAD especially in the young.

Other equally important factors are a positive family history of CAD, sedentary habits, lack of regular exercise, adverse/stressful conditions at home and/or at work, and the personality/behaviour of a person concerned. There are certain personality/behaviour characteristics called coronary prone personality/behaviour (CPP/CPB) responsible for CAD. This point will be taken up later under primary prevention of CAD. Although as age advances, some hardening of coronary arteries does occur, yet the above factors hasten the occurrence of atherosclerosis, leading to a premature death.

Besides genetic factors, the size of coronary artery /ies that may differ from race to race is responsible for the incidence of CAD. Narrower the caliber of coronary arteries greater the chance of its blockage leading to CAD.

Another notable risk factor in the development of CAD, is the use of oral contraceptives in women. Great caution is required, and a regular check-up by the physician is essential to keep their side-effects away. Their unchecked/continuous use may cause increase in blood pressure, blood sugar, various blood lipids, as well as an increase in weight of the body. Hence the various untoward effects of the use of oral contraceptives are the important risk factors causing CAD. Besides CAD, oral contraceptives may also cause other vascular diseases like a stroke where the same factors and pathogenesis are operating. Even the coagulability of blood may also be increased with the use of oral contraceptives, thus enhancing the chances of CAD.

Hence, women, especially those who are already suffering from high blood pressure, diabetes, high blood lipids, etc., should avoid the use of oral contraceptives. These may be used by younger women, say below 35 or even earlier, with necessary precautions, and that too if no risk factors are involved.

There is an interesting point, that the incidence of CAD increases after the natural menses of women stop, i.e. when they enter the menopausal period, or when as a result of surgical intervention, menses stop, called surgical menopause. Hence chances of CAD increase in all menopausal women, and they should be cautious and follow the various preventive measures (mentioned later) strictly. Higher levels of high-density lipoprotein (HDL) cholesterol and lower levels of low-density lipoprotein (LDL) cholesterol may protect females till menopause. The belief that a woman before menopause cannot get a heart attack is not true. Such a misconception can kill the woman, especially if the symptoms of heart attack are not typical, and time is wasted at home and specialist care or emergency treatment is not initiated immediately. Needless to say that all the risk factors need to be cared for in all age groups in females too. Women are at greater risk if they smoke while taking oral contraceptives.

Detection of occult/asymptomatic cases of CAD

As mentioned earlier, the disease starts in early childhood and remains asymptomatic till the third or fourth decade of life. It means, prior to this, irrespective of exertion, no symptom of the disease occurs, and unless the symptom occurs, the patient does not seek medical advice. However, tests like resting electrocardiogram (ECG) and/or exercise ECG do help in detecting early asymptomatic cases of CAD.

Besides detection of early hidden cases of CAD, detection of various risk factors responsible for CAD, like high blood cholesterol/uric acid/sugar, etc. is equally important. Those who have a positive family history of CAD, are addicted to smoking, suffer from high blood pressure, are overweight, sedentary workers, have a coronary prone personality/behaviour (see later), women on oral contraceptives, or during their menopausal period, are all open to risk and need a periodic follow-up for the detection of CAD.

By and large, ECG is essentially required of all persons to see whether CAD exists or not. In case a resting ECG is normal, and especially if the person has one of the risk factors, or has a doubtful history of chest pain even in the past, an exercise ECG should also be carried out.

It is important that in all asymptomatic persons both resting and exercise ECGs must be read by a specialist for an early diagnosis of CAD. A wrong label of CAD may prove highly damaging to the person, especially psychologically.

However, if resting and exercise ECGs are normal in a person, irrespective of age, he should not take it for granted that CAD can never manifest itself or does not exist. The disease may still be in infancy so that the blood supply to the walls of the heart is not affected even on exercise, accounting for the normalcy of exercise ECG. However, both resting and exercise ECGs may have to be repeated periodically, especially in high-risk cases, or even in all middle-aged persons, for the detection of CAD at the earliest possible.

In case, exercise ECG is negative, and the patient is still suspected of suffering from CAD, or one likes to be very sure of the existence of CAD, or one's profession is such that the elimination of CAD is a must, the next alternative would be to undergo thallium stress test (see later). Coronary angiography, being an invasive test, cannot be carried out for the detection of CAD in all asymptomatic cases. (See page 34 for CT Coronary Angiogram test).

It is stressed again that a periodic check-up of the heart/related factors will go a long way in timely detection of CAD, and many of the conditions/factors may be preventable right in infancy.

It is only with the co-operation of the public, especially those people who are prone to suffer from CAD, or those who have entered middle age, that we can detect CAD in many asymptomatic cases, and save the person concerned from its serious consequences. At least all middle-aged persons or those who are in the risk of getting CAD, must report to their physicians for a check-up as and when advised, so that an early diagnosis of CAD does not remain missed, when the patient is still asymptomatic.

Is every pain in the chest related to the heart?

Certainly not; every pain in the chest is not always related to the heart. There are several other causes of pain in the chest. But since a pain in the chest, if related to the heart, could be even fatal, therefore, whenever there is even the slightest doubt clinically, a pathology of the heart must be included to be on the safe side.

One must be aware that there is a great variation in the manifestation of pain in chest relating to the heart or CAD, and therefore, for practical purposes the possibility of cardiac/heart involvement must be kept in mind. Even if a pain in chest does not seem to be related to the heart clinically, an ECG is the least which should be done in each and every case.

Some of the causes of pain in chest not related to the heart may be cervical spondylosis in which the neck of a person is involved, inflammation of the food-pipe (oesophagitis), pleuritis i.e. inflammation of the pleura (membrane covering the lungs), pain as a result of a pathology in the bony cage i.e. ribs, sternum and spine (i.e. portion of the spine related to the chest). Similarly, a lesion in the abdomen may cause pain in the chest as well like gastritis or peptic ulcer (i.e. inflammation/ulceration of stomach or duodenum), cholecystitis/cholelithiasis (i.e. inflammation of gallbladder/gallstones), pancreatitis (i.e. inflammation of pancreas), including some diseases of the liver (Fig. 3).

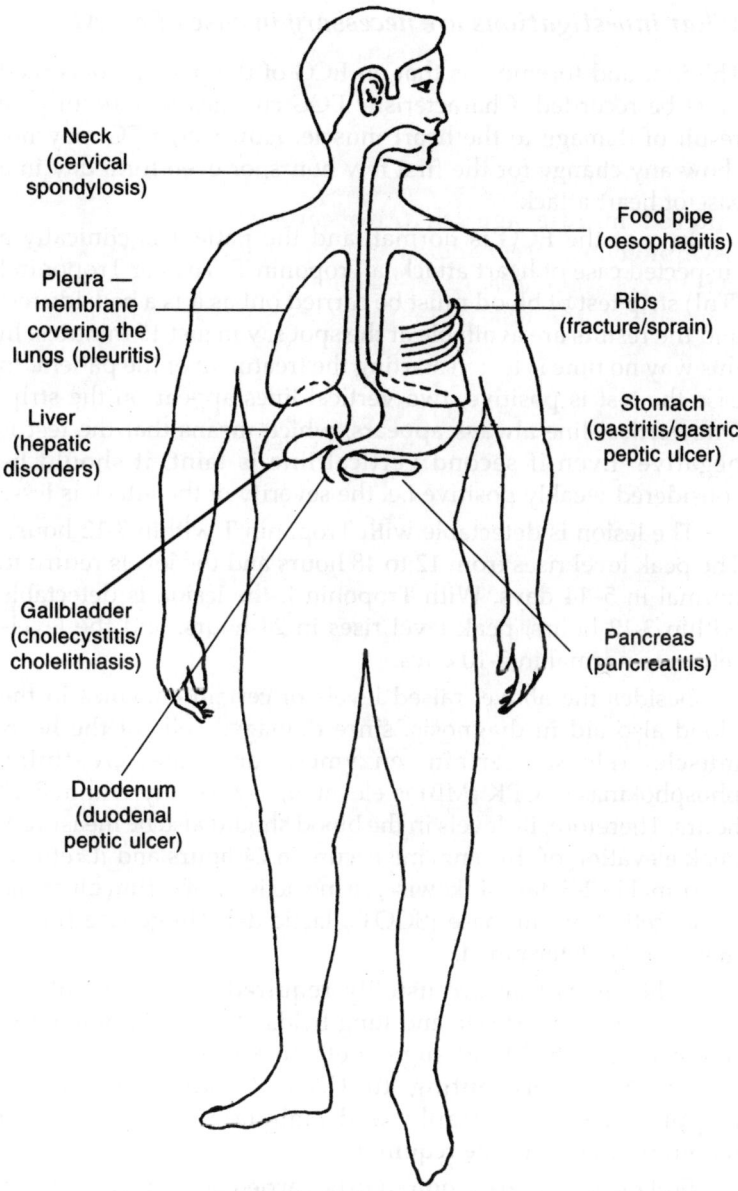

Fig. 3. A diagrammatic representation of the various causes of pain in the chest — not related to the heart.

What investigations are necessary in case of a CAD

The first and foremost is that an ECG of the patient concerned must be recorded. Characteristic ECG changes may occur as a result of damage to the heart muscle. However, ECG may not show any change for the first few hours, or even for a day in a case of heart attack.

In case the ECG is normal, and the patient is clinically a suspected case of heart attack, a Troponin T (TnT) or Troponin I (TnI) strip test of blood must be carried out as it is a bedside test and the results are available at the spot say in just 15 minutes. In this way no time is lost in starting the treatment of the patient. In case the test is positive, two vertical lines appear on the strip. One vertical line always appears, which means that the test is negative. Even if second vertical line is faint, it should be considered weakly positive i.e. the severity of the attack is less.

The lesion is detectable with Troponin T within 3-12 hours. The peak level rises from 12 to 48 hours and the levels return to normal in 5–14 days. With Troponin I, the lesion is detectable within 3-12 hours, peak level rises in 24 hours, and the levels return to normal in 5-10 days.

Besides the above, raised levels of certain enzymes in the blood also aid in diagnosis, since damaged cells of the heart muscle release certain enzymes, and the creatinine phosphokinase - CPK (MB) is elevated, say usually within 3-12 hours. Therefore, its levels in the blood should also be measured. Peak elevation of this enzyme occurs in 24 hours and it returns to normal in 2-3 days. Likewise, rising activity of serum glutamic oxaloacetic transaminase (SGOT), lactic dehydrogenase (LDH) may also be determined.

Other tests that are usually required are X-rays of the chest, both for heart size and lung fields. A fasting lipidogram, blood uric acid, blood sugar help to know any associated risk factors contributing to CAD. In addition, colour Doppler echocardiography and ambulatory ECG (Holter) monitoring may also be required.

Still more tests are required to be carried out which are given below :

Diseases of the Heart

Treadmill stress test (TMT) or exercise ECG test

It is a very important test, and is carried out in almost all cases of CAD. This test reveals the response of the heart to the stress of exercise. The patient is connected to the ECG machine, and is asked to walk on a treadmill. The recordings of ECG indicate the response of the heart during exercise. If the muscle of the heart is getting less supply of blood during exercise, the same will be evident in the ECG. The patients who cannot exercise because of disorder of knee joints or any other musculo-skeletal disease or breathlessness on exertion or those who are not used to exercise may undergo stress test with dobutamine that is used in place of exercise. Same is true for stress echocardiogaphy (mentioned later).

Since a normal resting ECG does not rule out CAD, the stress test may prove valuable in the detection of occult/asymptomatic cases of CAD. This test is especially indicated when the person is suffering from one or more risk factors responsible for CAD like high blood pressure, high blood sugar/cholesterol/uric acid, etc. and/or when there is a strong family history of CAD.

Besides detection of hidden cases, a stress test is also indicated following a heart attack, in all cases. It tells about the extent of lesion, prognosis, including efficacy of treatment. In some cases, after a heart attack, only a modified treadmill stress test may be possible in which only a specific heart rate is achieved as the patient starts exerting.

In addition to the above, TMT must be carried out in all cases of angina pectoris. If it is negative, it may again be repeated after 1-2 months. If it is positive, it means there is a blockage in the coronary arteries/its branches, and the patient may need further tests like the thallium stress test or coronary angiography. In such cases all investigations, as in the case of heart attack, should be carried out for proper treatment.

Thallium stress test

In this test, thallium is injected intravenously while the patient is at peak exercise. Thallium goes through coronary arteries/branches and collects in the heart muscle. If the collection of thallium in the heart muscle is normal, it means that coronary arteries are functioning normally. Thus, it gives an indirect evidence of the functioning of coronary arteries. It is a non-invasive test and some prefer to carry it out before coronary angiography.

Computed tomographic (CT) coronary angiogram

Computed tomographic (CT) coronary angiogram by using the 64-slice CT scanner is a useful non-invasive test that detects the presence of coronary artery disease including its severity. In asymptomatic patients, changes in the coronary vessels can be detected and prompt preventive action can be taken. Narrowing/ blockage of the arteries, presence of different kinds of plaques (wall thickening) along the arteries causing narrowing of arteries can be easily evaluated by this method. Plaques may be soft, stable and unstable, and their rupture may even cause sudden death. The test helps in evaluating the type of plaque for timely treatment. It is also useful in follow up cases in determining if a bypass graft or stent is open and functioning or some blockage has started appearing. However, this test cannot be carried out in cases of cardiac arrhythmias and in those cases that are on pacemaker. Morbidly obese patients are also not able to undergo this test. The test takes only five seconds and the patients of heart disease can hold their breath for this period i.e. five seconds, which helps obtain a clear image. The patients are required to take a dose of beta-blockers the night before for controlling the heart rate that helps obtain the best possible images. If the patient cannot take a beta-blocker, an alternative is considered by the physician. An injection of x-ray contrast is used in this test.

Coronary angiography

Besides above tests, coronary angiography may also be required. In some cases even direct coronary angiography may be carried out without taking the help of the thallium study. It is a highly reliable diagnostic test.

In this test, a dye is pushed into the coronary arteries through a very thin plastic tube (catheter), inserted into an artery (femoral artery), located in the middle of the fold of the groin, and series of X-rays are taken. This study, as well as the extent of lesion in the coronary arteries, gives the correct picture of a particular patient. After carefully studying the report of angiography, a suitable treatment can be planned.

Stress echocardiography

Instead of the thallium stress test, stress echocardiography may be done to assess the viability of the heart muscle. It is a non-invasive test and can be done in remote areas as well. It may be carried out with exercise or dobutamine. Two-dimensional echocardiography alone is useful to determine regional wall motion abnormalities of the left ventricle as a result of ischaemia.

Ambulatory ECG (Holter) monitoring

Ambulatory ECG monitoring is recommended both in symptomatic and asymptomatic patients who are clinically suspected of high risk cases, for detection of degree of lesion so that appropriate treatment could be started in time and complications of ischaemia that include sudden cardiac death could be prevented.

What is the treatment of CAD?

If there is a blockage in a coronary artery or in its branches, as is evident from the report of the coronary angiography, coronary artery bypass graft (CABG) surgery, also called coronary artery bypass surgery may be required.

However, in early cases, angioplasty (ballooning) and stents are sufficient to clear the blockage, and allow a free flow of blood in the coronary artery or its branch/es involved; thus saving the person from further attack/s of CAD.

These procedures widen the caliber of the related blood vessel. The stent is like a flexible tube made of wire mesh. It is mounted on to a balloon catheter in collapsed form. The balloon and stent are guided across the lesion and once in the specific area, the balloon is inflated. This pushes the plaque against the artery wall. The balloon is deflated and removed. The stent remains as a permanent support, helping to hold the artery open.

Drug - coated stents in contrast to bare metal stents have further brightened the prognosis of the patients. The drug – coated stents have been able to reduce the rate of in-stent restenosis that used to occur with bare metal stents. As a result, fewer patients will now need to undergo stent implantation another time. The drug permits natural and normal healing of vessel walls and re-endotheliation (i.e. helps in restoring the inner lining of vessel wall).

In case the blockage is an old, calcified one, and the walls of coronary artery/ies or their branches have become thick, fibrosed, or when the lesion is a diffuse one involving a greater portion of the coronary vessels, or the blockage is severe, or there is obstruction/blockage in several branches of the coronary artery/ies, angioplasty/ballooning may not help and there remains no alternative except to go in for coronary artery bypass graft (CABG) surgery so that an adequate supply of blood to the heart muscle is maintained.

It is now recommended that patients with 1-2 vessel-disease with normal left ventricle function may undergo angioplasty. If there is a 3-vessels disease, or 2-vessel disease and one of the involved vessels is proximal left descending coronary artery, and ejection fraction is less than 50% i.e. left ventricle functions are impaired, or when left main coronary artery is involved or when the patient is suffering from diabetes mellitus CABG is recommended. With latest advances the coronary bypass surgery is getting less traumatic or invasive. The International Society for Minimally Invasive Cardiac Surgery looks up this very aspect. The incision on the skin is reduced and amount of blood transfusion cut down.

There is one bright side of the picture though. As people are becoming more and more aware/conscious of CAD, early diagnosis may be the rule in future, so that only angioplasty may serve the purpose in most of the cases.

Drug treatment: Drugs have a significant role to play in the treatment of CAD. They are given primarily to dilate the coronary arteries (called coronary artery dilators) so that the flow of blood in the coronary arteries is increased. Drugs which prevent the clotting of blood (anticoagulants) may also be given so that further blockage/clotting in the coronaries can be prevented. Some drugs may also be required even after the coronary artery bypass surgery, or after angioplasty.

Drugs are also indicated to control the associated factor/s like high blood pressure, high blood cholesterol/sugar/uric acid, etc.

Drug treatment is valuable in cases of angina pectoris. Surgery/ballooning may also be required in some of the cases of angina especially when medicinal treatment fails and the coronary angiography shows specific lesion/s.

Hence for the treatment of CAD, drugs, balloon/angioplasty followed by drug coated stenting or CABG surgery, together with the control of associated risk factors, if any, diet as well as restricted activity is required to keep the heart running normally as far as possible, and to prevent the recurrence of CAD. While on drugs, tests like ECG, echocardiography, blood lipid profile, blood uric acid, TMT (in selected cases) need to be carried out six monthly/yearly or earlier, as the situation warrants keeping watch on the status of the condition of the heart. Drug regime may have to be reviewed from time to time.

What are the steps of prevention of CAD?

Ideally, prevention should be our primary consideration so that the person does not at all suffer from CAD, either heart attack or angina. However, if the person has suffered from heart attack or angina, preventive steps should be taken so that the patient is saved from further heart attack/s and the angina remains well controlled. This is called secondary prevention.

1. Primary prevention of CAD

To achieve total prevention, a long-term national policy is required. Motivation of the people is the key to such a prevention. For this, one needs a multi-faceted approach/motivation involving primary health centres, inclusion of important aspects of CAD in school curricula, regular health education programmes, together with identification of occult/hidden or high-risk cases of CAD. All the medical and paramedical staff have got an important/vital role to play in such a campaign.

As a preventive measure, one should keep one's blood pressure within normal limits. The levels of serum cholesterol and other lipids, blood uric acid, blood sugar, if one is suffering from diabetes, should be kept in the normal range. One should not be overweight. Smoking and tobacco chewing have to be avoided. As to alcoholic beverages, if one drinks, one may consume it only in moderation (see also page 291, para 2). One's diet should be given due consideration. However, one should refrain from a heavy meal or a full stomach. All these factors are also described in the relevant chapters (or in appendices). Oral contraceptives should be avoided, or taken with caution, as already indicated. All menopausal women should also take all precautionary measures as they are more prone to CAD.

Sedentary habits should be curtailed as far as possible, and one should take regular exercises. At the same time, sudden/violent/unaccustomed exertion, especially after the age of 40, should not be undertaken. The author has 2-3 cases in view. In one of the cases, the patient suffered a heart attack when he started pushing his car vigorously and continuously when it went out of order on the road. All those persons who have a family history of CAD, or family history of various risk factors like diabetes, high blood pressure, etc. should be more vigilant in such situations. The parents who have had heart attack, diabetes, obesity or hypertension etc. need to pay equal attention to their children as they are at high risk due to familial tendency.

Coronary prone personality / behaviour (CPP / CPB)

There is one more important point in the primary prevention of CAD. There is a group of persons who are more prone to suffer from CAD, called CPP/CPB. Such persons work for long periods, take/enjoy no vacation. They may be highly articulate, hostile, aggressive, ambitious, competitive, impatient, tense/frustrated, etc. As a preventive measure, it is very difficult to change the personality of a man, irrespective of motivation. However, efforts must be made in this direction. It is seen that personality does change after a heart attack, but here we are talking of primary prevention. It is advisable that relaxation, by various means/techniques, including recreation, together with suitable exercise, are a must in life, irrespective of the amount of heavy work/tension. Sincere counselling given to such persons by family physicians may prove highly valuable.

About weather and CAD

As a preventive measure one should keep oneself warm in cold weather. Cold may precipitate an attack of angina/heart attack, and it may cause narrowing (vasoconstriction) of coronary arteries. Therefore anginal/heart attack/s are more common in cold weather. Ideally, all types of adverse weather conditions should be avoided.

Often, more than one or two risk factors may be present in a person, which must be considered for the prevention of CAD. But none of the risk factors may be present in many cases of CAD. In spite of this, however, it is always advisable to keep the risk factors, if they are present, under control.

Since CAD starts developing in childhood, prevention should be taken from a very early age, even when there is a single risk factor, or a positive history of CAD in the family. This is the only sound way to prevent CAD.

Role of aspirin

Aspirin (acetylsalicylic acid) has got an antiplatelet action and thus it interferes with the clotting of blood. Hence, if this drug is taken continuously, it may reduce the incidence of heart attack or death rate as a result of CAD.

Although the drug is highly recommended in the treatment as well as further prevention of heart attack, its role in primary prevention of CAD is still being studied. That is, whether the drug should be given in the case of all asymptomatic middle-aged persons (when the disease is expected to be symptomatic) for the prevention of CAD or not, is yet to be seen, although some positive results have been reported. Further, it is also to be seen if daily use of aspirin is of benefit to persons who are suffering from 1-2 or more risk factors responsible for CAD.

However, aspirin as a primary prevention of CAD, is being used for many, and its efficacy varies from case to case, or on the severity of the risk factor/s involved. In one of the departmental seminars, at the Newcastle General Hospital, U.K., in which the author participated, while discussing the role of aspirin in various vascular diseases like stroke (involving the blood vessels of the brain) and CAD etc, the Registrar of the Department spoke in a lighter vein that his mother had been taking aspirin, half a tablet daily for the last several years, and that she had no problem at the age of eighty years!

What is homocystein (Hcy)

It is an amino acid derived from the break down of dietary methionine. Its normal fasting plasma level lies in the range of 5 to 15 mmol/L with a mean level of about 10 mmol/L. Hyperhomocysteinemia (HCA) is categorized 'moderate' if the value ranges between 15 - 30 mmol/L, 'intermediate' 30 - 100 mmol/L and 'severe' more than 100 mmol/L.

Higher levels of Hcy cause vascular injury leading to CAD. HCA occurs due to the deficiency of vitamin B6, B12 and folic acid. This deficiency is more in Indians and that could be attributed to the reduced intake of vitamins and prolonged cooking of vegetables as has been observed in some of the Indian houses in the U.K.

Hence multivitamin supplementation containing vitamin B6, vitamin B12 and folic acid could go a long way in decreasing Hcy levels and thereby offering potential benefits vis a vis mortality and morbidity. One study recommends 100 mgm of vitamin B6, 400 mcg of vitamin B12 and 650 mcg of folic acid for a period of 6 weeks. Increased consumption of green leafy vegetables and fruits that are rich in vitamins helps in such cases. Estimation of Hcy levels has been particularly recommended in young individuals who are prone to develop CAD.

2. Secondary Prevention of CAD

It means prevention from further heart attack/s after one has recovered from the first attack. In such cases, besides adhering to the various steps of primary prevention of CAD, described above, one should take medicinal treatment regularly. Angioplasty/surgery i.e. CABG should not be delayed unnecessarily, whenever indicated. This is an important step of secondary prevention.

Sex and CAD: In secondary prevention, a usual question is asked by the patient about the performance of sex. One may lead a fairly normal life in this regard, of course with precautions. However, it depends upon the severity of the lesion of CAD. As a rough guide, following a recovery from a heart attack, if the patient is able to climb one, preferably two full flight of stairs without any feeling of discomfort, he may indulge in coitus. More precisely, the heart rate should not be more than 120 per minute during the period of sex, and the patient should have no pain/discomfort.

To avoid additional stress, sex should be avoided immediately after meals, and even extra-marital sex should be abstained from. If suitable precautions are not taken, or the lesion happens to be more severe, an attack of angina may be precipitated during sex, and one may have to keep a quick-acting coronary dilator i.e. glyceryl trinitrate under the tongue (or chewed). If severe pain occurs during sex, follow the steps of first-aid treatment for heart attacks. Although rare, an unaware patient may even die in orgasm, i.e. during the climax of a sexual excitement, the so-called coital death. It is more likely to occur in extra-marital sexual intercourse. The idea of writing this is only that such type of exertion should be kept in mind by the concerned patient. It is an important step of secondary, or even primary prevention, especially in high-risk cases. In any case, the patient should not feel hesitant to ask any questions in this regard from his physician/family doctor. He should also not feel embarrassed to discuss with his physician, in case he has any problems during the performance of sex.

From the above account of prevention of CAD, it is evident that both primary and secondary steps of prevention are necessary to keep the fast-increasing cases of CAD under control, thus saving people both from morbidity and mortality.

Rehabilitation after heart attack

This aspect is of vital importance. Gone are the days when the patient was given prolonged rest, say at least six weeks, for a heart attack. Whenever a heart attack occurs, the patient or his relations should not feel frightened. Even now, home treatment has been advocated in uncomplicated cases of heart attack. Treatment is simple, easy, as long as no complication/s occur. In such cases, about two weeks of rest is essentially required. Even on the second day of the attack, the patient can walk round the bed, and may gradually increase his walk, and in about two weeks' time, he can walk 400-500 yards.

Unnecessary prolonged rest is not at all in the interest of the patient. He becomes markedly weak. There is loss of strength as well as efficacy, i.e. the capacity to work decreases markedly. However, prolonged rest has to be given if the patient has developed complications, or if the patient's condition becomes more serious as a result of the heart attack.

Climbing of stairs needs special mention/precaution in the case of a CAD after recovery from a fresh attack. The patient is advised to initially climb stairs once a week, and the difference of pulse rate should not be more than 20 before and after the climbing of stairs.

The patient must be encouraged to resume his work/normal life-style as soon as possible, whenever he is declared fit by his physician. He may be advised light work and his daily duration of work may be reduced in the beginning. The patient may even need psychological assistance. It is also good for the patient to take light regular exercises. However, sports requiring heavy exertion should not be undertaken. The patient in any case should not overexert himself, should take good rest/sleep, and should feel happy and contented. Emotional outbursts, undue anxiety or depression, etc. must be avoided as far as possible.

In a nutshell, all aspects of the patient must be looked into, including the economic aspect, if possible, by all concerned. And it is only with the co-operation of all that we can hope for a comfortable lifespan for such patients.

Recapitulating the topic of CAD, it may be emphasised that since the disease process starts right in childhood, and though clinical manifestations appear around middle age, various preventive steps should be observed from early in life. The child must be made aware of the various preventive aspects of CAD. It is easier to mould a child for a specific lifestyle, including the behaviour pattern, and it must be seen that such a cultivated manner/pattern of life continues throughout life. Besides, the general public must be made aware of various aspects of CAD through the media, talks, camps, seminars etc., from time to time, and all hidden cases of CAD must be unearthed. This is the only way to curb the incidence of this fatal disease. Undoubtedly the medical fraternity ought to keep abreast of latest technique so that it could provide the best to the patients as well take part in awareness programmes.

2. *Rheumatic fever (RF) and rheumatic heart disease (RHD)*

Both RF and RHD are linked together as RHD is one of the important manifestations of RF.

What is RF ?

It is a disease of children/adults, and is characterised by fever and painful swelling of the joints, mostly of the limbs, especially of the ankles and knees. The notable feature of the painful swelling of the joints is that it is fleeting in nature i.e. the swelling of the joints travels from one joint to another. Simultaneously/soon, in acute stage, the heart may also be involved.

Diseases of the Heart

Hence, early diagnosis, or suspicion of the disease is necessary for proper treatment, especially to save the heart from damage. Hence, the warning signal of RF is that whenever fleeting pain/swelling occurs in the joints, the physician must be consulted for a precise diagnosis. This signal should be recognised by parents/teachers especially, and adults should know about such diseases as a matter of routine.

A number of joints may be involved at one stage, and the other joints may also be involved before swelling/pain in the earlier involved joints disappears. The swelling in the affected joints starts regressing in about a week, and the joints may become normal in 3-4 weeks' time.

The most important point is that the disease may be self-limited i.e. it may subside without any treatment. If such attacks continue to occur, although the joints heal completely during each attack, the most vital organ of the body i.e. the heart, may be damaged permanently (see later).

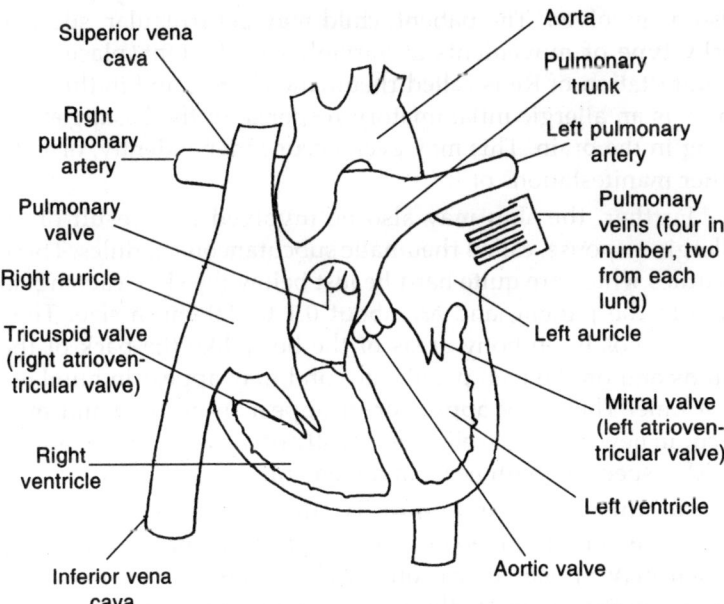

Fig. 4. A diagrammatic representation of the heart showing the chambers, the blood vessels and the valves.

What is the cause of RF?

The disease occurs as a result of sore throat by a specific organism called group-A beta haemolytic streptococcus (GABHS). There is no direct extension of infection from the throat or from upper respiratory tract, either to the joints or to the heart. Both the joints and the heart are involved as a result of abnormal immune response due to streptococcal infection in the throat, after a latent period of 7-10 days, during which antibodies to streptococci develop/appear in the blood. It is thus an immunological disease, and of course, occurs in susceptible individuals.

Since the infection in the throat is caused by a specific organism, i.e. GABHS, all cases of sore throat may not result in this type of serious problem or disease. Further specific strains (like serotypes 1, 3, 5, 6, 18) are associated with RF.

What are the other parts of the body where the above allergic response occurs?

Besides the joints and the heart, the central nervous system may also be involved. The patient/child may get irregular, sudden, jerky type of movements at variable time/extent/place. This manifestation of RF is called rheumatic chorea, and in this case there is an allergic inflammatory response of the basal ganglia lying in the brain. This may even occur independently, or with other manifestations of RF.

Further, the skin may also be involved as a result of an allergic response, called rheumatic subcutaneous nodules. These nodules which are quite hard lie just below the skin, causing no pain to the patient, and are about 0.1 to 2.0 cm in size. They appear mostly on bony areas of the body like the back of the hands and on the feet, patella etc., and may appear in numbers at a time. They may appear or disappear in no time and may recur in new areas as well. They mostly occur with other features of RF, especially with heart involvement.

Another manifestation of RF, though rarely seen in the tropics, is an allergic skin rash called erythema marginatum, which may appear in various circles. These circles may join giving various shapes to the lesion. The rash may also be fleeting at times, i.e. it may travel from one part of the skin to another, leaving no sign of involvement in the affected part. Like subcutaneous nodules, it is also mostly accompanied by cardiac lesion of RF. Both the subcutaneous nodules and rash may occur in the same patient. The rash/es disappear completely as soon as the acute stage of RF is over. It occurs usually on the back of the patient and upper parts of both the upper and lower limbs.

Hence, from the above, it is clear that the various manifestations of RF, i.e. joint, heart, central nervous system, skin etc. involvement may occur independently, or in various combinations, and hence both the patient and the physician have to be quite vigilant in suspecting/early diagnosing the condition.

As regards a sore throat, it may not help in the diagnosis, as the manifestations of the disease occur after 7-10 days (latent period) of a sore throat, and even a history of sore throat may not be in the notice of the patient.

Diagnosis of RF

The diagnosis of RF at times becomes difficult, especially when the various clinical manifestations occur either independently, or in varied combinations. In such a situation, other points need to be considered, like presence of fever, pain in joints (arthralgia) i.e. when typical painful swollen joints were not present in the patient earlier or any of the manifestations of RF/RHD. Some laboratory tests may also aid in the diagnosis like ECG (prolonged PR interval), and various blood tests like raised erythrocyte sedimentation rate (ESR), presence of C-reactive protein and raised leucocyte count (leucocytosis).

The above-mentioned are only minor criteria for the diagnosis of the RF. The major criteria for diagnosing RF remain the painful swelling of various joints (polyarthritis), involvement of heart (when on examination the physician finds murmurs, pericardial rub or signs of pericardial effusion i.e. fluid in the pericardial cavity surrounding the heart), including other major clinical features of the disease like rheumatic chorea/nodules, erythema marginatum, described earlier.

If any one of the above-mentioned major criteria is present in a patient, and it is associated with any two of the minor criteria, the patient is in rheumatic activity, and needs urgent treatment. Alternatively, if the patient has the two major criteria, with or without any minor criteria, an acute stage of the disease should be considered. Recent evidence of infection in the throat by GABHS further helps in the diagnosis. Tests like throat culture for GABHS, blood tests for group A streptococcal antibodies like anti-streptolysin O, anti-deoxyribonuclease B, and rapid antigen detection test may be carried out.

The idea is that early diagnosis should not be missed in any case, and the patient, if an adult, or the parents of the child, should be careful enough to keep the physician in touch with the various symptoms of RF.

In addition to the above criteria, if in a patient some evidence of infection of the specific organism, i.e. GABHS is available, that further helps in diagnosis, and therefore, blood examination for antibodies to streptococci, or a throat culture may be carried out, if possible. However, there are no precise tests for the diagnosis of RF, and it is only through the overall clinical picture and a few general tests that the diagnosis can be reached. Other tests, like echocardiography, radiographs may also be required, depending upon the case.

Why is early diagnosis vital?

The most severe complication of the recurrence of various attacks of RF is that the heart may be damaged permanently, called chronic RHD, requiring surgical intervention to improve the functioning of the heart. The other manifestations of RF like involvement of joints etc., disappear completely even if the disease is recurrent. It may look astonishing to the readers that the joints which become adversely affected as a result of the disease, making the child/adult incapacitated, on recovery, become perfectly normal without any sign of impairment left in the joints. But this may not happen so far as the heart is concerned. Each attack of RF may damage the heart, and this damage may be added during each recurrence of the disease. One may say in a lighter vein that the disease only frightens the joints, but severely beats/damages the heart.

The prevention of RHD lies in the early diagnosis and treatment of acute RF. In the heart, it is the valves that are permanently damaged, as a result of recurrent allergic effects on the valves. Once the patient has been properly diagnosed, further attacks of RF/RHD can be prevented by the prophylactic use of antibiotics for sore throat (see later), and hence saving the heart from permanent damage.

RHD

As already mentioned, out of various manifestations of RF, it is the heart, particularly its various valves, that get deformed/ scarred as a result of repeated attacks of RF/RHD. The intensity of the damage to the valves of the heart increases, as the frequency of the attacks of RF/RHD increases. Even RHD may occur independently, without any associated joint activity/ pathology. It may or may not be associated even with other clinical manifestations of RHD e.g., skin lesions etc., and even a history of sore throat may not be available.

Out of the various valves of the heart, there may be involvement of the mitral valve causing mitral stenosis (MS) and/or mitral regurgitation (MR), and similarly the aortic valve may be damaged leading to aortic stenosis (AS) and/or aortic regurgitation (AR). Both mitral and aortic valves may be involved at the same time (Fig. 4). The mitral valve is involved first and repeatedly.

Various irregularities in the rhythm of the heart may also occur called arrhythmias, like atrial extrasystole, flutter or fibrillation, including various blocks like bundle branch block.

Prognosis

The prognosis of the disease depends upon the age of the patient. Hence if the disease starts right in childhood, and is not properly treated, repeated occurrence of the disease may go on damaging the heart. If the disease starts in the later age group, say near puberty, chances of recurrence will be less, and moreover the heart involvement will also be less at this age.

If no treatment is given to a patient of acute RF, it may take about 3-6 months for the whole condition to subside. However, it entirely depends upon the severity of the disease. Such untreated cases will have further recurrence as well, being even devoid of prophylactic treatment. Hence the value of both proper diagnosis and treatment, for better prognosis of the condition, cannot be denied.

Treatment of acute RF/RHD

As the chances of heart involvement always exist in a patient of RF, especially in children, bed rest must be given till all the clinical manifestations disappear. Strict bed rest is a must, particularly when clear signs and symptoms of heart involvement are present.

The patient is daily assessed, especially for the condition of the heart. The physician regularly checks up/auscultates the heart for the character of heart sounds, any occurrence/change in the murmur/s of the heart, enlargement of heart or any sign of congestive heart failure. The pulse rate during sleep is also a useful sign for the rheumatic activity of the heart. A weekly ECG and ESR are also done in such cases. The duration of bed rest depends upon the condition of the patient. It may vary from a few weeks to a month, or more. Besides rest and daily assessment of the patient's condition, the physician prescribes a set of drugs to tide over the crisis. Oral penicillin V in doses of 500 mg twice

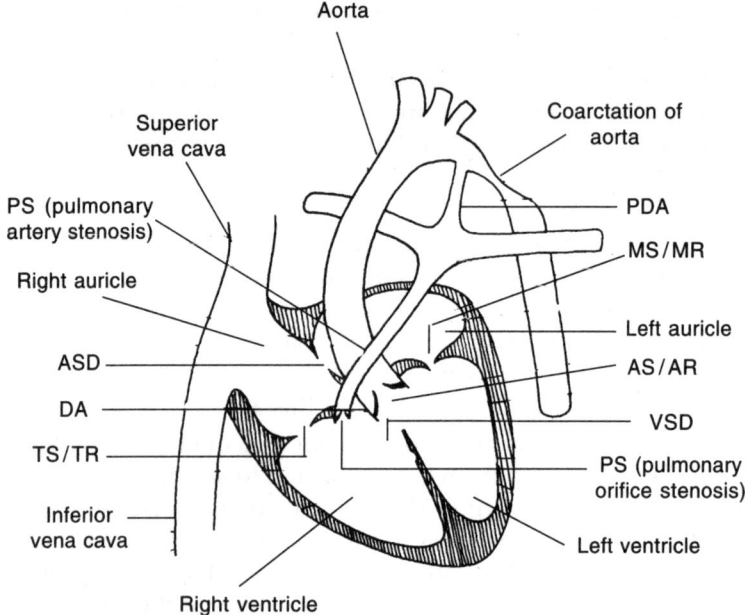

Fig. 5. A diagrammatic representation of the various congenital lesions of the heart.

a day or erythromycin 250 mg four times a day for a period of ten days needs to be prescribed for throat infection even when throat culture is negative. Alternatively, a single intramuscular injection of benzathine penicillin of 1.2 million may be recommended. This will also serve as the first dose meant for secondary prophylaxis (see later).

Treatment of chronic RHD

As stated earlier, once the valves of the heart are damaged, besides medicinal treatment, the patient may need surgery for the proper working of the heart. However, in early and selected cases angioplasty (ballooning) may serve the purpose, and the patient may be saved from a major surgery.

Prophylaxis of RF/RHD

RF/RHD has always been considered to be a preventable disease. Since the disease occurs primarily as a result of sore throat, through a specific group of organism i.e. GABHS therefore, prophylaxis of RF/RHD means prevention of sore throat. But the prevention of sore throat is not so simple as it may appear to be. There are a large number of cases of sore throat, and most of them are viral in nature, and out of the bacterial infection only a small number may be related to the specific organism i.e. GABHS responsible for RF/RHD. Approximately 3% to 20% of sore throats may be of streptococcal infection and out of these nearly 0.3% result in RF. A recent study shows that almost 90% of cases that get RF develop RHD. GABHS can only be identified if a throat swab is taken of each and every child for culture of the organisms. It may not be feasible in a disease like sore throat which is so commonly prevalent and subsides even without treatment in many of the cases, i.e., it is a self-limiting disease.

Due to the above reasons, it is not possible to detect the occult/hidden cases of sore throat as a result of GABHS in a mass survey/check-up of children, as for example in various schools and colonies etc., because throat culture takes 48-72 hours, and there is no kit for quick detection of cases.

However, as a general prophylaxis sore throat should be immediately treated, irrespective of the causative organism, especially in children/adults for the prevention of RF/RHD. Doctors, especially paediatricians, can play a significant role in explaining to parents, especially mothers, for immediate treatment of sore throat in their children whenever it occurs. Teachers in schools also play an equally important role in this respect. Oral penicillin for a period of 10 days or one injection of benzathine penicillin may suffice in most of the cases. However injectable procaine penicillin twice daily for 10 days is recommended in cases of recurrent sore throat or when a case of RF has been reported in the community recently.

A long-term drug prophylaxis should be given to all children/adults, who once suffered an attack of RF/RHD, for the protection of the throat against the above mentioned streptococcal infection. Drug prophylaxis is important as RF has a tendency of recurrence, and each fresh attack leads to further damage to the valvular tissue making the disease further worse. No doubt the drug prophylaxis may decrease the chances of further attack, but it cannot prevent the initial damage caused by RF.

The duration of prophylaxis differs from case to case, as the incidence of the disease decreases as age advances. This drug prophylaxis may be given till the child reaches the adult age, or for five years after the last attack of RF/RHD. Once the prophylaxis is withdrawn, great vigilance is required, and the child/adult should take proper treatment for sore throat as and when it occurs. However, drug prophylaxis may be required almost forever/lifelong, especially in cases which exhibit permanent signs of valvular/rheumatic heart disease. These damaged valves need foolproof protection against infection, and due to this reason, drug prophylaxis is given continuously. Long-acting antibiotics, like benzathine penicillin, is given in such cases every month; some advocate it every three weeks. In the case of children, the concerned parents must see to it that the child is strictly administered a regular course of antibiotic, as explained/motivated by their physician.

Also, all cases of RHD should take a short course of antibiotics (besides the long-acting antibiotics they are taking monthly) before undergoing any operative procedure, either minor or major, as for example dental extraction etc., as more virulent bacteria are likely to enter the blood from the area of operation leading to gross infection of the already damaged valves of the heart, called subacute bacterial endocarditis (SBE), which requires emergent measures to save the heart from damage. In that case strong antibiotics will be required to tide over the crisis.

As a part of prophylaxis, it is also important that the warning signals of rheumatic fever, already mentioned, must be known to all, especially parents/teachers and those at the rural level. Unless the people, particularly the parents, know that a sore throat can cause RF and RHD, it is most unlikely to be attended by a doctor and treated. The children should be immediately treated on the very first attack of RF, and drug prophylaxis i.e the use of penicillin to eradicate streptococci should be started without any delay.

Above all, since the disease occurs as a result of the infection of throat, proper hygienic conditions must be maintained for the prevention of sore throat / RF/RHD.

This is the reason that people living in overcrowded/highly-populated, damp colonies/slums etc. become highly prone to this disease. Good food is also necessary for the prevention of this disease.

Summing up, it may be said that in order to achieve everlasting prevention, socio-economic factors as a whole, including especially the living conditions as well as the nutrition of the people, have to be improved, particularly among the lower strata of society. The people are required to be educated through various media regarding the dangerous consequences of sore throat, and that any sore throat must be treated promptly whenever it occurs. Of course, an early detection/treatment of cases which have already picked up the disease will be essentially required. For this all, we need a national strategy/programme, and only then we can hope to prevent this disease which is still one of the major health hazards in many developing countries. It is earnestly hoped that a anti-streptococcal (GABHS) vaccine will soon be available, which may indeed prove to be a breakthrough in the prevention of this disease.

3. Congenital heart disease (CHD)

For general awareness of CHD, one is required to know about the anatomy of the heart for practical purposes (Fig. 5).

The heart is a four-chambered organ. The upper two (small) chambers are called auricles and the lower two (larger) are called ventricles. The auricles on each side are connected with their respective ventricles through an orifice/opening, the left one is called mitral orifice and the right one is called tricuspid orifice. The orifices are guarded by valves (called the mitral valve and the tricuspid valve) so that blood flows in one direction only i.e. from auricles to ventricles, on each side.

The left side of the heart contains pure or oxygenated blood. After oxygenation, the blood comes from the lungs to the left upper chamber i.e. the left auricle through the pulmonary veins. From the left auricle, the blood goes to the left ventricle through the mitral orifice, and from the left ventricle, the blood is pushed/pumped into the aorta (through the aortic orifice, guarded by the aortic valve) i.e. the main blood vessel which supplies blood to the entire body through its several branches.

From the body, the blood has to return to the heart for further oxygenation. This blood enters into the upper right chamber of the heart (right auricle), through superior vena cava which returns the blood from the upper half of the body and through the inferior vena cava, which returns the blood from the lower half of the body. The blood then goes to the right ventricle through the tricuspid orifice. The right ventricle further pushes the blood through the pulmonary orifice (guarded by pulmonary valve) into the pulmonary trunk, which divides into right and left pulmonary arteries for carrying the blood further to the right and left lung respectively, for oxygenation.

It is obvious from the above that the left side chambers contain oxygenated blood while the right side chambers contain impure blood. The right and left side chambers of the heart are not connected in any way, so that there is no mixing of pure and impure blood.

What are the areas of the heart where congenital defects occur?

The main pulmonary artery/trunk which carries blood from right ventricle to the lungs for oxygenation may be involved. If this vessel is stenosed, called pulmonary stenosis (PS), the whole blood from the right ventricle will not be able to go to the lungs for purification. This defect may be associated with a septal defect either between the two auricles called atrial septal defect (ASD) or between the two ventricles called ventricular septal defect (VSD), or both, so that impure blood goes to the left side (as in such cases pressure is more in the chambers on the right side), i.e. into the left auricle or the left ventricle.

In this way, left side chambers of the heart instead of containing pure oxygenated blood, contain mixed blood i.e. both pure and impure blood. This mixed blood is supplied to the body through the aorta, so that the body instead of getting pure oxygenated blood, gets mixed blood, and hence each organ/tissue of the body suffers, and the child may be born blue/cyanosed, or becomes blue with a slight exertion.

If pulmonary stenosis (PS) is associated with VSD with resultant right ventricular hypertrophy (RVH), and the aorta also gets connected with the right ventricle (as a result of VSD), called dextroposition of the aorta (DA), the condition is called tetralogy of Fallot (PS, VSD, RVH, DA). And when tetralogy of Fallot is associated with ASD, the condition is called pentalogy of Fallot. In such cases the child is expected to be markedly blue (cyanosed) right from birth i.e. a blue baby may be born (Fig. 5).

What are the early symptoms / warning signals of the above-mentioned congenital defects in the heart—tetralogy / pentalogy of Fallot?

Such a child soon after birth or may be a little later (during infancy), depending upon the area as well as severity of the lesion, gets attacks of breathlessness. The growth of such a child will not be proper, and the child may become blue (cyanosed) with a little exertion. If the child is born blue, the condition of such a child is considered to be very serious.

In all such cases, immediate diagnosis at birth is important for the proper planning of the treatment, including surgery. Early diagnosis may be missed, especially in cases when the child is not blue at birth, and becomes blue only on exertion while the child is growing.

Hence in the case of any child who becomes blue while playing and sitting down, and cannot play any longer with children of his age, or gets palpitation and/or becomes conscious of some abnormal sound (murmur) in the chest, the parents should immediately get him or her examined by a cardiologist for any congenital lesion in the heart which may need immediate surgery.

What are 'late cyanotic (blue)' cases of congenital heart disease?

In the group of cases, described above, i.e. tetralogy/pentalogy of Fallot, since more than one or two congenital lesions in the heart are present at the same time, the child may be born blue, or becomes blue in infancy/childhood, and therefore, the diagnosis may become obvious early. However, parents' awareness in such cases is of utmost importance.

But in cases where the congenital lesion is a solitary one i.e. ASD or VSD, or there is a congenital communication between the aorta (carrying oxygenated blood) and the main pulmonary artery/trunk (carrying impure blood to the lungs), called patent ductus arteriosus (PDA), the cyanosis will be much later i.e. in adulthood or in middle age or even later.

In ASD, there is a congenital communication between the two auricles, so that blood flows from the left auricle to the right auricle, because the pressure in the left auricle is normally higher than in the right auricle. Similarly, in VSD, there is a communication between two ventricles so that blood flows from the left to the right ventricle. In PDA, the oxygenated blood will flow from the aorta into the main pulmonary artery/trunk, which carries impure blood to the lungs for oxygenation.

Since in the above congenital lesions of the heart, it is the pure or the oxygenated blood which gets mixed up with the impure blood, the patient will not be much affected, especially in the beginning, and more so when the defect is minor. Such cases may remain hidden for years together, or may be detected in a routine check-up, say on joining service, etc. I have seen a female patient in whom such a congenital lesion remained undetected in spite of the fact that she had gone through two deliveries normally.

The earliest possible diagnosis is required of such cases. If such a lesion in the heart of the patient is not detected in time and the defect is not corrected surgically, the patient, slowly, say over a period of years, will develop pulmonary hypertension. With the result of this, the flow of blood will get reversed i.e. the blood will start flowing from the right to the left side through the congenital lesion concerned. Thus there will be a mixing of impure blood with the pure blood, and the patient will become

Diseases of the Heart

blue (cyanosed), first on exertion and later even while at rest. This point is of utmost importance that once pulmonary hypertension has developed and the shunt has reversed, the operation will not be possible, and one can imagine the debilitating condition of the patient. It is, therefore, in the above said group of cases that an early diagnosis should be the rule. Such cases where surgical intervention is not advisable have to be on constant medication, and still their life may not be completely comfortable.

The author would like to report one of his cases, of a middle-aged male who was diagnosed as a case of ASD. The patient was investigated for the possibility of an operation of his heart. This case proved to be too late, and he could not be operated because by then pulmonary hypertension had developed. It is really astonishing that his congenital lesion in the heart, could not be detected earlier. Incidentally, the patient is still alive, but his life is very debilitating, and he often finds it difficult to breathe, gets blueness/palpitation of heart. He is almost confined to bed. Had this case been detected and operated right in his childhood, he would have lived almost a normal life, and would have been spared the heavy medication he is now taking, which also accounts for a good deal of expense, especially in old age. Therefore, early/timely diagnosis is the only key to give a comfortable span of life to such patients. As a general principle, women who are suffering from cyanotic congenital heart disease, pulmonary hypertension should avoid pregnancy and may even go for tubectomy after medical consultation.

What are the other congenital lesions of the heart?

Not all the cases of congenital lesion/s of the heart cause cyanosis/blueness. There is also a group of conditions which are equally important, and cause marked symptoms except cyanosis. Such cases need a good deal of medicines, and also require early surgical intervention.

One of the lesions in this group occurs when there is a congenital narrowing/stenosis in the upper portion of the aorta (usually near the ductus arteriosus) called coarctation of the aorta (Fig. 5). In this disorder chest X-ray provides important clues. It may reveal '3' sign appearance i.e. there would be dilation before and after narrowing of aorta. Further chest X-ray may show notching of the ribs as a result of collaterals. Echocardiography, Doppler studies, magnetic resonance studies are other tests relating to this disorder. The patient will develop hypertension in the upper part of the body. This will also find mention in Chapter 4 on high blood pressure. Such patients must be treated for raised levels of blood pressure so as to prevent the serious complications of high blood pressure. At the same time surgery and / or dilation (ballooning) of the stenosed/narrowed lesion in the aorta should not be delayed.

Other cases in this group would be when the mitral/aortic/tricuspid orifice is involved leading to mitral stenosis/regurgitation (MS/MR), aortic stenosis/regurgitation (AS/AR), tricuspid stenosis/regurgitation (TS/TR) respectively. Solitary stenosis of pulmonary orifice (PS) also comes under this group (Figs. 4,5). Early diagnosis and treatment, both medicinal and surgical, are necessary in such cases, so that the patient is relieved of his symptoms. In all such cases, the heart may get enlarged, and the patient usually feels breathless especially in advanced cases. In some of the selected early cases even angioplasty (ballooning) may be possible and thus save the patient from a major surgery.

What steps should be taken for detection of occult/hidden cases of CHD?

Since there are still a large number of occult/hidden/asymptomatic cases of CHD, especially of the late cyanotic or acyanotic (in which cyanosis does not occur) group, urgent steps are required to be taken for their early detection. Such cases can be detected in various camps, especially in schools/colonies, etc. However, in many of the late diagnosed cases, as described earlier, treatment/surgery may not be possible.

It will be appropriate if at the time of birth, a paediatrician examines all the babies for any congenital lesion of the heart, and if suspected, an echocardiography should be carried out so that the disease can be diagnosed right at birth, and necessary steps of treatment can be planned well in time.

It is not difficult diagnosing/suspecting/detecting various congenital lesions in the heart, say, in the general population. The physician, besides a detailed clinical examination, is mainly required to auscultate the heart of each child or adult, as the case may be, for heart sounds and murmurs. It gives a fair clue of various congenital lesions of the heart, although all the murmurs of the heart may not be pathological. There are also so-called innocent murmurs. However, once the disease is suspected, the diagnosis can be confirmed by various tests, especially echocardiography.

Even a rare/uncommon heart disease can be diagnosed with fair accuracy on clinical examination of the heart. Hence in various camps that may be proposed to be organized by various voluntary organizations, not much expenditure is likely to be incurred. Routine tests, like ECG and X-rays etc., are required when there is at least some clue on auscultation/clinical examination about the presence of CHD.

The case of a Chinese woman suffering from a congenital heart disease, rupture of sinus of valsalva, which is not very common, was reported in the *British Medical Journal* in its issue of 16th March, 1968. The same year, a similar case of an Indian patient was suspected clinically by the author. Advanced tests like echocardiography etc. were not available at that time. The patient was operated at Mumbai by Dr. K.N. Dastur, Honorary Cardiac Surgeon and Honorary Professor of Surgery, Topiwala National Medical College and B.Y.L. Nair Charitable Hospital. Dr. Dastur, confirming the author's diagnosis, wrote, "The rupture of sinus of valsalva was into the right ventricle as postulated by you."

Hence, a clinical examination/auscultation of heart will go a long way in detecting the subclinical cases of congenital lesions of the heart. And, therefore, a general realization of this fact is all that is required so that people themselves come forward for such routine check-ups of their children by their physician, or report in the various camps that may be held from time to time. Unless this is achieved, the desired goal can not be reached. And the people, especially the late cases who are not fit for operation, may go on suffering from the morbidity of the disease, which is chronic in many of the cases.

Prevention of subacute bacterial endocarditis

A word of caution! All cases of CHD whether operated or not must take a short course of drug prophylaxis, as and when they undergo any sort of operation relating to dental, gastrointestinal and genitourinary surgery and also while carrying tests like sigmoidoscopy or cystoscopy, so as to prevent the infection of the congenital lesion in the heart from the site of the operation/surgery. If this is not strictly followed, the patient is likely to develop gross infection of the heart, called subacute bacterial endocarditis, which is a medical emergency and may need very potent antibiotics to deal with the crisis. Besides drug prophylaxis, utmost oral and perineal hygiene are recommended.

What are the tests required in cases of CHD.

Tests like echocardiography, Doppler imaging, haemodynamic study, angiocardiography help in detecting the precise nature of lesion.

Prevention of congenital heart disease (CHD)

It is indeed difficult to deal with this topic. Not much is known about the various causes, for operating on a pregnant woman, in the first three months of pregnancy, during which period, development of the heart in the foetus is expected to be complete.

Under the above circumstances, the best thing would be that all pregnant women must undergo a routine ultrasonography, and if some abnormality is suspected, foetal echocardiography must be undertaken for the precise detection of congenital defect in the heart. However, the question of termination of pregnancy must be taken especially in consultation with a heart specialist, or one who is dealing with paediatric cardiac surgery. Many of the congenital lesions of the heart can be satisfactorily treated, though surgically. All aspects of the case must be studied like the number of children, and if the previous offspring have any congenital defect or not, or, if this pregnancy has occurred after a long period of time.

Heredity may play some role in the causation of the disease. If the mother has any congenital defect in her heart, the chances, though minimal, of a defect in the heart of the expected baby may increase. Genetic counselling may help in such cases before the pregnancy is planned.

There are some conditions worth mentioning which must be avoided by a pregnant mother, as there are some likely factors which may disturb the development of the heart in the foetus.

If the mother is diabetic, it must be properly controlled. Diabetes, and even prediabetes, is known to cause congenital defects in the heart. Similarly, if the mother is suffering from epilepsy, the teratogenic effect of antiepileptic drugs must be kept in mind. Therefore, in such cases foetal echocardiography is a must to assess the condition of the heart. Exposure to X-rays/radiation should also be avoided.

All pregnant mothers, especially in the first three months of pregnancy, must be prevented from contracting any viral infection, particularly infection caused by the virus of German measles. A good diet is also essential during pregnancy, and in case the individual is taking alcohol, it must be stopped altogether. It may not only cause a congenital defect in the heart, it may also affect the general development of the foetus, especially the brain.

A drug like thalidomide, which is a known teratogenic, and one used in psychiatry, i.e. lithium, should also be stopped.

However, in spite of taking best possible precautions, as mentioned above, the child may still be born with some congenital lesion in the heart. Therefore, as stated earlier, a routine ultrasonography and if need be, foetal echocardiography, is a must for all pregnant mothers in their first trimester. This will help them know the exact position of the heart of the foetus they are carrying and whether the pregnancy should be terminated, or continued, though there may be a little congenital lesion in the heart which can be treated/taken care of after the child is born.

It may be concluded that although prescribed precautions must be taken by a pregnant mother, yet detection of a lesion in the heart of the foetus during the period of pregnancy, or after the child is born, or during childhood (if the case has remained undetected earlier), as well as timely treatment/surgery, will help a lot in improving the overall healthy span of life in such cases. And for all this, a mass consciousness is essentially required for successful completion of this aim.

3
DIABETES

Diabetes is one of the occult diseases which needs widespread awareness among people. It must be diagnosed as early as possible, especially in the persons who have a family history of diabetes, are obese (body mass index-BMI ≥25 kg/m^2), in women who have given birth to overweight/stillborn/abnormal babies, and/or have elevated blood sugar, or pass sugar in urine during the period of pregnancy, have polycystic ovary syndrome (PCOS), in people who are inactive, hypertensive, have deranged blood lipids levels and have suffered from vascular disease. Such persons are called prediabetics and are at high risk of developing type 2 diabetes mellites (see below). An effective control of the disease is of vital importance so that prediabetics do not become diabetics and those who are suffering from diabetes are able to keep their blood sugar levels normal.

The only way to detect the problem is to check the blood sugar levels of all persons irrespective of their age. The reasons being that the duration of diabetes has a cumulative effect, adding to the complications of the disease later. An early detection helps control the disease immediately, and various complications can be prevented or reversed through timely detection and treatment.

Diabetes mellitus is of two types — type 1 and type 2 diabetes mellitus (DM).

Type 1 DM occurs when the body's immune system destroys insulin-producing cells (called beta cells) that are present in the pancreas. Insulin is produced in the beta cells of the pancreatic islets. It is interesting to note that normally the body's immune system fights off bacteria/viruses that invade the person. In type

Diabetes

1 DM body's immune system starts attacking its own beta cells leading to partial or even total deficiency of insulin hormone.

Type 2 DM occurs as a result of varied disorders that lead to variable degrees of insulin resistance, decreased insulin secretion and increased glucose production. There may be genetic and metabolic defects in some cases leading to type 2 DM.

Although type I DM usually occurs in younger age group say before the age of 30 years and type 2 DM commonly manifests as age advances, both the types of DM can occur at any age. Type 2 DM is fast occurring due to rising state of obesity and reduced levels of activity.

Since the disease has no symptoms in the beginning, as in the case of hypertension, and in many other diseases, mass surveys of the population, for checking blood sugar levels, are of the utmost importance for diagnosing it in time.

This holds true in other parts of the world as well. Diabetes is a world-wide problem, and the author is reminded of an incident while he was in New York. He noted a crowd at a public place/crossing where blood sugar levels of all passersby were being checked with the help of a tiny blood glucose meter. It can be successfully applied in mass checking, for quick results. The author also conducted similar check-ups, by holding medical camps for early detection of diabetes, hypertension, various cancers, etc. and recommends that such camps are organized by various physicians/voluntary organizations/institutes so as to curb the menace right at the beginning.

A fasting, and preferably postprandial, i.e. 2 hours after meals called 2-hour postprandial glucose test, is required for finding out hidden cases of diabetes. The results of blood sugar estimation are required to be interpreted by the biochemist/ physician as these are likely to differ depending upon the sample of the blood used for the test, i.e., whether venous whole blood, capillary whole blood (finger prick blood) or venous plasma, has been used. Similarly, the results are bound to differ with the method/kit applied for the test.

However, one simple way would be that if a sample of urine, taken two hours after meals (the person should be advised to evacuate/empty the urinary bladder before taking meals to avoid the mixing of previously collected urine with the urine which is stored within two hours after taking the food), shows the presence of sugar, it is a good indication that the blood must be tested for establishing a diagnosis of diabetes.

A strip may be used for immediate testing of sugar in urine. It is a small strip, the end of which is coated with testing material. The coated end is dipped in urine which gives instantaneous reading of the changed colour. One may even just wet the end of this strip while passing urine. Care should be taken that the reagent on the strip is not washed away with the force of the stream of urine. The last drops of urine should be enough for just wetting the reagent part of the strip. Such strips are readily available with different names like Diastix, etc. The detailed instructions are provided for the ready reference of people.

There is another method for testing urine for sugar which needs to be interpreted carefully for early detection of cases of diabetes. In this test, in a 5 ml of Benedict's reagent 8 drops of urine are added in a test tube. The tube is put on a flame to boiling point. The normal colour of the solution is light blue. Any change in colour of the solution is noted. It may be green, greenish-yellow, yellowish-red, red, depending upon the level of blood sugar/severity of the disease. It is mild when the colour is green. It may be cautioned that this green colour may also appear when the patient is taking drugs like aspirin, vitamin B complex, vitamin C, etc. However, a blood sugar estimation will clear the diagnosis of diabetes.

In more susceptible cases, especially in prediabetics, a glucose tolerance test (GTT) may be required in which five samples of blood as well as urine are taken to establish the diagnosis. In this procedure, after taking a fasting blood sample, usually 75 g of glucose (in adults) is administered orally, after dissolving it in 250-300 ml of water. The patient has to drink it within 15 minutes.

Alternatively, a fasting blood sample and blood sample, two hours after having oral glucose, just mentioned, may suffice in many of the cases, called 2-hour postchallenge glucose test. This test is more accurate than the 2-hour postprandial glucose test, since the different constituents in a meal, the time availed of in taking meal, and above all, the absorption of food, may vary from person to person.

For labelling an individual diabetic, great care is required both on the part of the clinician and the biochemist. Laboratories are required to provide a precise interpretation of the test for immediate attention of the physician. A wrong label of diabetes may unnecessarily traumatise the person for the whole of his life. He/she may follow uncalled-for dietary and other restrictions, and may not feel comfortable in social gatherings. Since it is a hereditary disease, all the members of a family will naturally always feel suspicious of being prediabetic.

Blood test/s for detecting early cases of diabetes are required to be performed with utmost accuracy, and detailed instructions prior and during the test must be observed to avoid false reports. In GTT or in the 2-hour postchallenge glucose test, a good preparation is required before the test is carried out, since some factors like stress, anxiety, infection, smoking, drugs like oestrogens, corticoids, etc. are likely to impair glucose tolerance. All these factors are required to be borne in mind. Even the regular diet and activity of the person in question needs consideration. At least 72 hours prior to the above test, the person should be on his normal diet (he should not be dieting particularly on carbohydrates), and he should be busy in his routine work as usual (undue rest should be avoided). The duration of previous fasting also has a bearing on this test, which is required to be performed in the morning after an overnight fast of 10-16 hours. However, water may be taken during the fasting period.

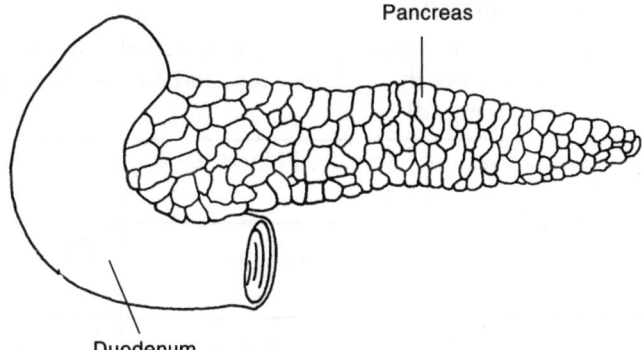

Fig. 6. The pancreas. Islets of Langerhans, present in the pancreas, secrete insulin.

Particular attention is needed during the two-hour period of the above test. The patient is required to sit calmly and should not undertake any type of exertion. Smoking should never be permitted during this period as it is likely to raise blood sugar levels.

It must be seen that the person undergoing the above test stops all such drugs which are known to influence or affect blood sugar levels. It is very important to avoid an incorrect label of diabetes. Many years back, I came across a case who was wrongly diagnosed as a case of diabetes. His blood sugar was found elevated as he was on corticoids. When I told him that he had no diabetes, he was highly relieved, and till today he remembers the episode. Such cases may not be uncommon, and need to be reinvestigated. It is best if some of the factors, mentioned above, are also kept in mind by all concerned, at least by those who have a family history of diabetes. In fact, such a difficulty particularly arises while detecting early/borderline cases of diabetes.

Normal fasting blood sugar (FBS) levels are less than 100 mg/dl. It is important that overnight fasting should be at least of 8 hours duration. The normal 2 hours post- parandial (2-h PP) blood sugar levels (i.e. levels 2 hours after intake of 75 g of glucose) are less then 140 mg/dl.

FBS levels are stated to be impaired if the values are 100 or more than 100 (=> 100) and less than 126 (<126) mg/dl. 2-h PP impaired levels would be 140 or more than 140 (=> 140) and less than 200 (< 200) mg/dl.

The individual is labeled as a case of diabetes in case FBS values are 126 or more than 126 (= >126) and 2-h PP 200 or more than 200 (=> 200) mg/dl.

Normal blood sugar levels	Impaired blood sugar levels	Diabetes
FBS < 100 mg/dl	FBS= > 100 and < 126 mg/dl.	FBS => 126 mg/dl
2 – h PP < 140 mg/dl.	2-h PP => 140 mg/dl < 200 mg/dl.	2 – h PP => 200 mg/dl.

Table: Showing various blood sugar levels for detection of diabetes.

Diabetes

What is glycosylated hemoglobin (Hb AIC) test? It is a test that measures the average blood sugar levels over preceding 90 days. Normal values are < 7% and preferable values are < 6%. This test is carried out for the diagnosis of DM especially in pregnancy and routinely in all patients of DM every 3 months.

Besides the estimation of blood sugar levels, an ultrasonographic examination, especially the magnetic resonance imaging (MRI) of the pancreas may also be required to exclude or confirm the pathology of pancreas which can be responsible for the presence of diabetes. Groups of insulin-producing cells, called the islets of Langerhans, are present in the pancreas (Fig. 6). Insulin is the main hormone for the control of the blood sugar levels. It may be noted that a genetic/family history of diabetes has an important role to play in the causation of diabetes. It is usually more frequent among overweight/sedentary workers.

Warning signals of diabetes

The various complications/warning signals of diabetes are as follows:

    (i) Excessive hunger and thirst, and urination.
    (ii) Sudden loss of weight.
    (iii) Loss of vision — cataract, especially in the young, retinal detachment, etc.
    (iv) Myocardial infarction (heart attack), angina pectoris. Diabetics are more prone to myocardial infarction and its recurrence than non-diabetics.
    (v) Stroke, i.e., paralysis of a part or whole limb or both limbs of the same side, or loss of speech/vision.
    (vi) Kidney failure, urinary tract infection, etc.
    (vii) Non-healing of injuries/boils/carbuncles/ulcers of the skin, fungal infection of the skin/nails, itching on vulvae/penis, loss of sweating, etc.
    (viii) Paresthesias (tingling sensations) in lower limbs.
    (ix) Impotence, intermittent diarrhoea.
    (x) Hypertension.
    (xi) Unconsciousness (diabetic coma).

Either one or a combination of varied complications can occur in a patient.

How to control diabetes

When so diagnosed, the disease must be controlled energetically so that its complications are either prevented or treated. While treating diabetes, one must keep in mind that control of diet and exercise are two important tools in conquering this serious problem.

Patients are advised to take low-fat, low-calorie, sugar-free/ restricted and high-fibre diet. A low-fat diet has been mentioned in Chapter 6 on high blood cholesterol. A low-fat diet is especially required when one has higher levels of blood cholesterol. In general also, a low-fat diet is recommended for preventing the complications of diabetes, especially coronary artery disease/ stroke. It may be mentioned that diabetes is a disease of the blood vessels.

In addition to a low-fat diet, the patient should avoid sugar, sweets and very sweet fruits. However, he may use some sort of artificial sweetener like 'Equal', manufactured by RPG Life Sciences Limited, Ankleshwar. This can be added in tea, milk and even in sweets, ice-cream, etc. The idea is that a diabetic should lead a normal healthy life, and may take even sweets using a harmless sweetener, described above. Aspartane is contained as sweetener in 'equal'. World Health Organization (WHO) has found that aspartane is suitable sweetener. It is all sweetness but no calories. It is sweetener in diet Coke and diet Pepsi. One may design one's own sweets and drinks with pure aspartane.

A high-fibre diet, which diabetics are advised to take, consists of green vegetables—cooked/salad, whole wheat, cereals, unpolished rice, etc. It is the outer covering of grain i.e. bran, which helps in the control of diabetes. Green vegetables, besides being a high-fibre diet, also contain very low calories, and hence can be used by diabetics in larger quantity so as to satisfy their appetite.

As regards exercise for the control of diabetes, diabetics are advised to take exercise according to the recommendation of the physician. If a diabetic is suffering from any one or more complications of the disease, especially coronary artery disease, he/she should take only limited exercise for its control. In uncomplicated cases, especially in young age, even vigorous exercise can be taken. Ideally, light exercise, especially walking after meals, is very useful for most diabetics, as blood sugar is raised after taking food, and walking will control its higher levels, reducing or completely eliminating the use of antidiabetic drugs. However, walking should be taken in a pleasant atmosphere, say in the evening/night after food, and should not be taken after lunch, especially in summer.

Special care is required if the diabetic patient is overweight (see Appendix III).

In case diabetes is not controlled by diet and exercise, only then drugs i.e. insulin (administered by injection) or oral drugs should be started in minimal dosages, and the patient should be again detailed about the diet and exercise, as it will reduce the

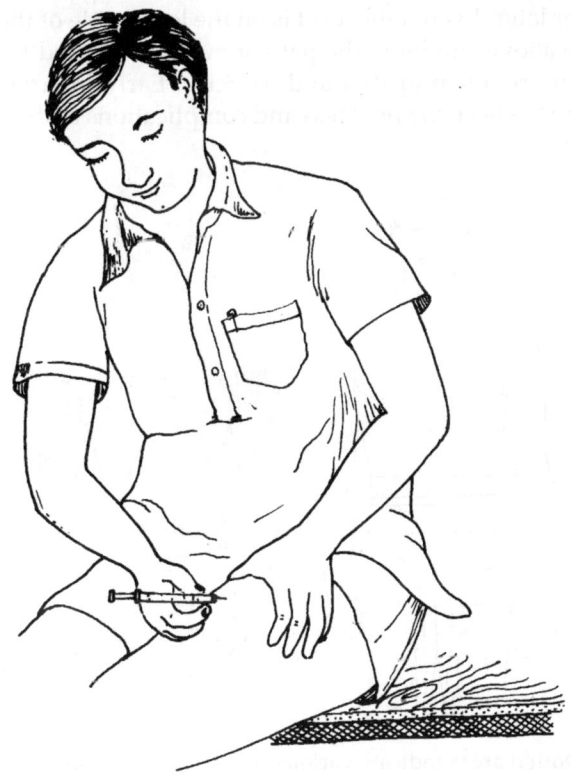

Fig. 7. A diabetic patient taking a dose of insulin by injection.

dose of antidiabetic drugs. It is important to point out that the dose of antidiabetic drugs should be properly adjusted to avoid low blood sugar, causing unconsciousness. However, a diabetic may also become unconscious when the level of blood sugar is markedly elevated, say above 400 mg/dl.

It is worth mentioning that even if the glucose tolerance test (GTT) is impaired (i.e. the level of the test does not indicate a case of diabetes), particularly if the range of the level of the test is close to the diabetic level, the patient must be advised regarding the value of diet and exercise so as to correct the impaired glucose tolerance (IGT). Small dosages of oral antidiabetic drugs may have to be advocated in cases where the diet and exercise regimen fail. If this step is not carefully followed, cases of IGT are likely to become regular diabetics sooner or later. Even if the level is on the lower side of the range, as in the above situation, the patient must be advised to strictly follow the regimen of diet and exercise. Early intervention is necessary to check the progress and complications of the disease.

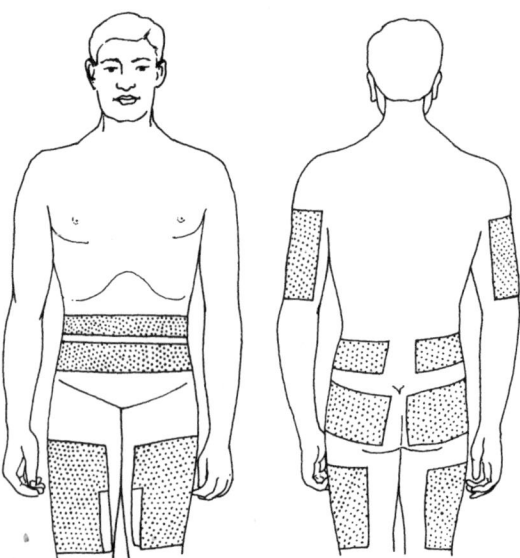

Fig. 8. Dotted areas indicate various sites for taking insulin injections; it is advisable to leave the area of abdomen, where one ties trousers/pants etc.

General instructions for diabetics
1. Daily estimation of blood sugar levels

Daily estimation of blood sugar levels is necessary in all cases of diabetes — three times a day i.e. fasting, before lunch and dinner. However, at least twice daily measurement of blood sugar levels must be taken — fasting and before dinner. All diabetics are advised to use a blood glucose meter at home for a regular checkup of their blood sugar levels.

If a diabetic finds more/elevated sugar in his blood, he should analyse as follows:
- (i) What has he been doing for the last 2 hours? He may be under stress.
- (ii) Did he eat more?
- (iii) Did he get less insulin/oral drug?

He should act as follows:
- (i) If the result is mild sugar, do exercise, jump, walk; the sugar will thus get consumed or dissipated.
- (ii) Avoid stress.
- (iii) If the quantity of sugar is high, he should regulate his subsequent diet, exercise and drugs.
- (iv) If the sugar is alarmingly high, he should consult his physician immediately.

2. Self-insulin injection

If the patient is on insulin injections, he should preferably learn the technique of self-injecting insulin into the various sites of his/her body, as shown in Figs. 7, 8. In such cases one should know about the proper sterilization of syringes, needles, or preferably use disposable syringes as well as needles which are available particularly for injecting insulin. A device such as NovoPen 3, like a pen loaded with penfill (refill containing enough insulin which can be used for many days depending on the need of the patient) can also be used for administering the daily dosages of insulin, under the direction of the physician. The penfill can be replaced when exhausted.

3. Prevent diabetic coma

A diabetic should avoid fasting. Even if a diabetic is getting diarrhoea/vomiting/both, he should take the insulin/oral drug along with glucose/sugar dissolved in water as soon as the situation permits. In advanced cases, referral to a hospital is important for glucose therapy along with parenteral insulin. If the above is not strictly followed, it will lead to diabetic coma which is a medical emergency.

4. More about diabetic coma

It occurs when the blood sugar level becomes below normal (hypoglycaemic coma) or very high (hyperglycaemic coma). In the former case the patient may have taken more than the prescribed dosages of antidiabetic drugs in over-enthusiasm to make the blood sugar levels normal, or he may have taken meagre food with the same dosages of antidiabetic drugs. In the latter case, the patient either misses the drug, or takes heavy food as well; the chances are much more when there is some infection in the body.

The symptoms/signs of both the above types of coma are different. In hypoglycaemic coma, the skin is moist with profuse perspiration which can be noticed even by a person standing nearby. All diabetics should be aware of these symptoms and as soon as they start perspiring, they should start taking sugar cubes which every diabetic is required to keep in his pocket. In hyperglycaemic coma, the skin is dry. To meet this emergency efficiently, diabetics are required to keep a card in their pockets indicating that they are diabetic, so that on reaching the hospital, the doctor on duty can immediately ascertain the cause of coma and start treatment.

5. Care of feet

A diabetic is required to be extremely vigilant about his feet. The elevated blood sugar primarily damages the nerves of the feet, the condition called peripheral neuropathy. In early cases, symptoms like numbness, tingling, burning etc. appear. If not cared for complete loss of feeling /sensations may manifest leading to injury to the feet. At the same time elevated blood sugar may also narrow small blood vessels of the feet leading to peripheral vascular disease. Accumulation of cholesterol decreases the caliber of blood vessels resulting in less blood supply to the feet. The feet become cold, there may be pain in calves on walking. Due to loss of sensations including poor blood supply to the feet, the uncontrolled and long standing diabetics are prone to foot infection. Non-healing of foot ulcers caused by shoe pressure, heat, and cold or by a sharp object is the basic foot problem faced by diabetics. Further, due to reduced sensations caused by nerve damage, injuries remain silent. In many of the cases, the patient reports with foot ulcer or gangrene in such an advanced stage that there is no alternative except to go in for an amputation which leads to permanent disability. Hence the need for caution. The following should be strictly followed:

(i) The feet should be properly cleansed with soap and water. These should be properly dried, especially in between the toes.

(ii) If the feet tend to sweat, apply any powder, especially in between the toes.

(iii) Injury to feet should be avoided. If injury occurs, it should be dressed using alcohol or mercurochrome. Do not bandage tightly and avoid adhesive tape. Local antiseptics which are likely to irritate/burn the skin should not be used. Oral antibiotics are required to combat infection.

(iv) Do not use hot water bottle or heating pads on the feet.

(v) Do not soak sore feet in hot water.

(vi) Avoid tight shoes. New shoes should be comfortable. They should be broad at the tip so as not to jam the toes.

(vii) Socks with a tight elastic band should not be used. In winter, warm stockings are preferred.

(viii) If your feet ache, remove shoes and sit with legs elevated to hip level. This should be done regularly.

(ix) Never walk barefooted.

(x) Nails should be cut straight across and filed carefully to avoid rough ends. They may be cut after a bath when soft. If they tend to crack, leave them for the doctor's care.

(xi) Corns should not be cut. Do not apply corn remover. The doctor should be consulted.

(xii) A careful examination of the feet is required by the physician. The feet should be regularly examined for any injury, loss of temperature; inter-toes area must be looked into lest a hidden area of gangrene is missed.

(xiii) Tingling sensation in the feet, numbness or coldness of feet, change of colour of skin, like deep-red, or purple in between toes, toe-nails, and pain, tenderness, sepsis of feet are some of the warning signals. The physician should be immediately consulted.

6. Psychological aspect of diabetics

This aspect should be given equal weightage. If ignored, the diabetes may not be controlled. It depends on the patient's personality. Various disturbing factors for a diabetic may be dietary restrictions, self-injection, responsibility for self-treatment, hypoglycaemic/hyperglycaemic coma, fears about the future like marriage, children, complications etc. Psychological problems are more evident in juvenile/adolescent diabetics, being younger in age. To avoid psychological trauma, the co-operation of the whole family is required. A sympathetic approach both by the doctor and family members means much to the patient. This is an important aspect of treatment, since irritability, particularly in the case of a diabetic child, will lead to hyperglycaemia. This is vital to understand in the control of diabetes.

7. Other instructions for diabetics

(i) A diabetic should bathe regularly. Powder should be used frequently in areas of skin prone to excessive sweating.

(ii) Infection anywhere in the body should be promptly treated. Care must be taken to reduce the dose of antidiabetic drugs as the infection is controlled, otherwise hypoglycaemia may occur. During infection more dosages of antidiabetic drugs are required for the control of diabetes.

(iii) Injury to any part of body should be avoided.

(iv) Regular walks help both in the control of diabetes and in improving the circulation of blood in the limbs.

(v) One should not sit cross-legged for long periods of time, e.g. in cinema halls, air journeys, etc.

(vi) Avoid underpants that are tight around the thighs.

(vii) Stress in general should be avoided.

(viii) A diabetic should know the drugs of common usage which increase blood sugar, like oral contraceptives, corticoids, etc. It is important to know this to control blood

sugar while taking antidiabetic drugs. One should also be cautious when one is on a diet/exercise programme to control diabetes.
(ix) A diabetic should see his doctor regularly. He should keep a schedule both for medicines and diet, and spare time for exercise.
(x) Besides frequently monitoring fasting and post-parandial blood sugar levels, estimation of lipids in the blood (i.e. lipidogram), 24-hour urinary assay for protein, eye consultation by the specialist particularly for retinae need to be undertaken once a year. It is after 10-15 years of this disease that one is prone to diabetic retinal disease.

8. Diabetic emergency kit

It is essential especially while travelling to carry a diabetic emergency kit. It should have a diabetic identification card, enough oral antidiabetic drugs and the doctor's prescription. If one is on insulin, extra syringes, needles, insulin vials are required. The kit must contain sugar cubes to meet the emergency of hypoglycaemic coma. Strips for testing urine sugar, preferably a blood glucose meter and other first-aid articles, like bandages, antibiotics, mercurochrome etc., should be carried.

The above guidelines, though not exhaustive, if followed, will benefit most diabetics. The idea is that a diabetic should enjoy a normal and healthy span of life.

Lastly, it must be said that detection and treatment of hidden cases of diabetes is the need of the hour, and to achieve this aim more efficiently and promptly, a diabetic ambulatory care service (DACS) is ideal, so that a house-to-house/area-wise survey of the general population can be done as a lasting solution to overcome this problem.

A word about the discovery of insulin

During the last century, two Nobel prizes were awarded to Banting and Macleod, 1923; Sanger, 1958 for research on insulin. The first patient treated was a 14 year old Canadian boy, Leonord Thompson. Today insulin is known the world over as a life saving drug for diabetes.

4
HIGH BLOOD PRESSURE
(Hypertension)

It is a common hidden disease. It has no symptoms. It can only be detected by measuring the blood pressure. If it remains undetected, fatal complications due to the involvement of the heart (myocardial infarction — heart attack), kidneys (kidney failure) and brain (stroke — paralysis) may occur. The eyes may also be damaged as a result of hypertension, and it may even cause retinal detachment/loss of vision (Fig. 9).

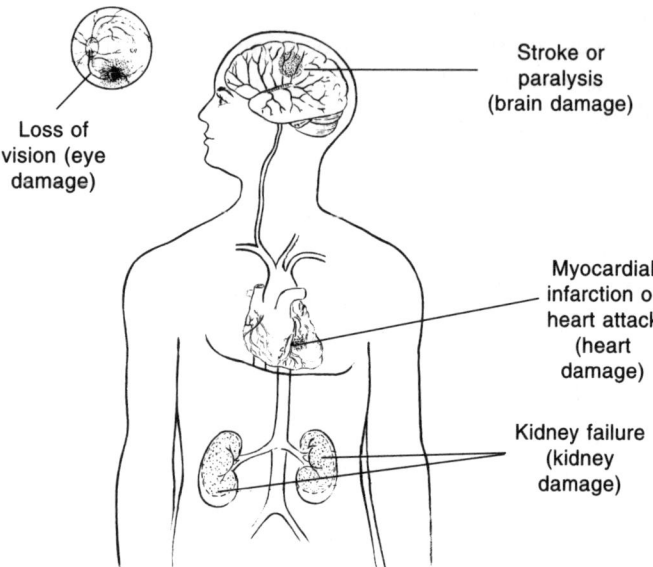

Fig. 9. The effects of high blood pressure on the heart, kidneys, brain and eyes.

High Blood Pressure (Hypertension)

The author organised various medical camps for the detection of latent cases of hypertension., and unearthed a significant number of asymptomatic patients suffering from this malady.

The normal blood pressure limit is 120/80 (120 mm Hg — systolic and 80mm Hg — diastolic). It may vary from minute to minute during various daily activities of life. It is the average of several readings, taken at various intervals, which is important. It is advisable, while taking various readings of blood pressure in an individual, to use the same blood pressure apparatus and same side of the upper arm and, ideally, the physician should also be the same. It is better to record blood pressure readings during a 24-hour period with the help of an ambulatory blood pressure recorder.

Some adults/middle-aged persons have a low level of blood pressure readings like 110/70 or even lower. Such a blood pressure is perfectly normal, rather, the person with such a blood pressure is very lucky.

It is equally important to keep an eye on the blood pressure of children.

The cause of hypertension is not known in the majority of cases, when it is called primary, essential or idiopathic hypertension. In about 20% cases, the underlying cause can be detected, and such cases are labelled as secondary hypertension. Out of the causative lesions, the defect may be either in the kidneys, or in the adrenal glands (located around the top of each kidney), or because of congenital narrowing of the main blood vessel (aorta) arising from the heart, called coarctation of the aorta. It is important to exclude such secondary causes, because if detected, the blood pressure can be controlled by treating the causative lesion. Some of the causes relating to adrenal glands may be listed as: aldosteronism, cushing's syndrome, pheochromocytoma.

Takayasu arteritis, a chronic inflammatory disease of aorta and other arteries may also cause high blood pressure. Renovascular hypertension i.e. high blood pressure due to narrowing/stenosis of the renal artery either on one side or both the sides needs special attention and tests.

Blood pressure also significantly rises as a result of taking oral contraceptives in females, and if it is so, the contraceptives should be stopped. Hypertension may also arise during the period of pregnancy, and should be treated urgently to avoid foetal/maternal mortality.

Also, the incidence of high blood pressure increases in persons who are addicted to smoking and/or tobacco chewing, as well as to alcohol. Further, obesity, hypercholesterolaemia and diabetes mellitus are associated with an increased incidence of hypertension.

A patient suffering from hypertension should be investigated thoroughly, both for determining the causative lesion and the extent of complications/damage which it has caused. Therefore, an electrocardiogram (ECG), renal function tests, a chest X-ray for heart size and for exclusion of coarctation of aorta, an ultrasonographic examination of the urinary tract and the adrenal glands, etc., must be done. A complete urine examination is equally important. A fundi examination by an opthalmologist is also required, in routine, to check the extent of damage caused to the retinae. Further, fasting blood sugar, lipidogram, echocardiogram and other tests may be required especially when secondary hypertension is suspected.

Those who are found to be suffering from early/uncomplicated hypertension should adopt the following non-pharmacological measures, i.e. measures without the usage of antihypertensive drugs to lower high blood pressure and to prevent its further rise. If these measures are strictly followed, a lower dose of antihypertensive drug may be sufficient, if required at all. Although control of blood pressure can be achieved by medication, i.e. by the administration of antihypertensive drugs, the drugs have got their own side-effects. Above all, it should not be forgotten that our ultimate goal is primary prevention of hypertension. The measures are:

(i) Low salt intake — Only 2-4 g of salt should be taken, otherwise the blood pressure will rise. We usually recommend that the patient takes minimum salt in each meal, preferably in one cooked vegetable only. It should be avoided in curd and salad. Avoid pickles, pepper, snacks, sauce, etc. as they contain a lot of salt.

High Blood Pressure (Hypertension)

(ii) More potassium, i.e. citrate fruits like orange, *malta*, *kenu*, *mousmi*, etc. should be taken.

(iii) Exercises like brisk walking/jogging should be followed under strict medical advice, because only limited activity is allowed in the case of persons suffering from severe hypertension, or its complications.

(iv) Reduction of weight is required, if one is overweight.

(v) A high-fibre diet (i.e. green vegetables, whole cereals, unpolished rice, etc.) is useful.

(vi) *Shavasana* — Regular *Shavasana* should be undertaken. It is highly beneficial for the control of hypertension. In mild cases the blood pressure may be fully brought down to normal levels, while in moderate to severe cases, doses of antihypertensive drugs can be brought down.

This *asana* is a conscious skeletal muscle relaxation exercise, and is strongly recommended for hypertensive patients.

In this *asana*, the patient is required to lie down straight on his back at a quiet place, limbs slightly apart and eyes closed (Fig. 10). He is then required to breathe slowly through his nose, and start relaxing his muscles from below upward. He may say the word of his choice, e.g. 'Om', 'God', 'Waheguru', 'Allah', everytime, while breathing out. It should be carried out once or twice daily for about half an hour.

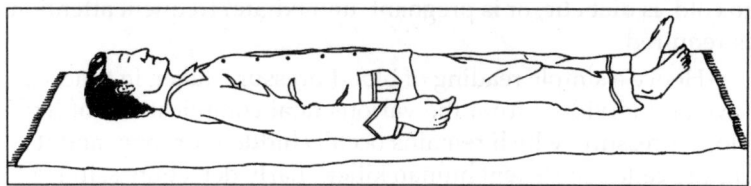

Fig. 10. A patient of high blood pressure undergoing '*shavasana*'.

The patient should remain awake and be alert during this therapy. It should not be undertaken immediately after meals.

It may be again said that if the above measures are religiously followed, this occult disease, i.e. hypertension, can be prevented in most cases.

Drugs should only be taken when the above measures of prevention fail. These should be given judiciously during pregnancy to avoid foetal complications. Most antihypertensive drugs, besides causing various side-effects, also cause postural hypotension. In postural hypotension, the patient is likely to fall down if he suddenly stands up after a long spell of sitting/lying down. To avoid this, the patient is required to stand for a while with support so as to be sure regarding his stability. A patient with this tendency should not pass urine in a standing position during the night. He should sit down to pass urine.

Needless to say, as is done in case of diabetes, the only way to diagnose hidden cases of high blood pressure is to have blood pressure measured in all persons, including children. Medical camps should be organized for the purpose. A single reading of blood pressure in a sitting posture is usually enough for population surveys. Blood pressure must be taken at least twice in childhood; adults should have their blood pressure taken every five years. Above the age of 40, it must be measured once or twice a year.

More frequent check-up of blood pressure is required, irrespective of age, if you have any of these conditions — a family history of high blood pressure, kidney trouble, a persistent morning headache. In all these cases, there is a need to be extremely watchful. Again, if you are obese, addicted to alcohol and smoking, a high-salaried person, a sedentary worker, the danger signal is always there. In addition, if a person is sensitive to cold, is diabetic, or is pregnant, immediate/frequent attention is required.

Hence a simple reading of blood pressure, taken in time, can save an individual from the various fatal complications of high blood pressure, which remains occult/hidden for long, and it is rightly called the 'silent human killer'. Early detection is, indeed, a boon, as one is able to take preventive measures in time and save oneself from ensuing complications, not taking into account the daily expenditure on medicines.

5
HIGH BLOOD CHOLESTEROL

Blood cholesterol is one of the most important constituents of the blood/body. It has varied bodily functions, and it builds up healthy cells. It is an essential constituent of the cell wall (membrane), and if the level of blood cholesterol falls below normal, the walls of the red blood cells (RBC) are likely to rupture, thus causing a severe fall in haemoglobin (Hb).

The source of cholesterol in the blood / body

Cholesterol mainly comes from the diet, i.e. from butter, ghee (saturated fat), egg-yolk, non-vegetarian food. Sea food/fish contains a low content of saturated fat. However, polyunsaturated fats like rice bran, safflower, corn, sunflower, soybean, and cotton seed oils, etc do not give rise to serum cholesterol levels in the blood. These are recommended both for prevention and treatment of high blood cholesterol.

Cholesterol is also synthesized/made in the body. It has got limited excretion. Some is passed in faeces/bile, but is mostly retained in the body. The level of blood cholesterol rises as soon as the person eats.

More about blood cholesterol

The normal blood cholesterol level should be less them 200 mg/dl, and if it is more than 240 mg/dl, it is considered a high level of blood cholesterol. Patients having a blood cholesterol level between 200-239 mg/dl are borderline cases. Both in high and borderline cases, repeated check-ups of blood cholesterol are required.

However, those with a normal level of blood cholesterol must get their blood checked-up, at least every five years, especially after the age of 40. In general, all adults above the age of 20 must get their blood tested to exclude high levels of cholesterol. Besides fasting serum cholesterol, such a screening programme includes low-density lipoprotein (LDL) cholesterol, high-density lipoprotein (HDL) cholesterol and triglycerides(TG).

In children above 2 years of age, blood may be tested for cholesterol levels in case they have a family history of high blood cholesterol/coronary artery disease/stroke.

Blood cholesterol level may increase when a woman is on oral contraceptives or is pregnant. The level tends to decrease after the pregnancy is over, or after oral contraceptives are stopped. It may take even 5-6 months to come to normal levels.

Screening for high blood cholesterol must be carried out through medical camps/house-to-house surveys to locate patients suffering from this malady, as they require immediate treatment. Significant importance is now being given to the levels of cholesterol among the general population. It is very important to know the level of blood cholesterol in a person at an early age. Sometime back, I treated a patient whose high blood cholesterol remained unchecked in childhood. As a consequence, at a very young age the patient developed coronary artery disease, and the deposition of cholesterol was also noted in some of the blood vessels of the brain. The skin also showed an even deposition of fat nodules (xanthomas), occurring on some parts of the body (Fig. 11).

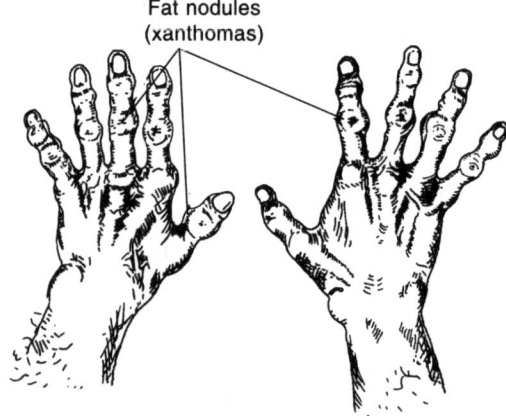

Fig. 11. Fat nodules (xanthomas) on the hands of an adult patient suffering from high blood cholesterol since childhood.

High Blood Cholesterol

Blood cholesterol can be tested at any biochemical laboratory, after recommendation from the physician. One must talk to one's physician about the testing of blood cholesterol. The cholesterol level should be checked while fasting in the morning, and if a person takes alcohol, he should avoid it for at least 48 hours before the test. Above all, the test must be carried out by an experienced biochemist. If the blood cholesterol level is high, it is advisable that a lipidogram be done.

Harmful effects of high blood cholesterol

High levels of blood cholesterol are dangerous for the body. They cause narrowing, and even blockage of the coronary arteries (blood vessels supplying the heart) and blood vessels supplying the brain, leading to heart attacks and strokes (paralysis, etc.) respectively. The chances of developing these diseases become higher if one has, in addition, diabetes, high blood pressure and obesity. The risk also increases if one has a family history of high blood cholesterol/heart attack. The danger is also greater in persons who are addicted to heavy smoking/tobacco chewing, and have sedentary habits. In females the risk is much more after menopause.

High levels of cholesterol may lead to gallstones, and may even be responsible for cancers.

How to bring back normal levels of high blood cholesterol

Higher levels of blood cholesterol can be lowered if one reduces the intake of saturated fat such as ghee, butter, cream, egg-yolk, etc. Only 20% saturated fats are permissible in such cases. One should use polyunsaturated oils (mentioned earlier), and they must be used in the minimum quantity necessary for cooking purposes. If onion or garlic or both are added to saturated fats, blood cholesterol does not rise, because they hinder the absorption of fats from the gut. This may be the reason for the practice of frying onion and/or garlic in 'ghee' for cooking vegetarian/non-vegetarian food.

In addition to the restriction of fats, one should take a high-fibre diet, i.e., whole wheat flour (bran to be taken along with it), whole pulses, unpolished rice and plenty of green vegetables — cooked/salad. Curd or yoghurt prepared from skimmed milk is said to be useful in lowering cholesterol. One should take only cottage cheese since it is prepared from skimmed milk.

Only low-calorie fruits are permissible, e.g. apple, orange, watermelon, muskmelon, etc.

The patient should also avoid routine dietary articles containing fats, like ice-cream, cakes, sweets, etc. Many a time the patient remains ignorant about the contents of fats in such items. However, taking an occasional sugary snack does not necessarily increase the level of blood sugar.

Exercise has got a very great role to play in lowering high levels of blood cholesterol. Depending on the condition of the heart etc., one should walk briskly, jog and do light exercises. It is well-established that exercise effectively lowers high levels of blood cholesterol. Drugs may be required in some cases where dietary restrictions and exercise fail to lower the level of high cholesterol. These may also be required when cholesterol levels are very high from an early stage. The patient may need either one, or a combination of two or three drugs. In some cases, a maintenance dose of the drugs may be required for some years, and in severe cases, even for the lifespan of the patient. While taking cholesterol lowering drugs, one has to stick to a very strict diet. This must be kept in mind.

From the above, therefore, one can realize that it is vital to detect high blood cholesterol at the earliest possible stage, so that its complications, especially heart attack, can be prevented and the disease can be treated by dietary restrictions and exercise alone. Drugs should be avoided as far as possible because they have their own adverse side-effects.

High density lipoprotein cholesterol — HDL-cholesterol (good cholesterol)

There is also 'good cholesterol' called HDL-cholesterol. HDL-cholesterol should be more than 40 mg/dl. HDL-cholesterol less than 40 mg/dl is called low HDL-cholesterol. Higher levels of HDL-cholesterol are useful for the body and they lower the high level of blood cholesterol. That is why they are called good cholesterol. The above 'good cholesterol' is produced within the body. The levels are increased in persons who take regular exercise and maintain a desirable weight and are non-smokers. Hence, obese people are advised to reduce their weight, and if

High Blood Cholesterol

one is smoking, it should be stopped, or at least reduced. A low to moderate intake of alcohol increases HDL-cholesterol. This point has been explained on page 291, para 2, in the Appendix on alcohol.

Persons with a higher level of HDL-cholesterol have much less chances of developing ischaemic heart disease. In females, HDL-cholesterol levels are usually high, and this may be the reason that women during the reproductive period have very little chances of developing ischaemic heart disease. The chances are greater when they enter the menopausal period.

Low density lipoprotein cholesterol — LDL-cholesterol (bad cholesterol)

It is called bad cholesterol because its higher levels are injurious to the body, like blood cholesterol. Its normal level is less than 100 mg/dl. 100 to 159 mg/dl is a borderline level, more than 160 mg/dl is high-risk level and more than 190 mg/dl is a very high-risk level. These are also released within the body and the levels are increased by a diet rich in saturated fats. The levels tend to increase in obese people. This 'bad cholesterol' (LDL-cholesterol), like a high level of blood cholesterol, is also responsible for coronary artery disease. Therefore, all the measures mentioned above should be taken to lower high levels of LDL-cholesterol, in the control of high blood cholesterol.

While going through a lipidogram test report, levels of triglycerides need equal attention. Normal values are less than 160 mg/dl. Higher levels need to be lowered without fail, as they are equally harmful like the raised levels of serum cholesterol.

American Diabetes Association mentions that in cases of diabetes mellitus, the levels of serum cholesterol are required to be 135 mg/dl, LDL-cholesterol less than 70 mg/dl and triglycerides less than 150 mg/dl since diabetic patients are more liable to suffer from vascular complications like coronary artery disease (CAD) and peripheral vascular disease (PVD).

To sum up, it may be said that if a person has more than 200 mg/dl of blood cholesterol, more than 100 mg/dl level of LDL-cholesterol, less than 40 mg/dl of HDL-cholesterol and more then 160 mg/dl of triglycerides, he requires the urgent attention of the physician for the control of the above cholesterols, so as to prevent the chances of his developing coronary artery disease, stroke, etc.

6
HIGH BLOOD URIC ACID

High levels of uric acid in the blood are as dangerous as high levels of blood cholesterol. The public does not seem to be much aware of the risk involved. A high level of blood uric acid is a pushing factor in causing coronary artery disease, like high levels of blood cholesterol.

High levels of uric acid should be detected as early as possible, especially in persons who are prone to coronary artery disease/heart attack, or have a family history of heart attack or even stroke. The estimation should be done more frequently if the patient is addicted to alcohol, or mainly takes a non-vegetarian diet. In all cases of stone, either in the gallbladder or in the urinary tract, uric acid must be tested. The testing of blood uric acid is highly valuable in cases of problems of the joints, backaches and even in cases of vague aches and pains. If this test is ignored and high levels of blood uric acid are not taken note of, the patient will continue to suffer from backache or vague aches/pains, and moreover, various other complications of high blood uric acid may also appear in due course.

Uric acid is one of the constituents of the blood. Its normal levels are 2 - 6 mg/dl.

Source of uric acid in the blood

Uric acid mainly comes from non-vegetarian food or its products, like soups, etc. It also comes from caffeine present in tea or coffee. Therefore, when a person takes either meat or tea/coffee, he adds to the uric acid in the blood. Other beverages like alcohol, beer, wine, etc. also contribute to the levels of uric acid in the blood (Fig. 12).

High Blood Uric Acid

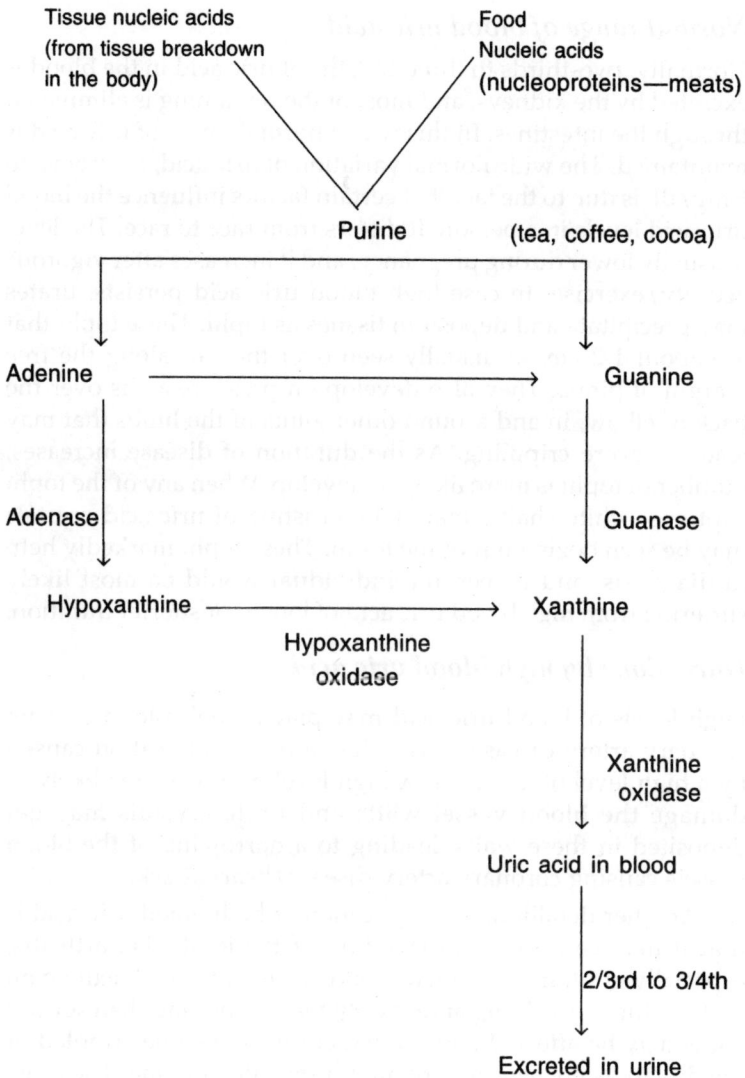

Fig. 12. A schematic 'formation' diagram of the uric acid in blood.

Besides food, uric acid is also added to the blood from various tissue breakdowns in the body. To some extent, the body also releases its own uric acid.

Normal range of blood uric acid

Normally, two-thirds to three-fourths of uric acid in the blood is excreted by the kidneys, and most of the remaining is eliminated through the intestines. In this way a normal range of uric acid is maintained. The wide normal variation of uric acid, i.e. from 2 to 6 mg/dl, is due to the fact that certain factors influence the blood uric acid levels in a person. It differs from race to race. The level is usually lower during pregnancy, and it increases after vigorous activity/exercise. In case high blood uric acid persists, urates may precipitate and deposit in tissues as tophi. These tophi that are about 1-2 cm are usually seen over the ear, along the free margin of pinna. They also develop on pressure areas over the back of elbow, in and around other joints of the limbs that may lead to severe crippling. As the duration of disease increases, number of tophi is more likely to develop. When any of the tophi ruptures, white chalky material consisting of uric acid crystals may be seen oozing out of the tophi. These tophi markedly help in diagnosis, and if seen the individual would be most likely suffering from high blood uric acid of longer or shorter duration.

Harm done by high blood uric acid

High levels of blood uric acid may play a vital role in causing coronary artery disease. It is a dangerous complication caused by a high level of uric acid. A high level of uric acid is likely to damage the blood vessel walls and urate crystals may get deposited in these walls, leading to a narrowing of the blood vessels causing coronary artery disease/heart attack.

Another debilitating complication of high blood uric acid is that it may cause painful swelling of the joints, i.e. arthritis, especially gout. In gout, there is a recurrent attack of acute pain and swelling, involving at first only the big toe, and then several joints may be affected and the patient may even be crippled, if the disease is not arrested/treated/prevented in time. The exact cause of high blood uric acid in gout is not known. The heredity factor in such cases cannot be ruled out.

As already said, vague aches/pains or backaches may be the result of high blood uric acid.

In addition to the above, kidneys may also be involved due

to constant elevated levels of uric acid in the blood. Since uric acid is excreted by the kidneys, and the excretion is much more if the levels are high in a person, the kidneys may be damaged as a result of excess excretion of uric acid through them. There may be a crystallization in the kidneys leading to uric acid stone, and if the excretion continues to be excessive, the kidneys may even be damaged markedly, requiring more drastic measures to maintain normal kidney functions. However, if high blood uric acid is detected and treated early, kidney damage may be reversed. Hence there is a vital need to detect high levels of uric acid well in time.

Even gallstones (cholelithiasis) are likely to form as a result of high levels of blood uric acid. Gallstones may cause infection in the gallbladder (cholecystitis). It is well known that both cholelithiasis and cholecystitis can lead to cancer of the gallbladder. It is, therefore, advisable that the gallbladder should be removed surgically in all cases of cholelithiasis (gallstones either as a result of high blood uric acid or due to some other reasons) or cholecystitis (inflammation of the gallbladder due to any cause), to prevent the cancer of the gallbladder. Early detection of high blood uric acid helps prevent gallbladder stones/infection, and finally cancer of the gallbladder.

High blood uric acid—as a result of various diseases/drugs

High levels of blood uric acid may also occur during the course of various diseases. For example, if kidneys are damaged even due to some other cause, say as a result of chronic infection or prolonged high blood pressure, or in acute cases, like acute nephritis, blood uric acid levels will rise, because the kidneys will not be able to maintain the normal levels of blood uric acid. And, in such cases, both kidneys and high blood uric acid require equal attention.

In some other diseases also, e.g. when a person is suffering from leukaemia, malignant tumours, polycythaemia, psoriasis, cyanotic congenital heart diseases, pernicious and haemolytic anaemias, during the administration of anticancer drugs, blood uric acid is likely to get raised as a result of excessive tissue breakdown. Again in such cases, care of both the primary disease and high level of blood uric acid is required so as to save the patient from additional complications due to high blood uric acid.

Besides the above, blood uric acid can also rise in other diseases which may be listed as: myxoedema, hypoparathyroidism and hyperparathyroidism, acromegaly, diabetes mellitus, rheumatoid arthritis, etc. Hence, in such disorders also, blood uric acid is required to be measured. If found elevated, it should be treated simultaneously.

Further, starvation and prolonged exercise may raise levels of blood uric acid. Even some drugs, especially aspirin, if taken more than 2 g/ day, may lead to a rise in blood uric acid levels. Some antihypertensive drugs, specially chlorthiazide, may even enhance it.

High blood uric acid and syndrome X

High blood uric acid is associated with syndrome X. It is a metabolic syndrome that includes various metabolic disorders like type 2 diabetes mellitus (DM) or impaired blood sugar levels either fasting or postparandial due to insulin resistance with increased insulin levels (hyperinsulinaemia), high blood pressure, high blood uric acid, dyspilidaemia (increased cholesterol, low density lipoprotein –LDL cholesterol, low high density lipoprotein-HDL cholesterol and elevated triglycerides-TG) and abdominal obesity and accelerated coronary artery disease. It is possible that high blood uric acid may precede the onset of (i) coronary artery disease, (ii) high blood pressure and (iii) type 2 DM in patients of syndrome X. Therefore it would be advisable to screen as well as treat all cases of high blood uric acid for any accompanying disorder of syndrome X.

How to control high blood uric acid?

Patients are recommended to take mostly vegetarian food and refrain from non-vegetarian diet, because nuclear/cell protein of non-vegetarian food add to the uric acid in the blood. Since caffeine is also responsible for high levels of uric acid, therefore, patients are advised to take a minimum quantity, or no tea, coffee, cocoa, etc. Due to the same reason, alcohol, beer and wine should also be avoided.

High Blood Uric Acid

The patient should take a lot of water so that high levels of uric acid in the blood are washed out by the kidneys.

In short, all cases of high blood uric acid should stick to a vegetarian diet with an ample quantity of water, no alcoholic beverages, and a minimum intake of tea and coffee, if, at all these are taken.

In case the high levels of uric acid are not controlled by the above-mentioned dietary measures, only then should the patient be put on drugs. The most commonly used drug is allopurinol (zyloric). In more severe cases even the maintenance dose of this drug may be required for a long period, besides dietary control.

However, if one gets an acute attack of gout, more drastic measures are required to control the attack. Drugs like colchicine, indomethacin, phenylbutazone, or even ACTH can be tried to control the attack. Once it is over, all preventive measures should be taken so that the attack is not repeated and the patient is saved from this debilitating disease. Those who have a family history of gout need to be aware of taking preventive steps to ward off this condition.

In case some underlying diseases/drugs have been detected as responsible for raising levels of blood uric acid in the blood, both the underlying disease and the drug should be watched. The drug responsible for high levels of uric acid should be discontinued. In selected cases, especially those patients who are receiving anticancer drugs, allopurinol is usually given. It is true in cases of luekaemias and likewise other conditions.

It needs to be emphazised again that the early detection and treatment of high blood uric acid goes a long way in warding off the serious complications resulting from high levels of uric acid, especially coronary artery disease and stroke, which are fatal in nature.

Urgent tests in childhood

Tests for blood sugar, cholesterol and other lipids, uric acid, thyroid function tests, etc. must be done, at least once, in childhood – more frequently in case of family history of such disorders, Likewise, blood pressure must also be checked. Obese children need more care.

7
STROKE, EPILEPSY, POLIOMYELITIS
(Diseases of the Nervous System)

Diseases of the nervous system can also be prevented, like diseases of the heart, if the right steps are taken at the appropriate time. If ignored, the disease can result in fatal consequences such as brain haemorrhage, in the case of stroke. A massive stroke is a grave emergency of the nervous system, and if the patient survives, his life is likely to be most miserable and handicapped as a result of paralysis, either of one half of the body, or of one of the limbs, or loss of speech/vision, etc.

Compared to a heart attack, general awareness about a stroke, more precisely brain stroke, which is even more debilitating, is very limited. Most of the people either are not aware of the symptoms of a stroke or, if they are aware, they do not know as to how to cope with this emergency.

General awareness/orientation is urgently needed by all concerned, so as to prevent the menace of various diseases of the nervous system. Specific guidance is vital for the prevention of the progress of such diseases. This will help the person take necessary steps, at an early stage, and also report to the physician for the treatment, before it is too late.

1. Stroke

Stroke/apoplexy commonly occurs as a result of disorders of cerebral/brain circulation, called cerebral vascular accident (CVA). It results in unconsciousness, paralysis either of a part or one half of the body (hemiplegia), or loss of speech or vision or balance of the body. As described earlier, it can be very serious.

The word 'stroke' has been used since long implying that it has occurred like a bolt from the blue without any specific reason.

In this condition, there could be either thrombosis (clotting) called ischaemic stroke or haemorrhage called haemorrhagic stroke in one of the blood vessels of the brain, leading to the above-stated manifestations. This can be best checked by the same factors which are required for the **primary prevention** of coronary artery disease. This includes proper control of diabetes, hypertension, high blood cholesterol, high blood uric acid, and by taking a proper diet and exercise commensurate with any of the above disease(s) one is suffering from. The various steps for the control of various disorders have been mentioned already in the respective chapters and there is an appendix on diet, as well as on exercise. In case one is overweight, reduction in weight is also essential for the prevention of stroke. Similarly, if one is addicted to smoking, tobacco chewing, and/or to excessive drinking, all these are required to be tapered off and finally stopped. (Refer to Appendix I, II, III). Family history of stroke, regular intake of oral contraceptives, ageing process itself are other predisposing factors.

It should be known to all that sometimes there may be even warning signals before the occurrence of stroke. These are termed as 'transient ischaemic attacks (TIA)'. In these attacks, the flow of the blood is momentarily hampered in one of the blood vessels of the brain, causing transient spells of loss of vision/speech/ paralysis of a part of the body/vertigo, etc., depending on the involvement of the vessel of the brain, supplying a particular part of the brain responsible for the above transient lesions.

Since the blood supply is only stopped/slowed for a while, the part of the body involved immediately returns to normal. If such attacks occur, especially in middle-aged persons, one should immediately report it to the physician/neurologist for proper diagnosis and prevention of a possible full-fledged stroke at a later stage. Such transient attacks may even occur repeatedly, in some cases, before the person gets a stroke causing complete paralysis. Once it occurs, i.e. complete paralysis, recovery is usually incomplete, and if brain haemorrhage occurs, it becomes a medical/surgical emergency.

Hence a stroke should be given weightage comparable to a coronary artery disease or a heart attack. Both are dangerous and need equal attention, and they also have common factors for their prevention. And, if a person seriously controls the above-stated factors, like diabetes, hypertension, etc., he will certainly bear the least risk of suffering from these disorders. Public education in this respect is essential.

Caution: As soon as the stroke occurs, the patient should be immediately taken to the hospital for advice/treatment, as the first three hours from the occurrence of stroke are vital for

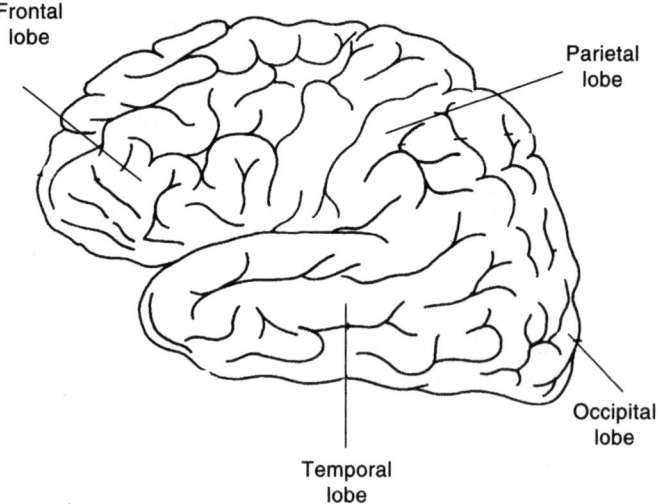

Fig. 13. A diagrammatic representation of the lobes of the brain (on lateral aspect of the cerebral hemispheres). Broadly speaking, the centre for motor function, various sensory centres (i.e. of sight, hearing, smell, taste, etc.), and other centres are located in these lobes.

treatment. In these three hours, is the time taken for transportation, urgent tests in the hospital, like computed tomographic (CT) scanning/magnetic resonance imaging (MRI), etc. Therefore, awareness of this limited period should be known by all so that not a single minute is wasted in dealing with this emergency. 64- slice CT scanning is a useful test for fast assessment of stroke cases. It offers the speed and image resolution required for rapid examination of the blood vessels in the brain, enabling the physician to make a quick diagnosis and determine the extent and type of lesion. It should be clearly understood that 'the therapeutic window' is ideally open in the first three hours only. It may be added that once a stroke occurs, it is very difficult to salvage the brain. Hence immediate recognition/diagnosis of the condition and prompt treatment are very important. Undoubtedly, prevention is most vital.

Secondary preventive measures
The important preventive measures that need to be followed once the patient gets the stroke are called secondary preventive measures. These are extremely important to be followed so that another attack of stroke may not be precipitated. Besides caring for above-mentioned preventive measures like control of high blood pressure, sugar, cholesterol etc., drugs like aspirin and other anticoagulant drugs need to be prescribed so that clot formation could be prevented. Aspirin is also recommended for primary prevention, more so in cases that have long standing one or more risk factors like high blood pressure, sugar etc.

2. Epilepsy

Epilepsy is one of the common diseases that we see in everyday life. It is not uncommon to see a person getting an epileptic fit/convulsions in a public place or to see parents/teachers rushing to the physician to report such cases in children.

In epilepsy, there is a sudden transitory disturbance in brain, leading to sudden generalized convulsions of the whole body, involving all the four limbs, including the face, all at once (i.e. disturbance in motor function of the brain — Fig. 13), called generalized/major/grand mal epilepsy. Or, there is convulsion of a part of the body, e.g. one of the limbs, or a part of the limb, say an arm, hand, foot, etc., or muscles of the face/eye only. In some cases, however, these convulsions may spread first on the same side of the body, followed by similar symptoms on the other half of the body. In which case, the whole body gets involved, and this is called focal or Jacksonian epilepsy.

In many cases, especially in children, there may be only momentary/transitory unconsciousness (i.e. disturbance of consciousness in the brain) called petit mal epilepsy.

Likewise, some disturbance may occur to affect special sensations in the brain, i.e., sensation of sight (when the patient experiences dots or momentary bright lights), of hearing (when he hears odd noises), of smell or taste (i.e. abnormal/unpleasant sensations of smell or taste etc.) (Fig. 13). Even sensations in the internal organs (visceral) may be involved in epilepsy, and the patient may feel discomfort in the upper and middle part of his abdomen (epigastrium), and this may also be associated with nausea/vomiting. Sensory sensations may also be involved, and the patient may feel pricking, burning, tearing etc. sensations in any part of the skin of the body.

In still other cases of epilepsy, say temporal lobe epilepsy, there may be emotional disturbances so that the patient may feel markedly frightened or terrorized etc. Or, there may be a disordered sense of the body, so that he feels as if one of his limbs, such as his arm, is getting smaller and smaller. He/she may even feel that the whole limb has disappeared. Likewise, the patient may feel that a part of the body is becoming larger and/or appearing in different forms/shapes. There is a feeling of unreality, depersonalization and the patient may sink into a dream-like state. There may even be hallucinations of smell or taste in a case of temporal lobe epilepsy, which is one of the common focal epilepsies.

In general, any of the above clinical manifestations relating to the involvement of special senses or consciousness etc. may occur alone, or may be quickly followed by generalized/focal convulsion/s, involving the motor function of the brain.

When such manifestations occur immediately before an attack of convulsions these serve as warning, or aura. These clinical manifestations are highly significant as they give a clue to the involvement of a specific area in the brain represented by them. The patient must in such a case be questioned, and symptoms must be confirmed so that the lesion in the brain can be diagnosed clinically. It is often seen that when convulsions occur, these important symptoms get masked, and the patient may remember the convulsions only, they being a major manifestation. Hence, awareness of such symptoms is of great importance so that the patients themselves reveal such vital information to facilitate the physician's task.

In a nutshell, in epilepsy, there is a disturbance in various functions of the brain relating to motor function, consciousness, sensation, emotion etc., and its various clinical manifestations occur when any/some of the above functions are disturbed. And once one function is disturbed, disturbance of other functions may follow, depending upon the resistance/threshold of the patient concerned.

The resistance/threshold of the patient plays an important role in the involvement of various functions of the brain relating to epilepsy. In case the threshold/resistance is very high, none of the functions of the brain may be disturbed, i.e. there will be no attack of epilepsy, although the person is prone to epilepsy. However, in case the resistance is moderately high, only one function of the brain may be involved with no involvement of any other function of the brain. When the threshold/resistance is low/very low, disturbance of a function of the brain may quickly be followed by the involvement of other functions of brain, i.e., there may be an involvement of the functions of sensation, consciousness, motor function, etc. almost at the same time. The patient, after experiencing some disturbance relating to special senses (sight, smell, hearing etc.) may become unconscious, followed by generalized convulsions of the body (i.e. disturbance of motor function).

Details of attacks of various types of epilepsy and mass awareness

It is very essential for everybody to be aware of a detailed account of the attack of major (or grand mal or generalized), focal or Jacksonian and petit mal epilepsies. At times, tests like electroencephalogram (EEG) and/or computed tomographic (CT) scanning may be normal in a case of epilepsy, and, therefore, it is only the evidence of the eyewitness, who is in a position to report the details to the attending physician, when the patient is brought to the hospital. As an emergency case, a clinical diagnosis of epilepsy can be made on the spot. Moreover, such cases/emergencies need immediate treatment, and the tests, even if they are conducted, take their own time.

In major (or grand mal or generalized) epilepsy, after momentarily experiencing an 'odd sensation in the head' or a 'sinking feeling' (the various types of auras/warning signals already described earlier are often absent), the patient loses consciousness instantaneously, and he collapses all at once. And if unluckily, the place is odd, e.g., a patient is coming down the stairs or standing near a fire or on a hill top, he may injure himself badly.

Following the fall, all the muscles of the body, i.e. all the muscles of the limbs, abdomen, chest and even face become rigid/stiff. Due to the spasm of the trunk/respiratory muscles, breathing almost stops, and as the muscles of the face are also involved, the mouth gets firmly closed, and the teeth get clenched. The patient then experiences acute agony, and is close to death. But within a few seconds, all the muscles relax, breathing is regained, and the patient starts getting convulsions of the whole body, which usually continue for about 1-2 minutes, and thereafter, the whole body gets relaxed or becomes absolutely limp.

During such convulsions, the tongue moves repeatedly inside the mouth, and together with the repeated movements of the jaws, the saliva in the mouth gets stirred, and frothing occurs. The tongue may also be bitten when it comes in-between the teeth, and sometimes bleeding may also occur, causing a blood-stained froth. The patient may pass urine (and rarely faeces) during this phase of convulsions. It should be remembered that tongue-bite, frothing, passing of urine are important clinical features of an attack of epilepsy, which must be noticed carefully by the eyewitness, for the information of doctor.

The patient may sleep for hours following an attack. However, he may be awakened after a reasonable time when he may complain of a marked headache and pain in all the muscles. When awake, he may or may not have recollection of his severe fall or convulsions. He may be able to remember the aura, i.e. transitory symptoms that he may have experienced before the onset of the attack of epilepsy. However, as mentioned earlier, this information about the aura has a great significance in clinical diagnosis, and, therefore, the patient must be coaxed again and again to elicit the required information.

The patient may even get the attack during sleep, and in such cases, tongue-bite or passing of urine in bed should help in the diagnosis. The patient may even die due to suffocation if he happens to turn over during this nocturnal attack of epilepsy, with his face buried in the pillow.

Attacks of grand mal epilepsy may occur many times a day. However, the occurrence of attacks of epilepsy are quite variable to the extent that the patient may not have any further attack during his/her whole life. And hence the value of mass awareness about the clinical diagnosis of epilepsy increases because the treatment cannot be started when a single/first attack of epilepsy occurs, which remains doubtful due to the lack of evidence. On the other hand, the patient may get one attack after the other without regaining consciousness in between the attacks, called status epilepticus, which could be even fatal, if immediate medical aid is not provided.

The details of the attack of focal or Jacksonian epilepsy have already been explained. In this type of epilepsy, the intensity of the lesion in the brain is not marked enough to cause a major attack of epilepsy. The attack subsides within seconds/minutes.

At times, there is a transitory jerky movement of the limb/s, so that in case both the lower limbs are involved and the patient is standing, he may fall down all at once. This state is called myoclonic epilepsy. Sometimes the small muscles of face, eyes etc. may also be involved.

In petit mal epilepsy, which occurs often in children, there is an extremely transitory attack of unconsciousness. The child, if standing, does not even fall down, and if he/she is doing his/her home work, the child continues with the work as if he/she has had no interruption. The attack of epilepsy may occur repeatedly even 15, 20, 30 times a day. When the attacks are limited to 1 to 2 per day, or on alternate days or even less, the child may remain unaware of such an attack. And even if he/she brings it to the notice of the parents, it may be ignored altogether.

However, whenever a child brings the attack to the notice of his parents, they must take it very seriously, and tests like EEG, CT scan etc. should not be delayed. Therefore, the knowledge of symptoms of petit mal epilepsy is most important for parents, and even for teachers in schools, so that the disease may not remain undetected especially in early and occasional cases. However, in rare cases, the child may even collapse during unconsciousness. This is called an akinetic attack/epilepsy, and thus, in such cases, there is usually no difficulty in diagnosis.

The attacks of petit mal epilepsy may disappear altogether on attaining maturity, although the treatment will have to be commenced as soon as the diagnosis is confirmed.

It is urgent that all persons, particularly all members/friends/colleagues concerned with the case must keep in mind all the relevant signs and symptoms whenever the patient is to report to the physician for diagnosis.

Sometimes, in a doubtful case, one may think of starting antiepileptic drugs thinking that these drugs will both control the epilepsy and confirm its diagnosis. This may not be so, as the drug in question may not be a true drug for the type of epilepsy the patient might be suffering from. And in case these drugs have been administered to a non-epileptic patient, they may have their own side-effects, as the treatment of epilepsy is usually a long affair ranging from 3 to 5 years. All this happens when the EEG/CT scan etc. does not confirm the diagnosis of epilepsy. However, antiepileptic drugs may be started if the very first attack of epilepsy happens to be a serious one, and the patient suffers grave injury as a result of a fall. Such a therapy will safeguard the person against another major attack of epilepsy. In case the second attack also gives no definite clue, and has occurred after a few days of the first attack, the patient may be admitted to a hospital for observation, diagnosis and treatment.

It may be stressed that an absolutely clear diagnosis of epilepsy is necessary to establish it. Unfortunately, this disease still carries a social stigma in some communities, and a lot of disinformation has to be countered. For this, the mobilization of public opinion is of great help.

What is the cause of disturbance in the brain which leads to an attack of epilepsy?

In many patients, in spite of exhaustive efforts/investigations, no cause of epilepsy may be located. Such cases are called idiopathic cases of epilepsy.

However, an intensive drive is a must to detect any lesion in the brain which could account for an epileptic attack, the reason being, that if the cause of epilepsy is detected, it is usually treatable, and, therefore, the patient will be cured forever, and thus may not need a long course of antiepileptic drugs.

If, somehow, the cause remains undiagnosed/undetected, especially when the pathology is right in the brain, the disease will advance further, and besides the manifestations of epilepsy, other clinical features of the underlying disease will occur, making the patient a most complicated case for treatment. It may even prove fatal, if a lesion like neoplasm/malignancy/cancer in the brain remains hidden. This usually happens when detailed investigations have not been carried out, especially the most informative ones like CT scanning and magnetic resonance imaging (MRI) etc. These are costly exercises, but all factors must be taken note of.

A thorough search for the detection of brain tumour is needed, especially in an adult/middle-aged/elderly person, more so when epilepsy is not being controlled in spite of high dosages of various antiepileptic drugs, and the attacks are increasing both in number and intensity. In such cases MRI must be done, even if the report of the CT scan is normal, as the MRI is more effective in the detection of any pathology in the brain. In one of our patients of about 40 years of age, epilepsy was not being controlled in spite of heavy medication, and even the CT scan was normal. An MRI was done, which showed the presence of a tumour in the brain. This was immediately operated upon, and the patient's epilepsy was subsequently controlled.

There are many types of brain tumours, both benign and malignant, responsible for epilepsy, and their clinical manifestations, especially aura, i.e., the very first symptom of epilepsy, depend upon the location of these lesions in the brain (refer to page 7 under the head 'brain tumours').

It is very important to keep in mind that epilepsy may be the only and the first symptom of brain tumours, which may even continue for several years, before other manifestations of brain tumour appear. This usually happens when the tumour is a slow-growing one/benign in nature. Hence, whenever epilepsy occurs for the first time in an adult/middle-aged/elderly person, a tumour of the brain must be suspected, and the case should be thoroughly investigated so that the treatment is not delayed. An early diagnosed and treated brain tumour has a very high prognosis.

Another cause of epilepsy could be either a recent or an old injury of the head, which also needs a thorough check-up. This shall be duly discussed while dealing with 'head injury', giving an example (refer to page 304).

Also, trauma induced by an injury to the head of a newly-born during delivery (i.e. birth injury/injuries) is an important cause of epilepsy, and again, even in such cases of birth injuries, epilepsy may occur after many/several years of birth.

Further, epilepsy may occur when the brain function is disturbed due to the various other lesions in the brain called space-occupying lesions (brain tumours are also one of the space-occupying lesions), like an abscess, tuberculoma as a result of tuberculosis, infarction (i.e. damage of an area of brain as a result of occlusion of one of the branches of cerebral/brain vessels, responsible for the blood supply of involved/damaged area of the brain), and cysticercosis (i.e. a lesion in the brain which occurs due to ingestion of infected and insufficiently cooked pork), etc. Focal epilepsy following 'tuberculoma' in the brain is also seen, and one such case will be mentioned while discussing tuberculous meningitis (page 137) with the comments of Dr. William Boyd (Canada), a well-known pathologist.

Heredity also plays a significant role in some of the cases of epilepsy.

Other important causes of epilepsy are fever, withdrawal of drugs or alcohol, toxaemia, etc. which are likely to precipitate an attack of epilepsy. Epilepsy sometimes also occurs in a case of renal/kidney failure, and this aspect will be taken up in 'chronic renal (kidney) failure — CRF' with the comments of Dr. H.E. de Wardener (London), a noted nephrologist — page 208, para 7.

Irrespective of the cause of epilepsy, and including the cases of idiopathic epilepsy, where no reason for an attack of epilepsy has been detected, the nature or clinical manifestations of the attack of epilepsy remain the same.

Pitfalls in detecting occult/hidden cases of epilepsy in a mass survey

It is the most difficult survey that we have encountered so far. Even in various medical camps that we hold from time to time, history of epilepsy or convulsions are not forthcoming. On hearing the word 'epilepsy', especially in most rural or backward areas, where people are not so educated, the audience tend to remain tight-lipped, as if they are concealing something. Even in our day-to-day practice, patients do not like to label themselves as epileptic, and many a time, a bona fide patient goes on taking medicine from some outside practitioner, silently, so that no one gets to know about his disease, at his place of work. I have seen patients who developed an acute attack of epilepsy, at a public place, and on enquiry, they felt compelled to tell me that they had been suffering from this malady for quite sometime, taking haphazard treatment from one doctor or another. Even, patients well-known to me conceal their disease intentionally, and I only come to know about it when they experience a severe attack, and need my emergency services.

Patients are not always at fault; social factors come in their way. Several problems arise for them or for their families, once it comes to be known that the person is epileptic. In any case, marriage is a big problem for the patient. If the patient is married, the problem may occur in respect of the marriage of his/her children, for though heredity has a limited role in this disease, the boy's/girl's family may think that the disease runs in the family.

If the patient is working in the private sector, he may not be assigned essential duties.

Similarly, a child may not feel comfortable in school, although he may be good in his studies as well as in sports. He may be refused entry in a team for competition. The child suffers both ways. If he does not take the medicine, i.e. he conceals his disease, he can hardly carry on with his studies, especially when the attacks are frequent. If his disease comes in everyone's knowledge, although he may take suitable treatment at an appropriate place and his attacks are also controlled satisfactorily, he may suffer due to the ignorance of others. He may feel isolated when classmates/teachers do not co-operate with him. Even at home he may, at times, find an adverse atmosphere.

It is for these reasons that a physician never labels a case epileptic, unless he is satisfied from all angles, i.e., clinical, investigations, etc. In a doubtful case, the diagnosis is never declared, or is withheld till the patient gets another attack of epilepsy. It is worth mentioning that a delay in diagnosis will not harm the person, but a false-positive diagnosis may, indeed, prove fatal.

Hence a massive awareness is required so that the patients themselves report for a check-up, and the disease is controlled in time. This will save the family and the patient from further misery.

Another important factor which poses a practical problem in such a mass survey is the lack of availability of eyewitnesses, since the diagnosis of the disease is a clinical one, and mostly depends on the information of a person who has seen the patient during the period of the attack. Therefore, in such a survey, the full co-operation of the whole area/place including family members/friends is required in identifying such occult/hidden cases of epilepsy.

The foremost task relating to mass awareness is that people should be guided about the treatable nature of the disease, through magazines, newspapers, radio, TV, pamphlets etc., emphasizing that the disease is neither a shame nor disgrace in society, and that it is only one of the common diseases. Once guided, people will themselves approach the physician for treatment, and even the eyewitnesses will fully co-operate. Till this is accomplished, no mass survey, however efficient, will be able to control the disease.

Childhood epilepsy

The disease is quite prevalent in children, and as many as 30% of all epileptics fall into this category.

It needs urgent awareness that, usually, there is an excellent prognosis of epilepsy in children. Hence there should be no unnecessary panic when a child gets an attack although detailed investigations will be required in each and every case. One such case of an Indian female child, aged 7, was discussed by the author with Lord Walton. The child suddenly started getting twitchings on the left side of her face, starting from the angle of the mouth towards the left ear. To begin with, the twitchings were transitory, and she suffered an attack per day for the first two days. On the third day she had three attacks. On the fifth day, the attack lasted for about 2-3 minutes. This female child was labelled as a case of focal epilepsy. The parents of the child were very co-operative; they did not lose much time, and showed the case to the author, and the patient, after necessary investigations, was put on a suitable antiepileptic drug, which continued for about 3 years.

The clinical data, along with the relevant investigation reports were sent to London to the reputed neurologist, Lord Walton, and he, after going through the case, labelled it as a case of 'benign focal epilepsy of childhood'. Later the case was taken up for personal discussion with Lord Walton during our meeting at General Medical Council, London. The overall opinion was that such cases have a very good prognosis, and if the full course of treatment is carried out uninterruptedly, it is very likely that the child may be free from attacks of epilepsy forever.

This patient had an uneventful course; the parents were highly convinced of the fact that their child would be free from trouble after three years of medication. That is exactly what happened, and now after a lapse of 6 years, the patient, taken off drugs, has had no attacks. Now this 16-year young girl is good in health, studies, as well as in sports.

It is, thus, clear that epilepsy is a curable disease, and the above case should serve to remove misconceptions about it. Therefore, one should not feel perturbed, irrespective of the age of the patient. Every patient is likely to recover, sooner or later. Some patients need drugs in high dosages for a longer period, i.e. beyond 3-5 years. This situation is dependent on the underlying pathology, threshold / resistance and severity of the disease.

A word may also be said about epilepsy in newborns/infants. In this case, the mother is the true eyewitness, and she should closely watch the child, especially when there is a history of epilepsy in the family. She should keep an acute eye on the movements of the newborn. There may be only unnoticeable signs like eye deviation, movements of swallowing, abnormal movements (smacking) of the lips, etc. There may be transitory generalized convulsions/jerky movement, as in myoclonic epilepsy. Being transitory, initially, these movements may be missed. However, whenever the mother notices any such abnormal movement(s)/convulsions in a child, a paediatrician/neurologist must be consulted for tests/therapy to especially save the brain from injury, and mental retardation at a later stage.

However, the parents should not become panicky at the start, as many of the transitory movements/disorders may look like symptoms of epilepsy, when the child, in fact, may be suffering from other disorders like breath-holding spells, or infantile syncopal (transient unconsciousness) attacks, as a result of a congenital heart disease. Hence the diagnosis of epilepsy in a newborn/infant must be made keeping all such considerations in view.

What are hysterical convulsions?

These convulsions are of a psychogenic origin, also called psychogenic seizures or psychogenic non-epileptic seizures. These should be differentiated from true epileptic convulsions; hence the value of an eyewitness for the precise diagnosis of epilepsy. Simple information, that the patient had an attack of convulsions, is not enough to attach the label of epilepsy. The physician needs to know the details regarding the convulsions and other associated factors, for the immediate treatment of the case. Hence convulsions, whenever they occur, need to be watched carefully.

Epileptic convulsions occur suddenly, and before that a specific aura/symptom may appear. On the other hand, hysterical convulsions are gradual and occur after vague symptoms/warnings. Moreover, hysterical convulsions have a strange look/style, and there is no sudden fall/injury during an attack of convulsion. Likewise, there is no tongue-bite or incontinence of urine, seen in cases of epilepsy.

After epileptic convulsions, the patient feels drowsy, and may sleep for hours, and he/she may be unable to recollect anything about the attack. In the case of hysterical convulsions, the patient may narrate the whole incident. It is significant to note that hysterical convulsions never occur during sleep. Further, hysterical convulsions are more common in young females, say in the age group of 20-30 years, and at times, it is observed that such patients have also a suicidal tendency.

Even while diagnosing childhood epilepsy, hysterical convulsions must be excluded, especially when the convulsions are generalized.

It may be said that one should not be perturbed whenever convulsions occur. Each convulsive attack needs to be analysed and diagnosed. In some patients, both types of convulsions, i.e., epileptic and hysterical, may exist. Therefore, in a case of epilepsy, if in spite of giving proper dosages of suitable antiepileptic drugs, the convulsions are not controlled, such convulsions must be again watched carefully for the associated hysterical convulsions.

However, it is both wrong and unfair to label hysterical convulsions hurriedly as epileptic convulsions, since the patient may feel insulted or injured. This may further increase psychogenic/hysterical convulsions, besides involve an unnecessary trial of antiepileptic drugs.

Other causes of transitory unconsciousness (besides petit mal epilepsy)

Since in petit mal epilepsy there is transitory unconsciousness as a result of disturbance in the consciousness region of the brain, the condition needs to be differentiated from other causes of transitory unconsciousness, i.e., syncope/syncopal attacks, described below:

1. Vaso - vagal syncope

The exact mechanism of syncope is still under study. In this condition, there appears to be a transitory fall in blood pressure due to the failure of peripheral resistance. This momentary fall in blood pressure causes a decreased flow of blood to the brain, leading to syncope, during which time there is a transient/brief form of unconsciousness, and the patient may fall to the ground, if he remains standing, i.e., does not sit, or lie immediately. Before his fall, he may feel some symptoms like nausea, giddiness, vertigo, disturbance of vision/hearing, blurring of vision or odd noises in the ears, body pallor, rapid respiration and sweating, etc.

If the attack is a prolonged one, in some of the cases, even twitching/jerky movements, or open convulsions may occur, thus creating some difficulty in diagnosing the condition clinically. Such attacks occur usually only in a standing/upright position. They do not occur when the patient is either lying down or sitting. The patient is not confused after the attack, although he still may be undergoing feelings of nausea.

This problem appears particularly in normal young adults, especially in females, with no obvious pathology which could account for these attacks. Such cases are usually seen in day-to-day practice, and can be embarrassing enough to cause anxiety.

The attacks are usually precipitated when a person keeps standing for a long time, e.g., as is sometimes seen in school students when they gather for their morning prayers (childhood syncope), or in older students standing for hours in various laboratories, and similarly in policemen and soldiers, when they happen to stand on duty at one place for a considerable length of time.

Also, the attacks are aggravated when a person suddenly stands up after lying down or sitting for a long period, or when the person gets up suddenly during his sleep at midnight/morning. Further, bad news or sight of blood, i.e., emotional shock, intense fear/pain, hot weather or a stuffy atmosphere, hunger, intake of excessive alcohol or loss of fluids, i.e., dehydration etc., may also initiate these attacks.

Recovery in vaso-vagal syncope occurs after the person lies down. As mentioned earlier, there is no underlying cause. There is only a failure of peripheral resistance which causes the various conditions mentioned above.

2. Cardiac syncope

Cardiac syncope, i.e., syncope as a result of some underlying heart disease, occurs suddenly, without any warning symptoms. In such cases, there is a sudden fall in cardiac output/blood pressure, as a result of various diseases of the heart, like arrhythmias, such as when the heart rate is very high (paroxysmal atrial tachycardia-PAT, atrial fibrillation), or in a heart block (Stokes-Adams attack) when the heart rate becomes extremely slow, or in advanced cases of aortic stenosis (aortic valve disease), which result in a decreased flow of blood to the brain, etc. Hence detailed tests like electrocardiogram — ECG (with a long rhythm strip), Holter monitoring (to detect arrhythmias), echocardiography (to detect aortic/other valvular diseases), etc., are required, besides an EEG, in some cases, for specific diagnosis and treatment.

3. Carotid sinus syncope

There are other causes of syncope like hypersensitive carotid sinus, which is located in a small, slightly dilated portion of the common carotid artery, at the level of the thyroid cartilage, just below the angle of the jaw, before this blood vessel bifurcates into internal and external carotid arteries. It is present on each side of the neck.

The carotid sinus is very important for controlling the heart rate of a person. In general practice, when a person comes with a very high rate, e.g. in a condition of PAT, when the patient feels marked palpitation, and is in acute distress, the physician may give a mild massage (about five seconds at a time) on the side of the neck, at the level of the upper border of the thyroid cartilage. This stimulates the carotid sinus (involving the cardioinhibitory effect of the vagus nerve), and the heart rate starts decreasing slowly. This method is so effective that if simultaneously the heart rate is not checked, carotid sinus may lower the heart rate to dangerous levels. It would be advisable to carry out carotid message in a well-equipped hospital under the supervision of a specialist physician.

One can imagine the role of the normal carotid sinus in lowering the heart rate with a simple massage, and if the carotid sinus is hypersensitive, a mere jerk/movement of the neck to one side may markedly bring down the normal rate of the heart, leading to the decreased flow of blood to the brain, causing syncope. The same may happen when there is a pressure on the carotid sinus from outside, i.e. from some lesions in the neck such as enlarged glands, etc. Or, this may happen when a person is wearing a very tight collar, etc.

Hence, every case of syncope needs a very thorough check-up for arriving at a definite conclusion, and besides, various investigations for detecting a lesion in the heart, when it is so suspected, tests may also be required to see the hypersensitivity of the carotid sinus, especially when other causes/possibilities are not contributory.

It is true that in spite of a thorough investigation in a well-equipped hospital, the cause of syncope may not be possible to detect. (The author happened to examine an emergency case of syncope in a 73-year old man, who as soon as he stood up from a chair, fell down suddenly. The patient was made to lie down, and when the author reached the spot he was fully conscious. He was then investigated extensively, but no cause of syncope could be determined, and the patient has had no such attack now for the last five years).

As stated earlier, rarely, in some cases, when an attack of syncope is a bit more acute, i.e., when the period of unconsciousness is slightly prolonged, even convulsions may occur. Hence, besides investigations for the heart, an EEG/CT scan, etc., may also be required for the exclusion of epilepsy.

4. Other causes of syncope

There are some other causes of syncope as well. Even a continuous fit of coughing may cause syncope, as a result of diseases of the lungs, like a severe type of chronic bronchitis. It is often seen in middle-aged persons, due to a low cardiac output (as due to prolonged coughing, there is a low return of blood to the heart, and so the heart output, accordingly, decreases), and hence less blood is supplied to the brain, leading to transitory unconsciousness. The patient recovers as soon as the bout of coughing is over.

Syncope may also occur while passing urine, due to the reflex action of the distended urinary bladder.

It is advisable that one should not immediately stand up while getting up from bed during the night, i.e., after a period of sleep or recumbency, for any reason, so as to avoid postural hypotension, which may also lead to syncope.

Again, syncope is likely to manifest itself due to the involvement/narrowing of the blood vessels of the brain, caused by atherosclerosis, say, when the involvement of the vertebro-basilar artery responsible for vertebro-basilar insufficiency occurs. Such attacks of syncope are called transient ischaemic attacks (TIA) — also discussed in stroke (page 91, para 2).

What are drop attacks?

These are thought to be due to the transient decreased flow of blood to the brain, and the patient while walking or standing, usually an elderly person, suddenly falls to the ground, and immediately gets up also. Such attacks do not come under the head syncope, as there is no loss of consciousness in such cases. In such attacks, the patient feels that something has gone wrong in his legs, that they cannot bear the weight of the body, and it occurs instantaneously without any prior symptoms/warnings/ aura, as in cases of epilepsy.

Does epilepsy cause deterioration of mental health?

Epilepsy, under usual circumstances (of course, excluding newborns/infants) does not affect the mental health of a person. Usually, patients who take regular treatment, with suitable drugs, under the guidance of a specialist, lead a normal life. It is said that Julius Caesar and Winston Churchill also suffered from this disease, and still continued to function effectively.

What tests are necessary for a case of epilepsy?

As described earlier, the only practical way to diagnose epilepsy (including its various types), entirely depends on a detailed account, or on an eyewitness account. Tests like EEG/CT scan can be even normal in a case of epilepsy, established clinically, but the importance of these tests cannot be undermined.

Electroencephalogram (EEG)

It is a useful test for the diagnosis of epilepsy, where the report of an eyewitness is not either completely available, or is not available at all. But, in such cases, a word of caution. The EEG must be read very carefully, and the guidance of a specialist must be obtained, so that a non-epileptic person may not be labelled as a case of epilepsy, which will be indeed very unfortunate for the patient.

In some cases, where the EEG is negative, and the patient is still strongly suspected to be a case of epilepsy, EEG recordings are done after showing a flash to the patient (photic stimulation), and/or asking the patient to deeply breath (hyperventilation), or the EEG is recorded when the patient is instructed to be awake the whole night before the test is taken (called sleep-deprivation EEG), as under these circumstances there is a possibility of a positive graph. But again, a careful analysis of the EEG is required by an expert to exclude false-positive results. In any case, if the EEG is grossly abnormal, risk of repeated attacks of epilepsy must be explained both to the patient and his family members, so that he remains under observation all the time till the attacks are controlled with specific treatment. An EEG is equally important for the diagnosis of childhood epilepsy.

In selected cases, a 24-hour continuous ambulatory recording of EEG may be taken on the same pattern as the Holter test, done in heart patients to see the various irregularities in the rhythm of the heart (arrhythmias). In such a continuous record of EEG, the chances of a positive graph increase, as the recording is for a considerable length of time, which increases the chances of detection of any abnormality in the graph. However, this test too has got its own limitations.

Hence, the value of clinical diagnosis and the true report of an eyewitness should be emphasized again.

Computed tomographic (CT) scanning

A computed tomographic (CT) scan is, indeed, a valuable, non-invasive test in detecting the causative lesions in cases of epilepsy, especially in cases of brain tumours (mentioned earlier). Besides tumours, the test is also useful in diagnosing other causes of epilepsy, like post-traumatic scarring/gliosis or porencephaly, i.e. cavity in the brain, tuberculoma (due to tuberculosis), cysticercosis (due to ingestion of infected pork), or cerebral infarction (due to occlusion/thrombosis of one of the vessels of the brain).

However, again a very careful interpretation is required for reading a CT scan for the diagnosis of a shadow/s, as it has been shown in various studies that following an attack of epilepsy, temporary shadows (disappearing in about 1-3 months) of varying sizes may appear in the brain. But such a diagnosis may not be free from danger, as such shadows may be pathological, more so, malignant, and, therefore, a close follow-up is necessary, and repeated scans may be required to check if the lesion is lessening, persisting or increasing, so that no time is lost in carrying out life-saving treatment. At the same time, unnecessary treatment/panic may be avoided.

Such lesions/shadows may probably be due to post-epileptic oedema/swelling of the brain.

However, for a neurologist, such lesions create no problem for reaching a precise diagnosis, and, above all, the picture is seen as a whole, i.e., all accounts/aspects of the case are taken into consideration — the clinical manifestation of an attack of epilepsy, age of the patient, EEG report, and follow-up reports.

In several hospitals, special epilepsy clinics are being run where a large number of cases are seen/followed up weekly/fortnightly and, therefore, with experience, such problems are tackled in a routine manner, but may create a genuine difficulty, at times, for a general practitioner who may need the urgent opinion of a specialist.

Magnetic resonance imaging (MRI)

As already mentioned, this test is more sensitive than a CT scan, and, therefore, in doubtful cases, it must be carried out, especially when a CT scan is not contributory, and there is no satisfactory improvement in the condition of the patient, in spite of a potent drug therapy for epilepsy.

Other tests may also be required, such as the examination of stools for worms, especially for pork tapeworm (Taenia solium), X-ray of both the calf muscles, below the knee, for the presence of calcified cysts of cysticerci, especially in places where the incidence of epilepsy is common as a result of taking infected pork. Worms in the gut, in general, irrespective of the type, may precipitate an attack of epilepsy, especially among children.

Needless to say that investigations have a definite role in suspected epilepsy, more so for the detection of possible lesions and their cure. Many of the cases of epilepsy are idiopathic, i.e., where no cause is available, requiring a long course of drugs, and in a very few, even a lifelong maintenance dose may be required.

Treatment of epilepsy

A few important points will also find mention in Appendix VI on first aid, regarding emergency measures that are required to be followed by an eyewitness who happens to be there when the patient gets a massive attack of convulsions as a result of epilepsy. To repeat, it should be ensured that the neck of the patient is straight, and his tie and other clothes should be loosened. He should be turned to one side, and a spoon should be placed in between the back teeth so that the tongue is not bitten. If there is any debris nearby, it should be removed so that the patient may not injure himself. The jaw, if tightly closed, should not be forced open to insert the spoon. It should be checked that there is no injury to the head.

At the same time, one should not try to hold the person and try to stop the convulsions, as once an attack occurs, it takes its own time to subside. In general, it is over within 1-2 minutes. It is also important that the patient should be duly cared for till he or she becomes fully conscious. He should be allowed to sleep after the convulsive attack is over, and he should not be disturbed unnecessarily, although he should be constantly kept under watch. However, an emergency / first-aid treatment at the spot, and shifting the patient to a hospital should not be unnecessarily delayed.

After the diagnosis of epilepsy has been established in a particular case, the next important step is the treatment of the condition.

An underlying cause of epilepsy, if available (a brain tumour, etc.), must be treated and given priority. However, drug treatment to control an attack/s of epilepsy remains the same, whether the patient suffers from a case of idiopathic epilepsy or symptomatic epilepsy, where though the cause has been detected, but nevertheless, drug treatment is needed.

As regards drugs, it is the rule that the patient should be given a single drug as a trial. The drug should commensurate with the type of epilepsy the patient is suffering from. In other words, the type/pattern of the attack of epilepsy decides the choice of the drug. It is highly important that the drug should be given in proper dosages, depending upon the age of the patient.

To begin with, a very minimal quantity of drug should be started, say even one-fourth of the normal dose required, and the dose should be increased gradually, say, weekly, or every 3-4 days, depending upon the severity of the disease. Otherwise, it is very likely that the drug may cause undue drowsiness in a person, and may be rejected by the patient, especially in the case of a child. However, it is usually well tolerated in most of the cases in due course of time.

Above all, continuity of the drug therapy for the full-length duration of the treatment plays a very significant role in the control of attacks.

By and large, a properly administered drug treatment works very well, and people with epilepsy get permanent remission after about 3 years of treatment, or may be more in some of the cases. Great patience is the key to success of monotherapy (single drug trial) in cases of epilepsy, and the parents/family members of epileptics, especially, as seen in the case of children, should not compel the physician for a quick control of the disease, or doubt the expertise of the physician, or the authenticity/potency of the drug prescribed.

However, there are some cases which do create a problem, when their attacks are not controlled with a single drug. Provided an appropriate drug has been started, it does work in the majority of the cases, though in a few the effect of the drug may not be up to the mark, so that the patient may get an attack of epilepsy, though much less in intensity as compared to the original attack, and the frequencies may also be reduced. In such cases, the physician or specialist makes his own judgement, and either changes or adds another antiepileptic drug, so as to give lasting relief to the patient.

The patient is also required to know about the details of the toxicity of the drug that has been prescribed, so that he can report to his physician well in time. In case the antiepileptic drug is being given to a pregnant woman, its teratogenic effect on the foetus, which may be responsible for congenital abnormalities in the newborn, should be explained to the woman. However, this may not happen in all the cases. It is advisable to seek a consultation with/or counselling from the physician before the pregnancy is planned.

Patient with first seizure

It should not be ignored. Besides history (say of epilepsy in the family, immediate withdrawal of alcohol/drug, recent/past trauma, fever, etc.), the statement of eyewitnesses, if available, EEG (if need be sleep-deprivation EEG), CT scanning/MRI should be carried out.

Status epilepticus

The emergency of status epilepticus occurs when the patient gets repeated attacks (2 or more) of convulsions without full recovery in between the attacks, or the attack remains almost continuous for at least 15-30 minutes, and can actually threaten the life of the patient.

This sudden problem occurs, commonly, when a case of epilepsy has not responded well to the antiepileptic drug, or the drug has been either stopped or reduced abruptly during the course of treatment. Or, it may be a manifestation of an underlying disease of the brain. However, in many of the cases, no cause can be ascertained.

The patient urgently requires immediate admission to a well-equipped hospital. In such cases, transportation of the patient to the hospital should not be delayed as the brain is likely to be damaged due to continuous attacks of epilepsy. And sometimes the brain damage may be of a very severe nature, if treatment is not started well in time.

In the hospital, prompt steps are taken to save the life of the patient, and in such cases, a combination of 2-3 drugs (polytherapy) is required to control the fits. A single drug therapy is never the rule, as there is no such ideal solitary drug which can control fits of such severe intensity and continuous occurrence. Other general measures, like the administration of oxygen, intravenous drip, catheterization of bladder, etc. are also taken in the hospital.

After the attacks have been controlled, the patient should be put on suitable long-term antiepileptic treatment at the earliest possible time, so that further attacks of status epilepticus can be prevented. Of course, a thorough search for the possible underlying cause has to be made for a precise diagnosis, by carrying out various tests, described earlier. An EEG, in this emergency, plays a vital role in the diagnosis and also helps to exclude the possibility of hysterical convulsions, which may still be suspected in some of the cases.

In some of the hospitals, there is a set routine to follow for such emergencies, so that no time is lost, and all steps are taken systematically by a team of medical/paramedical staff. Although the majority of the patients recover, around 10% cases may not survive.

As an immediate preventive measure, if in any patient with known epilepsy, the frequency of convulsions increases, besides reconsidering the underlying pathology, especially a malignant disorder, one should also consider that in such cases status epilepticus may be imminent and, therefore, urgent steps should be taken to control the frequency of attacks.

Refractory epilepsy

It means that the patient does not respond to drug/s administered. It is one of the serious problems relating to the treatment of epilepsy, and if it is not solved immediately, the patient will continue to suffer from troublesome attacks of epilepsy, or may even suffer terribly from the emergency of status epilepticus, described above. In such cases, look for the following:

(i) Is the diagnosis correct? It is possible that the patient may not be suffering from epilepsy at all. It should be taken seriously, and the whole diagnosis should be reviewed without delay.

(ii) Do hysterical convulsions exist simultaneously? In such cases, one has to make a close observation of the patient's convulsions.

(iii) Has a primary cause been missed? Hence all tests may be reviewed, and especially MRI, if not done, should be carried out, as it is more sensitive than the CT scan in detecting lesions of the brain.

(iv) Is the patient taking a suitable drug, and that too regularly?

(v) Is the patient taking the drug in proper dosages? The patient may need a regular estimation/monitoring of the blood concentration of the drug administered, as is indicated in such refractory cases. However, in routine/ usual cases of epilepsy, an analysis of the blood may not be necessarily required for adjusting the dosages of antiepileptic drugs, provided the clinical response of the drug chosen is satisfactory.

(vi) Has anything new, such as more consumption of alcohol etc., taken place?

(vii) Is there psychological stress?

The above are some of the reasons for refractory epilepsy relating to routine cases of epilepsy, but things become dark when the grave emergency of epilepsy, i.e. status epilepticus, becomes refractory to drugs. In such a situation the patient will suffer from repeated/continuous convulsions. There is no alternative then except to administer general anaesthesia. The patient may be administered intravenous thiopentone so that he goes into a coma and his muscles relax and the convulsions stop. However, all this is only possible in a highly-developed hospital/ medical centre.

Withdrawal of antiepileptic drugs

It must be ensured that the antiepileptic drug is withdrawn slowly, i.e. its dose should be reduced gradually, say, in six months or in one year, or even more. It is a very important factor in the treatment. In case the drug is stopped abruptly, or it is not withdrawn very gradually, it may precipitate an attack of epilepsy (even status epilepticus in some of the cases), and once an attack of epilepsy occurs, the patient may have to be given once again a full course of treatment for epilepsy for a period of about 3 years. Hence the importance of the slow withdrawal of antiepileptic drugs.

However, in case of a recurrence of an attack of epilepsy, when the drug is being reduced gradually, increase in its dose becomes necessary.

Can epilepsy be prevented?

Indeed, some of the causes of epilepsy are preventable. Utmost care should be taken at the time of delivery so that brain/skull injury to the newborn is avoided.

However, head injuries, at all ages, should be avoided, so as to prevent the occurrence of traumatic epilepsy, both following the injury or later. The use of helmets is advisable, especially while travelling on two-wheelers. However, while driving cars or any other vehicle, all precautions must be taken to safeguard against accidents.

Since the disease also occurs following the intake of infected pork, either one should abstain from taking pork, or take it when it is absolutely safe, and has been cooked properly and thoroughly.

Consumption of alcohol should be avoided. Epilepsy is said to be three times more common among alcoholics than in non-alcoholics. Both excessive drinking or even moderate drinking of alcohol may precipitate an attack of epilepsy.

There is a word of advice for alcoholics. For those who are addicted to alcohol for a long time, in such cases, alcohol must be withdrawn very gradually, otherwise it is very likely that an attack of epilepsy may be precipitated.

The same is true when someone is addicted to a sedative as a result of drug abuse. Such drugs should also be reduced gradually.

In all cases of diabetes, a strict control of blood sugar is required. It is seen sometimes, when a patient takes antidiabetic drugs in more than the required quantity, or takes reduced diet with the usual dose of the antidiabetic drug, there occurs a sudden fall in blood sugar (hypoglycaemia), which may cause in a small percentage of cases, generalized epileptic convulsions. Hence a proper control of diabetes is essential for the prevention of convulsions. In such cases, there will be no aura, i.e., warning signals/symptoms, before an attack of epilepsy is precipitated.

Fever in children should be controlled as a prevention of epilepsy. Convulsions as a result of fever constitute an important precipitating factor, and may necessitate a long-term course of antiepileptic drugs, especially in children who have a positive family history of epilepsy, and/or whose EEG findings are suggestive of the disease. Hence all care must be taken to control high fever in children as a preventive measure against epilepsy.

There are yet a few more precipitating conditions. An epileptic may be sensitive to light stimuli; therefore, as a preventive measure, such a patient should not face strong flashes/flickers. All epileptics recall that when their EEG was recorded, at one stage, the technician must have shown them a strong flash and recorded the EEG. The idea is to evoke epileptic response in the patient so that a positive reading can be obtained for the diagnosis of the disease. Photosensitive epilepsy is a common one and is found in almost 5-10% of all cases of epilepsy.

For the same reasons, an epileptic should be cautious while watching TV. He should not view it at a stretch, and the room should not be dark. A light in the room, preferably near the TV set, must be on so that the effect of a flash, if any, can be minimised. Besides flash, the patient may be sensitive to different intensity/shades of light repeatedly appearing on the television screen. However, the brightness/shades, etc. can be adjusted in any television set, the one suitable/pleasing for the patient should be used, and all the family members must co-operate with the patient who is watching TV at the same time.

Likewise, a child suffering from epilepsy may have difficulty in reading a book, and thus a proper light must be adjusted for the purpose. And if some print pattern in the book does not suit the child, or any epileptic, irrespective of age, it should be avoided, and the patient should be advised to read the book in bold print. If possible, the pattern of the print should suit him/her most. In other words, if a definite print pattern does not suit an epileptic, that should be preferably avoided so that an attack of epilepsy may not be precipitated. Parents have a vital role to play to guide their children in such matters. Similarly, if the patient is sensitive to a particular sound, however rough, loud or pleasant, it should be avoided.

General guidelines for a case of epilepsy

Falsely, a fear always exists in a patient that he may get a sudden attack of epilepsy anywhere and at any time. But this is not true, since in the majority of the cases the attacks of epilepsy are effectively controlled with proper medication, and the patient gets permanent remission after the treatment is over. Hence there is no reason that the patient should panic unduly. He should lead a normal life in all respects.

This uncalled-for apprehension of the patient can only be eliminated by the physician through constant counselling, and many a time the whole family may need to be guided about the true nature of the disease, in a particular case. This is of utmost significance in the treatment of epilepsy. The patient must be educated/motivated regarding all the aspects of the disease in detail, especially the preventive part.

As soon as the attacks are controlled with the therapy initiated, the patient should feel perfectly safe, although he needs to take the necessary precautions, depending on the profession of the person. A factory worker has to guard himself against injuries while working on various machines. Similarly, a labourer, or any other worker, has to be vigilant. Such professions may have to be avoided by the patient, to be on the safe side. However, it depends from case to case, and, above all, on the advice of the physician.

Similarly, a taxi driver/or any driver may find difficulty in continuing with his job. In some countries, driving is not permitted for six months, or even for two years after the patient is free from attacks. However, again, things vary from patient to patient.

Another important point to follow is that a patient of epilepsy should strictly follow his daily routine as regards his timing of food, work, sleep, etc. He should not keep awake the whole night, as may be required sometimes under certain circumstances, as far as possible. This point can be elaborated by saying that in some cases, for the diagnosis of epilepsy, when the usual EEG is normal, a sleep-deprivation (in which case the patient is instructed to remain awake the whole night) EEG is taken, which may be positive. This helps in the diagnosis of epilepsy. Hence the importance of good sleep for a patient of epilepsy.

There may be some cases of epilepsy in which attacks of convulsions occur during sleep only. In such cases, one person must sleep near the patient to avoid complications.

A patient of epilepsy should remain composed and avoid stress as far as possible. He should never feel excited.

There is no specific dietary restriction for an epileptic patient. All types of food can be enjoyed by them, unless particularly restricted by the physician due to some associated ailments, like hypertension or diabetes, etc. Hence epileptics should not worry too much regarding their food, including non-vegetarian food, although alcohol has to be avoided, as mentioned earlier.

A few words may also be said about epileptic children. Parents must boost them up. Children should never feel that they cannot study or achieve something in their life, as they have developed epilepsy. Mass awareness is essential in this aspect both for parents / teachers and fellow children/students. Such children should follow a set routine, both of study and sports. However, an epileptic child should participate in only light sports, since heavy physical exertion may not be suitable.

The children should get good hygienic food, and should have good health. Any type of infection, like a sore throat/tonsillitis or worms infestations should be avoided. The child must attend to his school duties regularly.

Before ending the topic of epilepsy, after elaborating the various ways and means to curb this so-called stigmatic malady, it needs to be stressed strongly that unless there is a mass realization that the disease is not a stigma and can be controlled easily with drugs, and that people should themselves come forward for its treatment, a desired goal can never be achieved. For this, grass-root arrangements are required right from the peripheral health centres, including the provision of a suitable team which can make a house-to-house survey for creating mass awareness, and for detection of hidden and uncontrolled cases of epilepsy, especially those who may be concealing their disease purposely due to the social stigma attached to it. It has to be an action-orientated team. Above all, both medical and paramedical staff should provide necessary counselling in various matters, so that epileptics can lead a peaceful life, with no myths in their minds.

3. Poliomyelitis

As the name of the disease indicates, there is an infection/inflammation of the grey matter of the spinal cord (Polios, grey + myelos, marrow + itis, inflammation), causing paralysis of the muscles of the body, especially of the limbs.

The disease is still common, although it can be prevented by vaccination.

How the infection of poliomyelitis occurs

The poliovirus is an enterovirus, i.e. the virus proliferates in the intestine (enteron, intestine) of the patient concerned.

The infection occurs by ingestion of food/water contaminated with poliovirus, and the faecal matter of a patient or a carrier (i.e. the one who carries the poliovirus in the gut, but does not show symptoms of the disease), is the true source of infection.

Flies may play an important role in the spread of the disease, so that epidemics of poliomyelitis may be more common in summer. However, sporadic cases are also seen.

Hence, upgrading hygienic conditions is an important aspect in the prevention of the disease.

The poliovirus may survive even for months in the sewage, i.e., in the waste matter in underground pipes or in various passages. Further, the virus may be passing out in the faeces of patients/carriers for many months, so that the source of infection remains almost continuous, especially during an epidemic.

How the infection reaches the spinal cord from the gut

The poliovirus multiplies in the gut of the man, and apart from passing out in the faeces, it reaches the spinal cord through the various nerves. Or it may enter the blood stream and infect the spinal cord.

The virus has got a particular affinity for the anterior horn cells (i.e. the motor nerve cells in the anterior horns) of the spinal cord, and inflammation/damage of these cells is responsible for the paralysis of the muscles of the body. Since the anterior horns of the spinal cord are involved, the disease is also called anterior poliomyelitis, and since the disease occurs abruptly, it is more precisely called acute anterior poliomyelitis.

In the whole spinal cord, two of its regions, i.e., the lumbar and the cervical are mainly/usually involved, and out of these two areas, the lumbar region is more involved, so that in a case of poliomyelitis, the legs are more involved than the arms.

Since only motor nerve cells are involved, there is no sensory loss/impairment in the involved limb, in any of the cases of poliomyelitis.

However, besides the lumbar and cervical portions of the spinal cord, the thoracic portion of the cord may also be damaged, leading to the paralysis of the muscles of the thorax, causing difficulty in breathing. Even respiratory paralysis may occur, and the patient may be in a state of grave emergency.

In addition to the spinal cord, the lower portion of the brain, i.e. the brain stem may be affected in some of the cases. This may cause paralysis of the muscles of the face, of the larynx and of the throat, so that the patient may have both difficulty in speaking and in swallowing. When this happens, the patient's condition becomes very serious, and treatment of such cases is only possible in a well-equipped hospital.

Incubation period

This is the period from the entry of infection in the body to the development of the symptoms of the disease. This takes about one to two weeks, in most of the cases.

Age of the patient

Since the disease occurs more often in children, it is also called infantile paralysis. But it can occur in older children, and also in adults.

What are the signs and symptoms of poliomyelitis?

In most cases, the patient may remain without any symptom. In others, the disease may pass off in about 3-4 days after a little fever, or upper respiratory tract infection, or a slight disturbance of the gastrointestinal tract.

In still another small group of cases, fever, headache, a stiff neck, vomiting (i.e. so-called meningitis) may occur. It is called the non-paralytic stage of the disease, or non-paralytic poliomyelitis, since in a few cases this stage may be followed by, in about 3-4 days, the next stage of the disease, in which paralysis of the muscles may occur. This last stage is called the paralytic stage of the disease, or paralytic poliomyelitis. Hence paralysis occurs only in a limited number of patients who are infected with poliovirus.

More about the paralytic stage of poliomyelitis

When the paralysis of various muscles, say of the limbs, is taking place, almost full recovery is the rule in most of the cases, as there may be only temporary involvement of the anterior horn cells. However, some permanent weakness may persist in some of the muscles. Therefore, during the acute phase of the disease, the patient and his attendants/family members must show patience. Once paralysis of the muscles has started, it continues for about a day, and may take more time in a few cases.

The extent of paralysis depends upon the degree of involvement of the spinal cord, i.e., of the motor nerve cells lying in the anterior horns of the spinal cord. And, therefore, the paralysis may be confined to only one small group of muscles of any of the limbs, i.e., only a part of the limb may be involved.

While in others, either the whole limb, or even all four limbs may be involved.

Further, the paralysis of poliomyelitis is a highly irregular or asymmetrical/variable, to the extent that in a particular patient, if on one side the foot is involved, on the other side, either the whole or part of the arm may be involved, etc.

As stated above, in spite of the full recovery of most of the muscles that have been paralysed, some residual paralysis can persist, leading to permanent paralysis of these affected muscles. The worst is that these muscles soon start wasting in about a week. Contractures in these muscles may develop, which become responsible for various deformities in a growing child.

Treatment of poliomyelitis

There is no specific treatment which can stop the paralysis of the muscles, once it occurs, or bring about the full recovery of the muscles that are going to be affected permanently.

Since in some of these paralysed muscles, contractures are likely to occur, and to begin with, one cannot say, which of the muscle/s will be permanently damaged, all the paralysed limbs or part/s of the limb/s must be kept in their proper positions.

Early mobility/physiotherapy is the most important part of the treatment, to avoid contractures. However, surgical intervention may be required in some of the cases, so that the paralysed limb can be used in the best possible way. Finally, orthopaedic appliances may also be required so that the person is able to live satisfactorily, as far as possible.

Vaccination

Besides maintaining strict hygienic conditions, vaccination is the key to the prevention of poliomyelitis. Although it is a routine affair to vaccinate every child for poliomyelitis, yet there are parents who are careless or negligent in this regard. I have seen a young girl who suffered from an attack of poliomyelitis, which caused paralysis of the lower limbs. Her mother confessed that she had purposely postponed the vaccination of her daughter, as in her view she had already attained adulthood, and, therefore, was unlikely to get this affliction. Hence, polio vaccination is of utmost importance in the case of a child, given well in time.

Country-wide campaigns called 'Pulse Polio Immunization (PPI)' programmes, including special/additional pulse polio drives focussing especially on those areas where poliomyelitis cases were still occurring, despite extensive PPI campaigns, were started in India, from 1996-97 to fulfil the target of zero poliomyelitis. In these camps oral polio vaccine (OPV) is administered up to grass-root levels to all the children up to the age of 5, irrespective of previous vaccinations, with the hope of eliminating this disease as far as possible. Great vigil and motivation are required in such programmes. Such camps are still being held. In spite of the best efforts of the organizers, some children may remain unvaccinated. Hence poliomyelitis may reappear, when and if unvaccinated cases manifest the disease sooner or later. Further, those vaccinated may require booster dose/s in subsequent years. Standard of vaccine ought to be maintained by storing it in proper conditions. Total eradication of this disease is a must throughout the world to avoid its recurrence. Such perception on the part of the parents can save their children from a possible attack in later years.

8
TUBERCULOSIS

Why is tuberculosis common in spite of the availability of highly potent drugs, and vaccination?

It is indeed a very tricky and difficult question, and for an accurate answer, one has to study the matter/subject in detail. One truly wonders that tuberculosis is still a common and fatal disease, in spite of the availability of a number of highly potent and specific antibiotics to fight it. Above all, immunization against this disease is almost the rule, after the birth of the newborn.

The frequency of the disease can well be imagined when separate hospitals called tuberculosis hospitals are seen at various places, and one finds the wards of these hospitals full of tuberculosis cases, with many patients in a highly serious condition, with fatal consequences.

Though there has been a substantial improvement in the control of this lethal disease, following sustained and vigorous research during the last few decades, no specific antibiotic was available for its treatment till nearly a century ago. The only way was to isolate the patients in various sanatoriums located at hills and to provide a good diet and tonics. One can, thus, think of the fatalities caused by this disease at that time. However, such sanatoriums are no longer required; now the disease can be treated even at home, with necessary isolation and prevention.

In spite of all this, i.e. great advances in its treatment as well as control, it is still a threatening medical problem all the world over, and is one of the important causes of death from infectious diseases. There are large number of deaths in a year from this disease in the world, and the death rate is much higher in developing countries. And every year, a substantial number of new cases of the disease are added the world over.

There is something wrong somewhere. That a disease which is absolutely curable and preventable, still takes such a heavy toll of life. It means that we will have to analyse the problem step-by-step to explore its nature.

What is the organism that causes tuberculosis?

This organism is known to all by now. The word TB gives the name of the organism, i.e. tubercle bacillus, more precisely called Mycobacterium tuberculosis, also commonly called acid-fast bacillus (AFB) (Fig. 14).

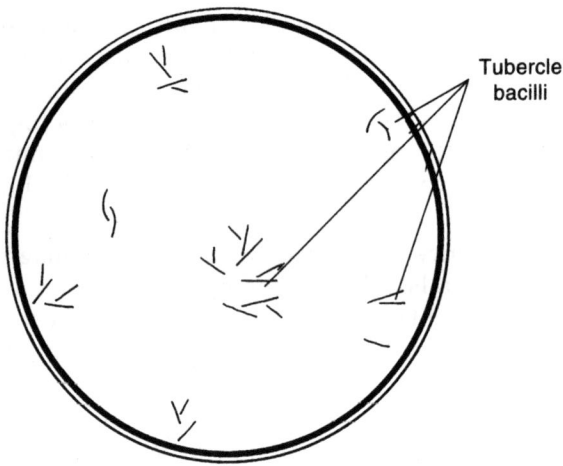

Fig. 14. The tubercle bacilli (which look like thin, straight/curved rods under the microscope) in the sputum of a patient of tuberculosis.

How do tubercle bacilli invade the body, and (some) remain dormant / hidden in the body?

When a person suffering from tuberculosis, coughs, sneezes, talks, especially loudly, laughs, spits sputum, etc., he throws out in the air tiny droplets of sputum laden with tubercle bacilli, when the patient has not covered his face with a piece of cloth or

Tuberculosis

handkerchief (Fig. 15). In this way, the air around the patient gets infected with enormous tubercle bacilli, grouped together in various tiny droplets of sputum. Any person, in close proximity of the patient is likely to inhale these tiny droplets. Many of these large size droplets may fall on the ground, and they may be inhaled later when they get dried and reduced in size further. They may survive in the soil for as long as six months. Hence the dust contaminated with tiny dried droplets

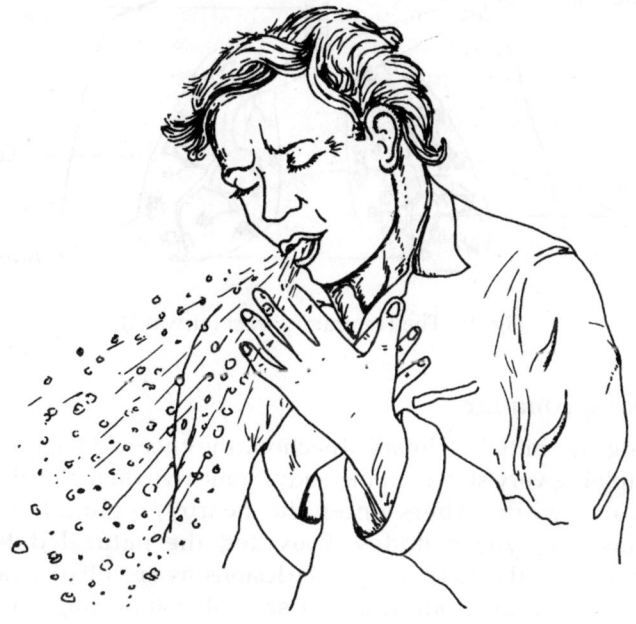

Fig. 15. A patient of tuberculosis coughing out droplets of sputum laden with tubercle bacilli.

of tubercle bacilli plays a great role in the transmission of the disease. Even the area/room, where a patient of tuberculosis has been isolated, remains potentially contaminated, as tiny droplets of sputum float in the air there.

Tubercle bacilli-laden sputum, in tiny droplets, enter into the nose and go through the air passages, and finally reach the tiny air sacs of the lungs (alveoli) (Fig. 16).

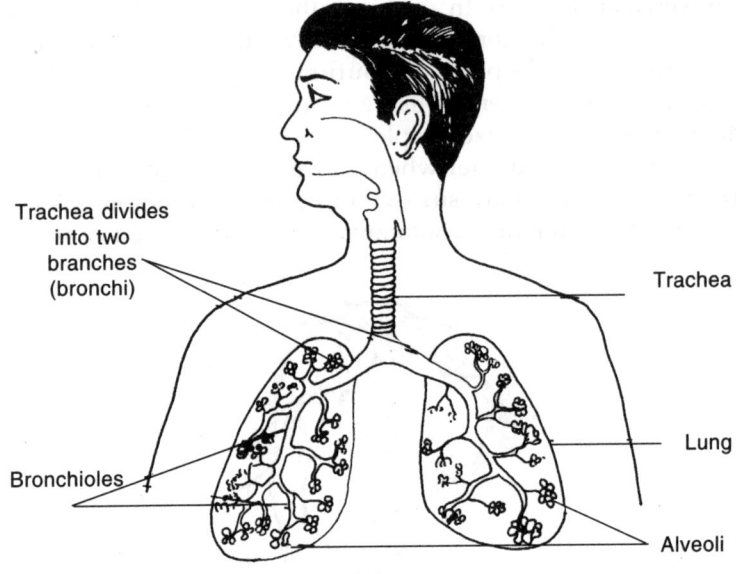

Fig. 16. The respiratory tract (airways).

Primary complex

During the initial/primary infection, the tubercle bacilli start multiplying very slowly in the body. Some remain in the air sacs (alveoli), while others enter the nearby/regional/hilar/mediastinal lymph nodes. Provided the natural defence mechanism of the body is good, the lesions, as a result of invasion of tubercle bacilli, both in the air sacs/alveoli or lungs, and in the glands, get healed and calcified. These two healed/calcified lesions, i.e., in the lung, as well as in the glands, together, are called a primary complex. It is understood that the patient will have hardly any symptoms during this infection. It will be of interest to the readers to know that this primary complex is supposed to safeguard the person against future/fresh infection of tubercle bacilli (explained later).

All persons in whom a primary complex has developed will be 'tuberculin skin test' positive, as the individual concerned would have developed hypersensitivity to the proteins of tubercle bacilli, known as 'tuberculins', which are used while performing this test. It is an important test, and is primarily meant to detect initial infection or a primary lesion/complex in an individual. This test has particular value in an epidemiological study to find out the infected cases of tuberculosis in a community, i.e., 'tuberculin test surveys'.

In case the natural defence mechanism of the body is poor, following primary/initial invasion by tubercle bacilli, the patient may suffer from frank tuberculosis.

Dormant tubercle bacilli

However, in some cases, following primary infection by tubercle bacilli, the bacilli may also remain dormant in the body, even for the whole life of the patient. This is the most dangerous situation, since the tubercle bacilli may become active at any time, say after one year or after many years, and start multiplying and triggering off the disease. They truly act like potential enemies in the body, and attack whenever the defence mechanism of the body is on the lower side/decreases. However, they may never become active, if the defence mechanism/resistance of the body remains strong.

Sites of infection of tubercle bacilli

The lungs are the most favourable sites for the multiplication/growth of tubercle bacilli, as the bacilli find suitable conditions for their development, including a good supply of oxygen. The kidneys, bones and brain are other places that favour the growth of tubercle bacilli. The tubercle bacilli reach these sites through blood from their lesion in various lymph nodes. Hence, tuberculosis may not occur in all organs of the body, as many organs/tissues may not be suitable for the growth of tubercle bacilli.

What are the circumstances/factors which lower the defence mechanism of the body and cause tuberculosis?

After the primary complex has been formed, i.e. when the patient is already infected, he gets additional protection against subsequent invasion by tubercle bacilli. This is the characteristic feature only of this bacterial infection. Hence, whenever tubercle bacilli invade a healthy person, who is previously infected, i.e., has a primary complex in his body, the tubercle bacilli, as they enter the lungs/alveoli/air sacs are likely to be killed by the various immune responses of the body. But this is not as simple as it looks like. On the contrary, tuberculosis does occur in many cases, since the defence mechanism of the body gets paralysed in one way or the other.

The defence mechanism of the body may be markedly impaired when a patient is suffering from a general disease like diabetes, occupational diseases of the lungs like asbestosis (due to inhalation of asbestos particles), anthracosis (due to coal dust inhalation), silicosis (due to inhalation of stone dust), etc. Similarly, AIDS is also known to be associated with tuberculosis, since in AIDS too the defence mechanism of the body becomes highly disturbed, and hence the disease is called acquired immune deficiency syndrome (AIDS).

Likewise, chances of tuberculosis increase in alcoholics, drug-abusers and in old people, or when a person is under acute stress/tension.

Further, chances of the occurrence of the disease increase, irrespective of the immunity of the person, if a person/s are in close contact with a tuberculous patient, such as among students/family members, or in places where living conditions are too much crowded, especially in poorly ventilated houses/slums. Such persons get repeated infections continuously from a patient of tuberculosis, living close by. Malnutrition further adds to the growth of the disease.

However, when the disease manifests itself, it is difficult to say whether the disease has occurred as a result of fresh infection, after the primary complex/infection, or is the reactivation of the previous dormant infection lying in the body. It could be the first infection in the body which has turned into a serious one, as the primary complex could not be formed, as may occur in infants due to their impaired resistance.

'Infection' and 'clinical manifestations' of tuberculosis

From the above, it is clear that there are two distinct clinical stages/entities of tuberculosis; one is only 'infection' of tuberculosis (in which case a primary complex develops with no symptoms) and the other is 'clinical manifestations' of the disease, in which case various signs and symptoms of the disease appear.

As stated earlier, the tuberculin skin test will be positive as soon as the patient gets an infection of tuberculosis.

Is tuberculosis a 'hidden' disease?

Yes, it is a hidden disease. The patient remains asymptomatic for long periods, and the disease is often diagnosed during routine tests, when a chest X-ray reveals the 'hidden' disease, i.e. tuberculosis. It has thus an occult/hidden character.

Detection of hidden cases of tuberculosis

In places where the incidence of tuberculosis is not marked, 'tuberculin test surveys' can be carried out among the general population, which gives an idea of the number of cases who are tuberculin positive, i.e. infected with tubercle bacilli (although the disease may be inactive in the majority of them). Those who have shown positive in the tuberculin test should be subjected to an X-ray examination of the chest, so as to find out hidden/symptomless, especially active cases of the disease — in other words those who are suffering from active tuberculosis, but still showing no symptoms of the disease, can be detected.

For an epidemiological survey, small X-rays may be taken through a special X-ray plant fitted in a van, which moves from place to place or village to village, or visits poor communities/slums. X-rays are taken in quick succession, one by one, of the various persons, who are made to stand in a queue before entering the van. They come out of the van after the exposure for the chest X-ray. This is called miniature mass radiography (MMR). These surveys were most common in the past when the disease was at its peak.

However, in places where the incidence of tuberculosis is high, all persons in such areas are expected to be infected with tubercle bacilli, i.e., they will be found as tuberculin positive. Hence the tuberculin test is of little value at such places, for epidemiological survey, and therefore, one can directly switch on to MMR study, for the detection of both hidden and active cases of tuberculosis.

It may, however, be noted that X-ray of the chest alone may not be always confirmatory of the diagnosis/activity of tuberculosis, either in a mass survey or in an individual. Hence, when the disease is suspected, other tests, explained later, must be carried out, including a detailed clinical examination, keeping the symptomatology of the patient in view.

Also, in the MMR study, small X-ray films taken may not give the true picture of the disease. And, there even may be variations in reading these X-ray films. Even if a tubercular lesion appears to be positive, it must be confirmed by a large chest X-ray, as well as by other tests. It is never wise to administer treatment of tuberculosis to a patient only on the basis of miniature radiographs.

The MMR study is now no longer widely carried out in places/countries where the incidence of tuberculosis is low, because too few cases may be found positive, involving the expense of a lot of time, money, and above all, at the risk of exposure to X-ray radiation for a large population.

However, even in these countries, routine X-rays must be taken to detect the active disease in those who are in close contact with tuberculosis patients. Also, in all those groups of persons who daily come in contact with a large number of people, such as the bus-drivers, conductors, teachers, and the entire medical staff, like doctors, nurses, attendants, technicians, radiographers etc., chest X-rays should be carried out because they comprise the high-risk groups. Spread of the disease has also been noticed in creches, schools, school-buses, hostels, and even in nursing homes, etc.

Similarly, the disease must be detected in servants, waiters in restaurants, salesmen, postmen, washermen, sweepers, barbers, cobblers, etc. People living in slums and shanty towns, chawls, etc. should also be checked for the detection of tuberculosis.

All efforts must be made to unearth 'hidden' cases of tuberculosis, as they are most dangerous to society. They go on spreading the disease for a pretty long time, till it is diagnosed and treated.

What is the tuberculin skin test?

This test detects the 'infected' cases of tuberculosis by eliciting a hypersensitivity reaction in patients who are already infected with tubercle bacilli. In this test, more precisely the Mantoux test, purified proteins isolated from tubercle bacilli called 'tuberculins' are injected intracutaneously on the upper surface of the forearm. Out of several tuberculin tests, the Mantoux is most commonly used, since by and large its results are highly reliable. As mentioned earlier, this test will have little value in places where there is a high incidence of tuberculosis, i.e., at such places almost every person can be expected to be infected with tubercle bacilli. However, it has value otherwise. Those cases which are tuberculin negative, may not be suffering from tuberculosis, and in such cases, one should think of other pathology in a concerned patient.

In about 48-72 hours, following the injection of the test, an allergic reaction occurs as a raised, hard red spot at the site of injection. The size of this area should be carefully measured, and an area of 10 mm, roughly about half an inch or more in diameter, indicates that the reaction is positive. Only the induration (raised area) should be measured with regard to its width. The redness around the raised area must be avoided while taking measurements. Ideally, a trained and experienced technician, especially one who specifically deals in carrying out tuberculin tests, is required. An induration of less than 7 mm is considered negative, while induration between 7-10 mm, may be considered a borderline or a doubtful case of tuberculin positive, and such cases need further tests, for exclusion, or for establishing a diagnosis of tuberculosis.

However, this test has its own limitations. Although a positive reaction does indicate that the person is infected with tubercle bacilli, it does not indicate whether the disease is active or not. Further, a false-positive reaction may also occur when the person has been infected with some atypical type of bacilli of this group, which have a close resemblance to tubercle bacilli. Furthermore, since now the BCG vaccination is given to all the newborns, especially in hospitals, all such children will be strongly positive for the tuberculin test. This considerably limits the value of the test in the diagnosis of tuberculosis. In a few specific cases, a false-negative tuberculin reaction may also occur, when the patient is suffering from some other disease at the same time, or the patient is on some drugs which are immunosuppressive in nature.

In a nutshell, this test may not have any value in detecting the hidden/symptomless, especially active cases of tuberculosis, when a large-scale screening programme is carried out; even though this test has its value in individual cases. Therefore, this test may not find a place in a national policy programme. However, an awareness about it is important since it is one of the routine tests.

What are the early symptoms of tuberculosis?

It is unfortunate that there are no specific early symptoms of the disease. Therefore, even apart from hidden cases of tuberculosis, it is not even possible to detect the disease when the symptoms appear, since early symptoms are vague, and both the patient and the physician cannot pinpoint or even suspect the occurrence of tuberculosis in a particular case.

The early symptoms are entirely of a routine type which may occur in any general infection of the body, like fatigue or tiredness, exhaustion, headache, irritability, night sweat, weakness, loss of appetite, low-grade fever, especially in the evening, mild shivering, loss of weight, etc. This may be associated with a mild cough, or the patient may have only a slight upper respiratory tract infection, or a 'cold' that has persisted. Or else, the patient may have pain in the chest due to the involvement of the pleura overlying the lungs. Even auscultation of the chest, i.e., examination of the chest with a stethoscope by the physician, does not help in diagnosing early cases of the disease.

However, blood in the sputum, i.e., spitting of blood (haemoptysis) is a relatively late sign. Hence, if it occurs, investigations of tuberculosis should be done immediately.

Is there any specific warning signal to suspect the disease?

In view of the vague symptoms of tuberculosis in early cases, the only suitable way is to adhere to some important signal/dictum. If a person has a cough for more than 14 days, with fever, loss of appetite and weight, tuberculosis must be suspected, and a chest X-ray and a sputum examination for tubercle bacilli must be carried out. If the X-ray examination of the chest shows an early tuberculous lesion, which is more common, at the upper part of the apex of the lung, ask the patient to cough, and if crepitations are heard/appear, it gives a strong clue of the activity of the disease; of course, this is the job of the attending physician/chest specialist who auscultates the chest to hear crepitations, i.e., crackling sounds from the lung/s, as a result of the infection of tuberculosis.

How to establish the diagnosis of tuberculosis?

As already explained, there are two entities of the disease, infection and clinical manifestations, i.e., when the disease is active. Hence, it is important to establish the activity of the disease, which is important for starting the treatment of tuberculosis. The treatment is a long one and needs a combination of 3-4 drugs in all the cases. The following tests help in establishing the activity of the disease. However, as one can see, all tests have their own limitations, and therefore, one cannot rely on a single test.

1. Sputum examination for tubercle bacilli

It should be carried out at least 3-4 times. Approximately 5,000 to 10,000 tubercle bacilli are required per ml of sputum for the detection of tubercle bacilli in a smear. Hence, repeated examinations of sputum are advised.

2. Sputum culture for tubercle bacilli

Although this test is more sensitive than the direct smear examination, it is more time-consuming, and requires about 6-8 weeks. Again, as in a direct smear examination, 3-4 cultures of tubercle bacilli may be required to obtain positive results. A well-equipped laboratory and trained staff is required for carrying out this test.

3. Chest X-ray

It should be carried out in all the suspected cases of tuberculosis. One should not rely solely on the chest X-ray report as proof of the activity of the disease. Other tests, including symptoms and signs of the disease, must be taken into account.

4. Tuberculin/Mantoux test

It has a limited value. However, a negative tuberculin test may prove to be highly valuable in some of the cases, to exclude the diagnosis of tuberculosis in a particular case.

5. **ELISA (enzyme-linked immunosorbent assay) test for tuberculosis**
It is one of the serological tests and detects antibodies against tubercle bacilli. It is highly useful to detect hidden cases of tuberculosis, especially extrapulmonary, i.e., when the lesion of tuberculosis is outside the lungs. The accuracy of this test is 90-95 per cent, and it does not become positive with the administration of the BCG vaccination.

However, like other tests, this test too has its own limitations. It may be false-positive, if the patient has an infection, with other types of organisms related to the group of tubercle bacilli, or due to some non-specific reaction. Similarly, the test may become false-negative when there are very low levels of circulating antibodies, due to suppression of the immune system of the body.

Hence, in view of the limitations of the test, this test should be interpreted keeping the clinical profile and other investigations in view.

Pleurisy or pleural effusion

The lungs are covered with two layers of pleura and the space between the two pleurae is called the pleural cavity/sac. Normally, there is about 10-30 ml of fluid in the pleural cavity, which remains spread in a thin layer.

Pleural effusion, as a result of tuberculosis, occurs within six months to one year after the primary/initial infection in the lungs.

It may astonish one that early pleurisy may remain completely hidden or asymptomatic. Besides tuberculous, the fluid could also be of a malignant nature, especially in elderly people, and this fact should not be overlooked for the early detection of malignancy.

The disease is so occult/hidden in early cases that even a clinical examination of the chest does not help, as only when the fluid is more than 300 ml can the physician elicit some of the physical signs. An ultrasonography is really valuable in detecting very early pleural effusion. An X-ray of the chest is also a useful test in such cases. Other tests for lung tuberculosis may also be carried out. Pleural fluid must be aspirated and examined for a precise diagnosis of tuberculosis or malignancy, so that a suitable treatment can be started without delay.

Extrapulmonary tuberculosis

The lungs are primarily involved as a result of tuberculosis. As already mentioned, other favourable sites for infection of tubercle bacilli are the brain, the kidneys, the bones, and the infection spreads to these organs through blood and / or from the lymph nodes/lesion in the lungs. Besides these organs, the genital tract, the intestine, including the peritoneum, the larynx, the various joints, say, the hip/knee joint, the pericardium, etc. may also be involved.

When the infection is acute, various organs of the body may be involved at the same time, called milliary tuberculosis, which is one of the medical emergencies.

Since the disease initially spreads by means of the lymphatics/glands, various glands of the body may also be affected. It is difficult to diagnose when the mediastinal glands, lying deep in the thorax, are involved. The glands of the neck, if involved, are easy to diagnose, since these can be palpated, and FNAC (fine needle aspiration cytology) of one of the glands can be easily carried out to confirm the diagnosis of tuberculosis.

Awareness about extrapulmonary tuberculosis is as important as that of lung tuberculosis as it is neither less common nor less dangerous than lung tuberculosis.

Tuberculous meningitis

Meninges, i.e. thin layers/membranes (3 in number, named from outside to inside, (i) the dura mater, (ii) the arachnoid mater and (iii) the pia mater) covering the brain may also be involved as a result of tuberculosis, and the disease is called tuberculous meningitis. In this case, the infection spreads from the brain to the meninges. Initially, a slow-growing tuberculous lesion called 'tuberculoma' develops in the brain, adjacent to the meninges, which ruptures in the subarachnoid space, i.e., the space between the second and third layer/meninx, causing infection of the meninges, leading to the signs and symptoms of tuberculous meningitis.

At the same time tuberculous antigen is produced by tuberculoma/s that cause marked inflammation in the subarachnoid space leading to the formation of a thick exudate which may surround the cranial nerves/blood vessels of the brain responsible for various neurological deficits as the disease advances.

It was sometimes thought that there is a true entry of the tubercle bacilli from this 'tuberculoma' into the subarachnoid space. The author discussed this aspect in detail with related case reports, with Dr. William Boyd (Canada), a renowned pathologist, who has also written *Text Book of Pathology* as well as *Pathology for the Physician*. In one of his communications to the author, while finally approving that there is indeed a rupture of tuberculoma into the subarachnoid space, he wrote, "Needless to say, I was most interested in your case of focal epilepsy followed by tuberculous meningitis. It seems to me that your idea of a tuberculoma rupturing and discharging bacilli into the subarachnoid space is the most reasonable one". In the case of the patient, discussed with Dr. Boyd, the patient developed focal epilepsy as a result of tuberculoma in the brain, and thus primarily presented the signs and symptoms of epilepsy, and later, as a case of tuberculous meningitis after the probable rupture of tuberculoma into the subarachnoid space.

An early diagnosis and treatment of tuberculous meningitis is most important in order to save the patient from various neurological deficits. It should be treated as a medical emergency. A delay in treatment could result in permanent disabilities. Initially, the patient gets vague symptoms like malaise, loss of appetite, a vague headache, irritability, and soon he gets the symptoms and signs of meningitis like a persistent headache, low grade fever, vomiting, neck rigidity/stiffness and lethargy etc. Stiffness and lethrogh of the neck is a valuable sign of this disease, and the rigidity of the neck gives the clinical clue to the diagnosis of tuberculous meningitis. Another important sign is that the patient cannot extend the leg after the thigh has been flexed, or brought close to the abdomen (called Kernig's sign). Of course, this is usually elicited by the physician/ neurologist while examining the case in detail.

It is important to recognize all the early signs and symptoms of tuberculous meningitis before the disease advances. All the relevant tests must be carried out to locate the lesion of tuberculosis in other parts of the body, especially in the lungs. An examination of the cerebrospinal fluid (CSF), including the computed tomographic (CT) scanning of the head, is also required for the diagnosis of tuberculous meningitis. PCR (polymerase chain reaction) for tuberculosis may also prove beneficial in such cases. Once diagnosed, the patient should be immediately put on suitable antituberculosis treatment in proper dosages, for a suitable period, so as to eradicate the infection of tuberculosis from the brain.

Should all cases of tuberculosis be put on antituberculosis treatment?

In view of the diagnostic limitation of the various tests of tuberculosis, especially to detect the activity of the disease, which is necessary to initiate the treatment, some of the guidelines have to be followed, and the ones recommended by the World Health Organisation are the most practical and suitable.

In all those cases, in which at least two sputum smears are positive for tubercle bacilli; or at least one sputum smear is positive, and the chest X-ray shows a classical picture of active tuberculosis; or the patient shows at least one sputum smear positive, which is also culture-positive for tubercle bacilli — antituberculosis treatment in all such category of patients is highly recommended.

Treatment of tuberculosis should also be administered where at least two sputum smears are negative for tubercle bacilli, but the chest X-ray shows clear evidence of active disease, of course, with the final approval of the physician as regards the full course of antituberculosis treatment; or when at least one of the sputum smears which has been found negative for AFB, but on culture shows positive results, i.e., culture-positive for tubercle bacilli.

As regards extrapulmonary tuberculosis, all such cases should be treated with antituberculosis drugs, where there is a strong clinical evidence of active extrapulmonary tuberculosis, but the physician takes the overall view regarding the administration of the complete regimen of antituberculosis therapy; or, at least one culture specimen from the extrapulmonary site is positive for tubercle bacilli, or if there is some histopathological evidence in favour of the disease, where again the physician forms his opinion regarding the duration of the administration of antituberculosis treatment.

What are the common drugs used for tuberculosis?

Isoniazid, rifampicin, pyrazinamide, streptomycin, ethambutol and thiacetazone are some of the common routine drugs for the treatment of tuberculosis.

Why is a long drawn out antituberculosis treatment with many drugs at one time required?

It is almost a 6-8 month regimen, and at least 3 or even 4 drugs are administered at a time. The reason for starting with a combination of drugs together is that the tubercle bacilli may be resistant to 1-2 drugs, and thus the drug therapy may fail. Usually, in the first 2 months of treatment, at least 3 drugs are given such as isoniazid, rifampicin, pyrazinamide, and in the remaining 4-6 months of treatment, isoniazid and rifampicin alone are recommended.

During the first two months of the treatment, an exhaustive therapy will lead to the killing of the tubercle bacilli, so that if the patient was sputum smear positive, he/she will become sputum smear negative and will be free from symptoms. The remaining months of therapy, when usually only two drugs are administered, will sterilize the whole respiratory tract by killing the remaining, if any, tubercle bacilli, and thereby eliminating the chances of the relapse of the disease.

How to assess the efficacy of the treatment?

In all the sputum smear positive cases, the sputum smear should be repeated after the first two months of initial treatment, followed by the same test at the end of the fourth month, and again at the end of the treatment for the 6-month regimen. This process should be repeated at the end of the fifth month as well, and at the completion of treatment for the 8-month regimen.

If the last two sputum smear examinations are negative for tubercle bacilli, the patient is said to be cured of tuberculosis. A chest X-ray is also required to be taken at the end of the treatment.

Likewise, in cases where initially the sputum culture is positive for tubercle bacilli, it should be repeated at the end of the second month, and finally at the completion of the therapy, so as to monitor the effect of the antituberculosis treatment.

Does long therapy by antituberculosis drugs cause toxicity?

Yes, and, therefore, it is always ideal if detailed blood tests like liver/kidney function tests, e.g. serum bilirubin, serum alkaline phosphatase, serum glutamic oxaloacetic transaminase (SGOT), serum glutamic pyruvic transaminase (SGPT), blood urea, serum creatinine, and also blood uric acid, total leucocyte count (TLC), differential leucocyte count (DLC), platelet count, etc., are carried out before the therapy is commenced, so that initial levels of these tests are at hand.

All the first three drugs which are usually administered, i.e. rifampicin, isoniazid and pyrazinamide are hepatotoxic (i.e., toxic to the liver), especially rifampicin. Therefore, one should keep a close watch on the occurrence of jaundice in such patients, and, if need be, liver function tests, like serum bilirubin, SGOT, SGPT, serum alkaline phosphatase may be repeated. If liver function tests are found impaired markedly, the combination already started may be modified, and usually rifampicin, which is the most hepatotoxic of all the three drugs, is replaced by another suitable antituberculosis drug like ethambutol.

Besides the above, isoniazid may cause peripheral neuropathy/neuritis, pyrazinamide may lead to arthralgia and raise levels of blood uric acid, ethambutol may cause both disturbance in vision and in colour vision—red/green colour. Likewise streptomycin may cause giddiness/vertigo and hearing disturbances. Thiacetazone may cause skin lesions like exfoliative dermatitis. All these side-effects should be carefully noted by the patient and brought to the notice of the physician/specialist so that either part or the whole combination of drugs is changed.

Ideally, all the patients before starting on the treatment for tuberculosis must be made aware of the above common toxic effects of the drugs, like jaundice or pallor of eyes, numbness/tingling/burning sensations on the lower limbs (peripheral neuropathy), pain in the joints, disturbance in vision, as well as difficulty in recognizing the red/green colour, giddiness/vertigo, including a problem in hearing. Only those side-effects, related to the drugs administered, should be explained to the patient, i.e. the side-effects of 3-4 drugs only, i.e. the combination which the physician has chosen for treatment in a specific case. The patients should be warned to immediately report to their consultants whenever they observe any of the toxic effects of the drugs, and laboratory tests, whenever required, should be carried out.

Prevention of tuberculosis

1. Improvement in socio-economic factors

Low socio-economic factors, i.e., poor/unhygienic living conditions like slums, overcrowding, lack of sunlight, poor diet, low resistance, etc. need to be looked into seriously for the basic prevention of the disease. Hence, good nutrition, better healthy conditions, including an improvement in the economy, are essentially required for the speedy control of the disease.

2. Detection of hidden/early/advanced unreported cases of tuberculosis

It is a very difficult task and needs to be tackled at the national level. In India, there is already a National Tuberculosis Programme (NTP) operating throughout the country since 1962.

Extensive awareness of the disease, including its danger of transmission in the community (including among one's own family members), should be brought to the notice of every person through various media like newspapers, pamphlets, TV, radio, etc. It can even be made a part of the school education programme. The idea of such an awareness programme is that people should report themselves to their physicians/health centres/hospitals for quick detection/treatment of the disease. Once this is achieved, a major task has been tackled.

Such awareness programmes should provide each and every detail of the disease, such as warning symptoms and signs of both early and late cases of tuberculosis, details of the investigations required, including the dire need of the uninterrupted administration of various antituberculosis drugs for the treatment of the disease, as well as vaccination of newborns against tuberculosis. Once the people are educated, they will follow the instructions in their own interest.

The other way of detecting hidden/open cases of tuberculosis would be through the NTP, which is a nationwide campaign for detecting and treating, both occult and open cases of tuberculosis, which works both at the district and rural levels. Mass miniature radiography (MMR)/X-rays, including an intensive campaign for the examination of sputum for tubercle bacilli, is required to be carried out to detect cases of tuberculosis. 'Tuberculin test surveys' may also be conducted in countries/ communities where the incidence of tuberculosis is low, before carrying out radiographical/sputum examination studies. However, in such countries, i.e. where the disease is not common, at least chest X-ray / MMR should be carried out for persons who are more prone to tuberculosis, like those who are in contact with an open case of tuberculosis, in cases of uncontrolled diabetes, and all those who daily come in contact with a large section of people like school teachers, bus drivers/conductors, etc., as already explained in detail.

It is obvious that early detection of the disease will help early isolation as well as treatment, and thus prevent the disease from spreading further.

3. Vaccination of the newborn

Vaccine against tuberculosis, known as Bacille Calmette-Guerin (BCG), discovered by two French scientists, Albert Calmette and Camille Guerin in 1922, has got its own limitations, and its efficacy is highly variable. Still the vaccine is recommended for administration to all newborns to protect them against pulmonary and extrapulmonary tuberculosis.

The newborn should not be denied this vaccination. If it is ignored, and the child is faced with a serious tuberculous infection, he may suffer from the active disease, before he develops the primary complex. However, if the infection is mild, a primary complex (page 128) will develop in a natural way, and the BCG vaccination will be of no value, as the child has already acquired natural resistance, of course under risk. As just mentioned, had this infection been a gross one, the newborn would have developed frank tuberculosis, leading even to death.

The BCG vaccination works on the principle that if a newborn is vaccinated (or already infected in a natural way), he will face the subsequent infection much better, and the tubercle bacilli on entering the lungs are likely to be killed. However, as already mentioned, the usefulness of this vaccine does not seem to be up to the mark.

In this vaccination, the strains of Mycobacterium bovis are weakened in their virulence (i.e. they become unable to produce the disease), and hence, when the BCG vaccination is administered, it will only cause an 'infection', and there will be no danger of the active disease.

Even if the BCG vaccination has been administered in a newborn who has immediately developed a mild infection/primary complex, for example when the child is born of a mother suffering from active tuberculosis, it will not cause any harm except that the local lesion/ulcer at the site of injection will be more marked. Hence the BCG vaccination is usually done in the first few days following birth, and before the child contracts the disease.

In highly developed countries like the USA, this vaccine is only restricted to newborns who are more prone to tuberculosis, for example, when the baby is born of a mother suffering from the active disease, or the child is in close contact with a highly infectious drug-resistant patient of tuberculosis. In such countries, the BCG vaccination is not administered, in general, to all newborns, on the plea that this vaccine makes the tuberculin test positive. Hence this test loses its value in identifying 'infected' cases of tuberculosis, in a specific community/population, as may be required in certain circumstances.

However, the BCG vaccination has little value in the case of adults, as reported in some studies. It has also been mentioned that the vaccination may prevent the reactivation of dormant/hidden tubercle bacilli (page 129), which may be lying in the body, but it may not prove helpful, when there is infection of tuberculosis from outside.

For vaccination of the newborn, 0.1 ml of the vaccine is administered intradermally in the uppermost part of the upper arm (deltoid). A crust is formed within 4 days approximately, which heals in about 4-6 weeks, and the child thus develops hypersensitivity.

4. *Chemoprophylaxis*

This is prescribed in certain situations to provide a constant preventive coverage of the disease. A single drug — isoniazid in dosages of 100 mg - 300 mg daily — is given for a period ranging from six weeks to about one year. Isoniazid is the recommended prophylactic drug for tuberculosis. It is a potent bactericidal drug, and is also used for the treatment of tuberculosis. The plea has been used that if this drug is used for treatment, it will at least give prophylactic cover to normal persons.

The drug is recommended in cases which need immediate preventive cover, e.g. all persons in the family or other attending persons who are in close contact with an active case of tuberculosis which has been recently diagnosed, especially when there are hardly any facilities for isolation at home. Similarly, it may be given to a child whose mother has the active disease. The drug is also indicated in all cases where the resistance has been lowered by the administration of corticoids or other immunosuppressive agents, those suffering from diabetes which is not controlled, or cases of AIDS, and even in cases of malignancies/leukaemias, especially when there is the danger of contracting the disease from a nearby patient of active tuberculosis.

However, the above prophylaxis is only a standby arrangement for special circumstances; it is, nevertheless, a perfect way of prevention. Moreover, it is unlikely to work if the person gets an infection of tubercle bacilli which are resistant to this drug. This drug is also sometimes used when a patient has an inactive tuberculous lesion in the lung, to safeguard against active tuberculosis.

5. Other measures of prevention

All patients of tuberculosis should be advised that whenever they cough, they should cover their nose and mouth with a mask/piece of cloth. All the attendants visiting the ward or the isolated room in the home must cover their nose and mouth to avoid inhalation of tubercle bacilli, which may be floating in the air in tiny droplets of sputum. The patient should always spit in specific containers containing antiseptic. A case of open tuberculosis should avoid spitting and/or coughing in front of anyone. All these factors must be strictly followed to prevent transmission of the disease.

What are the reasons for ineffective control of tuberculosis?

Under this head lies the answer to the very first question of the chapter, i.e. why tuberculosis is common in spite of the availability of highly potent drugs, and vaccination. It is true that the disease is still prevalent in both developing as well as developed countries.

At the outset, it may be said that there is still widespread ignorance about the details of the disease, including preventive measures; and very low socio-economic conditions always remain a constant basic threat, contributing to the spread of the disease.

The warning signal that if a person has a cough for more than 14 days, with fever, loss of appetite and weight, he must report to his physician for check-up and tests, for the inclusion/exclusion of tuberculosis, is hardly followed, and, even the symptoms are not known to all. The longer the disease remains undiagnosed, the more difficult it becomes to eradicate the infection. Even when it remains asymptomatic for sometime in many of the cases, when it presents itself, there may occur only vague symptoms of the disease. In such cases, either the above mentioned symptoms are missing or are not clearly recognized by the patient. All this further delays the treatment, and, therefore, the public is required to be highly vigilant and should have up-to-date and elaborate knowledge of early symptoms (page 134, para 1).

When the patient is late, and on top of it, he has taken some haphazard antituberculosis treatment, it will create a good deal of problem for the physician, to prescribe drugs, as the tubercle bacilli may have already developed resistance to some of the routine drugs for tuberculosis. Much difficulty arises, as is seen often, in most of the cases, because the patients do not know even the names of the drugs they have taken, and their prescription is often missing.

It must be known by all that drug resistance to tubercle bacilli is the major cause of failure to control the disease in any country. Once some routine antituberculosis drugs are not effective in killing tubercle bacilli, a great hope, for eradicating the disease, in a particular patient, is lost, because the second line of antituberculosis drugs is fairly costly, and one is never sure of their sensitivity to the tubercle bacilli in the concerned patient, and above all, they may not be easily available. Further, all patients are unlikely to benefit from them, and as such, the situation almost reaches a stalemate under these circumstances.

Tubercle bacilli rapidly undergo mutation or change their strains, which become resistant to the drugs administered. Since laboratory facilities for testing the sensitivity of various drugs are available only at a very few selected places, great caution is required in the treatment of tuberculosis to avoid drug resistance.

It, indeed, becomes a major issue in the control of tuberculosis, when the tubercle bacilli become resistant to various antituberculosis drugs, in a good number of cases, because such patients go on transmitting these multi-drug resistant tubercle bacilli to a large number of the population, making them all patients of multi-drug resistant tuberculosis, and these patients, even if they report themselves, are difficult to treat with routine drugs. These so-called multi-drug resistant tuberculosis (MDRT) patients go on spreading the disease like wildfire, which may be responsible for heavy casualties.

Such cases of MDRT become potential dangers to society / country, as their treatment, even if it is carried out, is not an easy one. It is one of the important tasks of NTP to pinpoint such cases, and all efforts should be made to treat them in hospitals. On discharge they must be educated to live in isolation at home and take preventive steps like wearing masks and avoiding crowded places, so that they do not transmit the resistant tubercle bacilli to other persons till they have been declared completely fit.

Close contact with family members, especially children, who may have a low resistance, must be avoided in the case of such patients. As more members of a family may contract this resistant form of the disease, it will not only add to the financial burden, but may also cause death/s in the family, if immediate steps for treatment are not taken. Undoubtedly, the threat of this type of resistant tuberculosis still needs a concrete solution, since fast-spreading cases of MDRT are a major obstacle for the control of tuberculosis, since these cases are neither easy to detect nor treat. When detected, they become a hard task for the specialist. It should be pointed out that unless this group of cases is dealt with satisfactorily, the entire programme of control of tuberculosis can never be successful.

Needless to say that the whole situation mentioned above is entirely due to human error on the part of patients of tuberculosis. If they report in time and take a full course of routine antituberculosis drugs, the problem will be largely solved.

But patients, even if they reach in time, may take the treatment during the first two months of therapy, when more than 2-3 drugs are given, but as during this initial period of treatment, they become free of symptoms, they hardly bother to follow the further course of four to six months, and thus a relapse occurs, and the patient goes on transmitting the disease to others. The patient, most likely, stops further treatment due to sheer ignorance, neglect or apathy. In any case such cases are a great challenge in the control of tuberculosis as it exists today. Multiple drug resistant tuberculosis societies are being formed to look after MDRT cases. Such societies are required to provide even financial help. Ideally there should be a government policy or budget provision for MDRT cases.

Although advances have been made to shorten the duration of treatment, and now only a six or eight-month regimen of treatment for tuberculosis is required, as against the previous two years, the present duration is still pretty high. It is hoped that with more advancement, the duration of treatment will be further minimized, and this will certainly help in dealing with this disease more effectively.

If the patient takes treatment for the entire length of the period in proper dosages, we can go much further in the control of tuberculosis, as inadequate treatment is one of the principal causes of failure of the treatment, which leads to drug resistance, throwing the whole task out of gear.

Also, in routine antituberculosis treatment, great vigilance is required in following up the case. The patient may become sputum smear positive after an initial sputum smear negative report, which shows that the combination of drugs prescribed has failed, and drug resistance has developed. Provided the patient, adhering strictly to the instructions of the physician, cares to visit the hospital/specialist regularly for getting the sputum specimen examined for tubercle bacilli, the whole combination or a part of it can be changed with another set of routine drugs, and the disease can still be controlled. But nothing can be done if the patient does not co-operate in the follow-up treatment, and apart from tests, even drugs, as stated above, are not being taken as per recommendations.

There is another side of the picture too. That is, many a time the patient loses heart and discontinues the treatment when he notices that he is not responding and his symptoms are not clearing up. He often leaves the hospital against medical advice or changes the physician, and sometimes a person from the lower rungs of society may even leave the community due to the stigma still attached to tuberculosis in some places. In such cases, the sputum smear remains positive in spite of giving 3-4 drugs in the right combination and dosages continuously for an initial period of two months. Although it shows that drug resistance has developed to the combination of drugs started, one can always start with an entirely new set of routine drugs, and follow up the case further.

Good counselling always prevails in such cases, and the patient must get proper treatment, both in his own and in the interest of his family, and above all of his community. If he leaves, as is sometimes seen, it may be due to financial reasons, as second set of drugs may not be affordable by the patient, or due to his illness, he may not be able to stay back from his work for so long. Whatever may be the reason, he will become a potential threat to society, transmitting most resistant tubercle bacilli both at home and outside, including his work area.

One of the strategies to combat this situation is that a regular watch must be kept, especially on such patients, by health workers/supervisors, particularly while the patients are taking their daily dosage/s of antituberculosis drugs. It is equally important to monitor the progress of these patients. This point has been duly emphasized by the WHO. All other aspects of the patients, including the financial ones, should also be looked into.

As regards the BCG vaccination for the control of tuberculosis, as mentioned earlier, its role in protection against tuberculosis is of a restrictive nature. Hence, it does not help in the overall control of tuberculosis.

In the end, it may be said that it is only with constant education/guidance/caution to the public/patients at each step, relating to the vital information/preventive measures indicated in this chapter, together with the availability of trained medical and paramedical staff, in a well-equipped (especially peripheral) rural health centre, with special facilities for Mantoux/tuberculin skin test, sputum examination for tubercle bacilli, MMR/X-ray, and the availability of a liberal, comprehensive range of antituberculosis drugs, that we can hope to uproot this disease, which is a great threat to humanity even today. Above all, an alternative to the BCG vaccination would be the real key to the prevention of the disease.

9
ALLERGY AND BRONCHIAL ASTHMA

Asthma is said to be more loyal than a wife. She may divorce you, but asthma usually does not. Such is the lingering characteristic of the disease.

Allergy and bronchial asthma are closely related. In an attack of asthma, as a result of allergy, there occurs an inflammation of the airways. Thus a swelling/narrowing of the airways manifests itself as a result of this inflammation.

Warning signals of asthma

The three notable early warning signs/symptoms are: cough, tightness in the chest / breathlessness and wheezing (whistling sound caused by difficult breathing through narrowed airways as a result of their inflammation / swelling). But these early warning signals are usually ignored by the patient. Since an early attack of asthma may pass off rapidly, and the patient feels normal in between the attacks, the physician is usually not consulted until the disease is at an advanced stage, when the patient feels marked breathlessness frequently. When the attack persists for hours, it is called status asthmaticus, which is a dangerous stage, and may prove fatal for want of emergency medical aid.

We cannot blame the patient either, because in early cases, after a little discomfort, i.e. cough and tightness in the chest for a while, the patient seems to get well even without medication and he/she hardly feels the need for consultation or treatment. This mild discomfort may not occur for several days/months. In children, these symptoms may appear only after exercise, and the disease is not suspected by the parents, because following some rest, the child usually becomes free of the symptoms.

Hence, the disease is highly unpredictable. However, those who have a family history of asthma, those who are heavy smokers, and those working in dusty places or in flour/saw-mills, bakeries, wheat/plastic/paint/cotton/glue industries, etc., must be alert, and keep in mind the early warning symptoms of asthma, for immediate medical attention. In some cases, there may be only a seasonal allergy, i.e. the patient gets attacks of asthma during a particular season only, as for instance, during the months of harvesting, threshing, etc.

Diagnosis of asthma/allergy

Once the disease is suspected and the patient reports in time, there is no difficulty in establishing a diagnosis of asthma. But another difficulty can arise. It is invariably seen that the underlying root-cause (allergen) responsible for the recurrent allergy of the airways, causing an inflammatory response in the airways, cannot be easily detected. Various skin tests for the detection of allergy have proved to be of limited value. Therefore, one has to be on drugs which give only temporary relief, and the patient is often dependent on drugs for his or her entire life. Such cases are usually perennial, i.e., they get attacks of asthma throughout the year. As soon as the drug is stopped, the patient gets an attack of asthma. This is agonizing for any person, irrespective of age.

A good deal of research work is being carried out all over the world to overcome this chronic disease of the respiratory tract, so as to give a permanent relief/cure to sufferers.

How allergy causes an attack of asthma?

The air passages of a person may become allergic/hypersensitive to any substance/s, and thus, whenever such a person gets exposed to the same substance/s, an attack of asthma will be precipitated. In other words, the patient acts like a loaded pistol, and the trigger of the pistol immediately gets pressed as soon as the patient comes in contact with the same allergic factor (Fig. 17). In chronic cases, the air passages undergo various pathological changes making the condition of the patient more and more miserable as time passes. There may be oedematous changes in airways and infiltration of various inflammatory cells like eosinophils, neutrophils and lymphocytes. Hypertrophy of mucous glands and damage of inner lining (epithelium) of airways may also occur.

Various allergic factors

1. Extrinsic factors

Besides some of the factors causing allergy/asthma in a patient mentioned earlier, other allergic factors are: (i) **house dust** (present in bedrooms, mattresses, pillows, rugs, curtains, woollen clothes, blankets, carpets, upholstered furniture, etc.), (ii) **moulds** (which grow in humid places, like where there is a leakage of water in walls, roofs, filters of desert-coolers or air-conditioners and places of poor ventilation like cowsheds, barns, etc.), (iii) **pollens** (from flowers, trees, grasses, weeds, etc.), (iv) **dandruff** from the skins of animals (i.e., scales from the outer parts of the skins of animals, like dogs, cats, cows, buffaloes, goats, sheep, horses, etc.), (v) **insect debris in the environment** (houseflies, mosquitoes, cockroaches, ants, butterflies, etc.), (vi) **feathers of birds** (pigeons, feather pillows), (vii) **various contactants** (like lipsticks, powders, soaps, perfumes, hair-dyes, shampoos, oils, creams, after-shave lotions, etc.), (viii) **air pollutants** (from ill-maintained engines of automobiles, like cars, two-wheelers, trucks, etc.)

Food allergy

Food allergy is also an important causative factor in many cases of asthma. Any food, like wheat, cereals, ice-cream, vegetables, non-vegetarian food, edible oils, fruits, milk, curd, ghee, eggs, coffee, cold drinks, etc. can cause allergy. Various condiments/spices used in the preparation of food may be the source of the allergy. Likewise, various preservatives used to preserve food articles may cause asthma. Colouring agents used in sweets, etc. too may prove harmful. Fermented food, like pickles, jams, beer, wines are other causes of food allergy. Even the metabolic by-products of ingested food may cause allergy. It is also seen that sometimes the patient is allergic to the outer covering of wheat, cereals, vegetables, etc. Hence a patient may be allergic to wheat, but not to *maida*, and similarly, one may be allergic to whole cereals, but not to the ones without outer shells, i.e. *dhuli dal*.

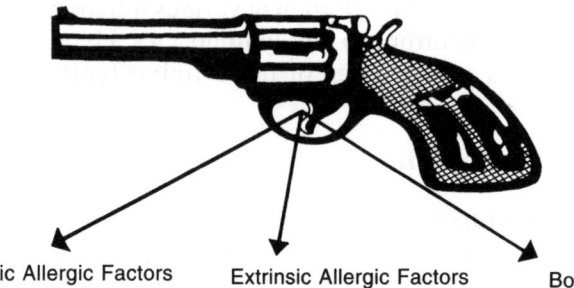

Intrinsic Allergic Factors — Extrinsic Allergic Factors — Both

INTRINSIC ALLERGIC FACTORS

— **GENETIC FACTORS**
  - Family History of Asthma

EXTRINSIC ALLERGIC FACTORS

— **FOODS,** like wheat, cereals, vegetables, non-vegetarian foods, edible oils, fruits, milk, curd, eggs, coffee, cold drinks, including condiments/spices, preservatives, colouring agents, fermented foods like pickles, jams, beer, wines; also the outer covering of wheat and cereals (i.e., allergy to whole wheat and not to *maida*, which is without the outer covering; allergy to whole cereals but not to *dhuli dal*, i.e., *dal* without the outer covering); fungus growing on sprouted food or on stale bread/cooked food, and even metabolic by-products developing during the process of digestion of food, may cause allergy.

— **PSYCHOGENIC FACTORS**
  - Emotional stress
  - Mental conflict
  - Depression

— **DUST,** like house dust, the occupational dust of flour/saw-mills, bakeries, wheat/plastic/paint/cotton/glue industries, etc.

— **SMOKE / INDUSTRIAL FUMES**

Allergy and Bronchial Asthma 155

— INFECTION ANY-
WHERE IN THE
BODY

— COLD/COLD AIR
AND STRENUOUS
EXERCISES

— HORMONAL
CHANGES IN THE
BODY
- Pregnancy
- Menstruation
- Thyrotoxicosis

— **MOULDS** (which grow in humid places like where there is a leakage of water in walls, roofs, filters of desert-coolers/ air-conditioners and places of poor ventilation like cowsheds, barns, etc.)

— **POLLENS** (from flowers, trees, grasses, weeds, etc.)

— **DANDRUFF FROM THE SKIN OF ANIMALS**, i.e., scales from the outer parts of the skin of animals, like dogs, cats, cows, buffaloes, goats, sheep, horses, etc.

— **INSECT DEBRIS IN THE ENVIRONMENT** (of house-flies, mosquitoes, cockroaches, ants, butterflies, etc.)

— **FEATHERS OF BIRDS** (pigeons, feather pillows, etc.)

— **VARIOUS CONTACTANTS** (lipsticks, powders, soaps, perfumes, hair-dyes, shampoos, oils, creams, after-shave lotions, etc.)

— **AIR POLLUTANTS** (from ill-maintained engines of automobiles, like cars, two-wheelers, trucks, etc.)

Fig. 17. 'A Loaded Pistol' acting like a patient of asthma. The trigger of the pistol is pressed automatically whenever the patient (pistol) comes in contact with any of the allergic factors (bad elements/ enemies in the case of the pistol) to which he/she is allergic/ sensitive, and an attack of asthma (bullet) is released/ precipitated.

(This figure was explained to viewers by the author in a TV talk on asthma in Canada)

Further, sprouted food like beans or any other cereals may cause allergy as a result of fungus in the food. Likewise, stale bread/cooked food may cause allergy when spoiled, as a result of fungus.

Therefore, it may be said that the various types of foods or related materials may cause allergy, and thus, sometimes it is almost impossible to identify the factor in the food causing the allergy/asthma.

2. Intrinsic allergic factors

Some of the factors present inside the body called intrinsic factors may be the precipitating factors causing such an allergy. The most important factors are psychogenic, such as emotional stress, mental conflict, depression. Children may suffer emotionally because of the parents having marital problems. Even parents who frequently scold their children may cause them emotional trauma.

Infection anywhere in the body contributes to the factors causing allergy in a patient. Even cold/cold air or strenuous exercises, like running, swimming, jogging, etc. may cause allergy.

As already mentioned, a family history of asthma is an important intrinsic factor. Hormonal changes in the body during pregnancy, menstruation, or in the case of diseases like thyrotoxicosis, may be responsible for an allergy.

Hence, an allergy in case of asthma is a very complex problem, and the patient may be suffering from more than one or multiple types of allergies at a time. Hence the difficulty in diagnosis and permanent cure.

3. Genetic factors in asthma

Asthma is known to run in families, and if one parent suffers from it, there is about 55% chances of the children developing asthma, and if both the parents have it, the chances increase to 70%.

Complications of asthma

Sometimes the patient continues to get mild to moderate degrees of asthma attacks, but does not take medicine, or takes inadequate/irregular treatment, with the result that he/she lands himself or herself in such a serious condition as a right-sided heart failure. It may be mentioned that this heart failure is the result of this disease of the lungs, and is different from coronary artery disease. Other complications of bronchial asthma may be emphysema, pulmonary infection, and even bronchiectasis and collapse of the lung (atelectasis).

What tests are required in a case of asthma?

A clinical examination of the chest, especially during an attack of asthma, is highly valuable for diagnosing asthma. Measurement of peak expiratory flow rate (PEFR) (see later) also helps in the diagnosis of asthma. However, an X-ray of the chest, and also various pulmonary function tests (besides PEFR), bronchoscopy, etc. may be required to see the extent of damage caused by asthma in a particular patient. Besides, other tests like sputum for tubercle bacilli/malignant cells, etc. may also be required in suspected cases for diagnosing any underlying pathology of the lung. Various skin tests for the detection of allergy are also carried out.

Asthma in the elderly

If an attack of asthma occurs in an elderly person, the involvement of the heart should be especially ruled out as the asthmatic attack may be the result of left ventricle failure in advanced age. In some old people, both lung and heart problems may be operating at the same time, requiring urgent steps to save the lives of such patients. Tests like electrocardiogram (ECG), chest X-ray, creatinine phosphokinase - CPK (MB), Troponin T/Troponin I are particularly useful to rule out heart involvement. More tests may be required at a later stage.

Prophylaxis of asthma

Ideally, if the allergen or irritant causing asthma is detected, the patient can take necessary steps to avoid such an allergen, so that his/her disease is completely treated and cured. This is the most successful method of treating this disorder.

But the difficulty is that the patient may suffer from the allergy of more than two or three types of allergens at the same time. In which case it becomes difficult to detect the causative allergen/s. It may be said that the 'detection of allergy is just like the detection of crime', and it is not possible to detect the causative allergic factor/s in many of the cases.

Under the above circumstances, the only way is to adopt some sort of general prophylaxis so that the patient may be relieved of asthma attacks, and so that the dosage of the drug is also reduced, and the patient feels comfortable.

Various general prophylactic measures

1. Extrinsic factors

One should try to avoid all the suggested factors/allergens which may be responsible for the attack/s of asthma, e.g.

(a) Dust should be avoided. Use a vacuum cleaner. Avoid upholstered furniture and use wooden/plastic furniture. Encase mattresses in zippered airtight covers, or use dust-proof clothes, if available. Cotton covers should be used for blankets and quilts.

Other measures to safeguard patients from dust, can be face masks (3-layered), room air-cleaners (if available), electrostatic precipitators (they attract harmful positively-charged particles present in the dust). Nasal filters are of limited value.

(b) One should avoid humid places, to protect oneself from moulds, i.e. fungal spores.

(c) Avoid pollens of flowers, trees, grasses, etc. Since these pollens attack in a greater degree when the temperature is low, i.e., early morning or late evening. Patients allergic to such pollens are advised to remain indoors.

(d) Avoid animals (like the ones already mentioned), so as to avoid the allergy of dandruff from their skins.

(e) One should live in clean places, and should ensure that there are no insects, i.e. houseflies, mosquitoes, cockroaches, etc., so as to avoid the allergy of insect debris in the environment. The places inhabited by insects should be regularly cleaned.

(f) Various contactants, already mentioned, should be avoided.

(g) One should avoid smoking including passive smoking, i.e., one should not be in the company of a smoker so as to avoid the inhalation of smoke from the smoker.

(h) One should refrain from food to which one is allergic. As a general rule, one should avoid overeating, fried, fatty, spicy food, and should take early meals both times of the day. Plenty of water should be drunk as it hydrates the respiratory passages and helps loosen sputum.

(i) An indiscriminate use of drugs is prohibited, as drugs often trigger off an attack/s of asthma. Beta-blockers used in the treatment of hypertension should not be taken by asthmatics as these drugs narrow the airways, leading to severe attacks in an asthmatic patient. In severe cases of asthma, tranquilizers including sedatives should not be prescribed under any circumstances to alleviate the anxiety of the patient as they may worsen the lung function leading to even respiratory arrest in some cases. Expectorants and/or mucolytic agents are not of much use both in acute and chronic cases of asthma.

(j) One should keep oneself away from the air pollutants of automobiles. The owners of the vehicles should be strictly warned to check that the engines of their vehicles do not emit air-pollutants. An anti-pollution drive in this behalf is urgently required.

2. Prophylaxis: Intrinsic factors

Besides the above, the prophylaxis of intrinsic factors is equally important. Psychogenic factors, like recurrent emotional episodes, mental conflict, proper treatment of depression must be looked into; and stress and strain should be avoided as far as possible. In the case of children, counselling their parents as well as the children will have a beneficial effect in the treatment of asthma. If there is persistent infection, it should be properly treated. One should protect against catching a cold, avoid over-exertion and strenuous exercises and keep away from cold air blasts.

3. Prophylaxis: genetic factors

When the mother is suffering from asthma, all precautions should be taken during pregnancy to prevent asthma in the newborn. Conception should be avoided during the particular season if the mother/father is suffering from seasonal allergy. The mother should keep herself away from passive smoking, and the home should be kept free from dust, insects and mites. She should not take the particular food to which she is allergic; and she should refrain from such food items both during pregnancy and breast-feeding. All pets should be removed, especially before the child is born.

The infant should be given only breast-feeding up to three months, and no solid food up to six months. Eggs should also be avoided. Such a child should not be sent to creches, so as to avoid infection and environmental allergy.

Drug treatment

Drugs should be used in the form of mists or aerosols, with the help of inhalers, so that the drug goes from the mouth to the various air passages immediately for quick action on the inflamed walls. With this therapy, a limited dosage is required, and the side-effects of the drugs are also the minimum possible. Spacehalers are also available, which are more effective as compared to inhalers (Fig. 18). In nebulizers, the drug in the form of mist is given to the patient, which can be easily breathed in. Dry powder inhalers are equally effective.

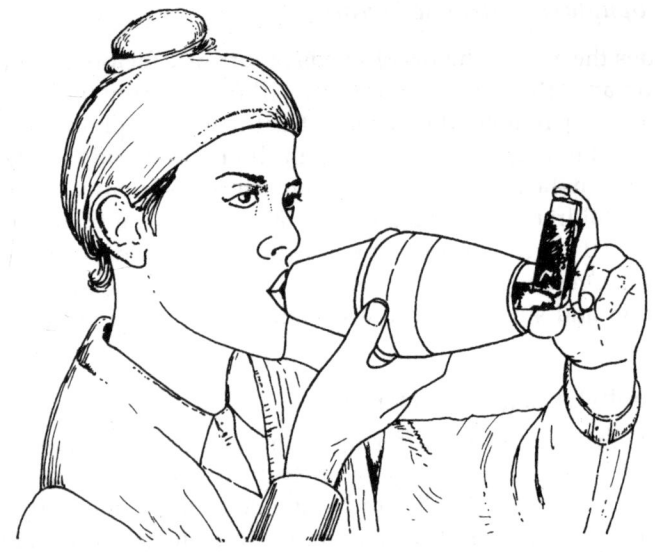

Fig. 18. A patient of asthma using a spacehaler.

It needs to be emphasized that inhaled steroids are recommended at the international level for the control of the inflammation of the airways. They are anti-inflammatory in nature, and inflammation is the basic lesion in airways in all such cases. They should be regularly used in dosages prescribed by the physician, and they have the least side effects in recommended dosages, unlike oral steroids. These can be used for a long period, so as to keep the patient comfortable. The current approach to asthma care aims at daily anti-inflammatory therapy with inhaled corticosteroids, and their dosages depend upon the severity of asthma. Needless to say that early diagnosed asthma improves faster with inhaled steroids than late cases where irreversible chronic inflammation of the airways has developed.

Bronchodilator inhalers, i.e. the drugs used in the form of aerosols, which dilate the airways, may also be used whenever required, in addition to inhaled steroids. The combination of an inhaled steroid and a bronchodilator may prove effective and add to the convenience of the patient.

Patients who are already on oral drugs should reduce their dosages and start aerosol therapy with inhalers. Later they may be able to completely stop the oral drugs. However, administration of drugs through injections, etc., will be required in severe cases of asthma, especially in status asthmaticus, when the patient gets several attacks of asthma at a time, so as to save the life of the patient. Massage on the back with any oil is also beneficial during an asthma attack.

Breathing exercises in asthma

An asthmatic is advised to do breathing exercises, like blowing into an air-pillow or the bladder of a football each day for about 10 minutes. In some countries, modernized devices are available for breathing exercises.

Peak flow meter (PFM)

It is a small instrument used to measure the peak expiratory flow rate (PEFR) in a patient of asthma. It is important to measure PEFR so as to follow up the disease and the patient's response to therapy. It is the simplest and most widely used pulmonary function test. The use of PFM in the management of asthmatics plays a role similar to the use of blood pressure apparatus in the control of a patient's blood pressure, or the use of a blood glucose meter for the assessment of blood sugar levels in the treatment of diabetes. Ideally, peak flow charts should be used so that the morning and evening reading may be plotted to see the effect of the drug. A decrease in the reading points out an impending attack of asthma, and calls for urgent precautionary measures. Since PFM readings may vary from instrument to instrument, patients are advised to purchase their own meter for regular monitoring (Fig. 19).

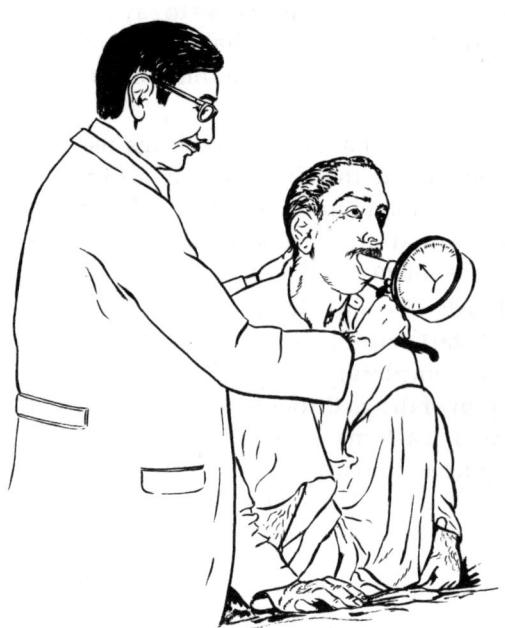

Fig. 19. The physician taking the peak expiratory flow rate (PEFR), with a peak flow meter (PFM) of an asthma patient.

Role of immunotherapy

Immunotherapy has a variable response in the treatment of asthma. Sometimes this therapy lessens the effect of the allergy, and so a reduced dose of the drug is required. In such cases, the patient will require a maintenance dose of immunotherapy, as well as the drug. However, a complete and lasting cure does not seem possible. Some people may be relieved of their problem for life, while others may again get attacks of asthma, though in reduced severity. Hence the role of immunotherapy is limited.

Outgrowing asthma

About 50% of children may outgrow asthma in their adulthood. However, it is not possible to predict whether an asthmatic child will outgrow asthma or not. Even adult asthma may improve or disappear with age. Irrespective of the onset of asthma, it is likely to disappear in old age.

Treatment of refractory asthma

Refractory asthma means that the patient does not respond to the varied drug therapy administered. In such cases, one has to look for the following:

- (i) Is the patient taking the drug?
- (ii) Is there psychological stress?
- (iii) Is there some underlying infection/pathology?
- (iv) Are there unidentified multiple allergens?
- (v) Is he suffering from sinusitis?
- (vi) Is there an inadequate drug response?
- (vii) Are there accompanying aggravating factors?
- (viii) Is the patient on drugs like ACE inhibitors, which are known to produce cough, and may worsen the condition of the airways?

All the above factors must be borne in mind while treating cases of asthma, so as to avoid unnecessary medication.

Epidemiological survey for detecting occult/hidden cases of asthma

It is imperative to detect early cases of asthma for immediate treatment. Therefore, an epidemiological survey would be of vital value in detecting hidden cases of asthma. Ideally, there should be a national screening programme for diagnosing occult cases of bronchial asthma, so as to save the patient from the morbidity/mortality of this disease. Besides, mass understanding regarding the details of this disease, including preventive measures, is urgently required.

10
DISEASES OF THE ABDOMEN AND ULTRASONOGRAPHY

Some diseases of the abdomen may also remain undetected for a long time. This is particularly true of gallbladder diseases — gallstones (cholelithiasis), inflammation of the gallbladder (cholecystitis), or even cancer of the gallbladder. As mentioned in the chapter 'Cancers and Their Prevention', (page 4, sr. 6), either gallstones or an inflamed gallbladder may lead to cancer of the gallbladder. Therefore, it is necessary to detect early cases of gallstones and inflamed gallbladder, so that once diagnosed, it can be removed surgically, and cancer of the gallbladder can be prevented.

It is a common finding that diseases of the gallbladder remain silent in the abdomen. Hence, all cases in whom the slightest clinical suspicion of gallbladder pathology exists must be subjected to ultrasonography, so that the disease can be detected at the earliest.

Ultrasonography has a significant role to play in the detection of subclinical diseases of the abdomen. This test is of vital value and has no radiation hazards. Before the availability of this test, it was at times impossible to detect diseases of the abdomen, and the last resort was to surgically open up the abdomen (laparotomy), so that the surgeon could see the suspected part and diagnose and treat the case. Sometimes, the diagnosis turned out to be quite different from what the surgeon thought it to be before he opened up the abdomen. Some doctors, therefore, used to call the abdomen a magic box. Thanks to ultrasonography, there is no such difficulty now.

An ultrasonographic examination, however, must be carried out by an experienced ultrasonologist, as this test is 'operator-dependent', i.e., the operator/ultrasonologist, before giving his/ her opinion, has to examine a particular organ from different angles, regarding the pathology of the concerned organ. A single casual view of an organ taken/recorded on an ultrasound film may not serve the purpose, and may even prove to be misleading altogether.

It is advisable that all persons, especially above the age of 40, undergo an ultrasonographic examination of the abdomen, so that various hidden diseases can be detected in time. The test must be carried out in all symptomless persons, irrespective of age. It should not be ignored or delayed if the patient has some symptoms relating to any of the organs of the abdomen. It is indeed an important test for detecting diseases of the abdomen. The author participated in an 'Ultrasound Update', so as to have an inside view of this vital investigation.

Besides gallbladder diseases, some liver disorders may also remain undiagnosed for long, especially cirrhosis of the liver, which may remain undetected, particularly in a chronic alcoholic. If this liver disease is not diagnosed in time, its treatment may not be possible. Similarly, early viral/serum hepatitis may remain undetected, since early jaundice/pallor of the eyes may not be noticed by the patient. If timely action is not taken, the patient is likely to be miserable at a young age. Besides an ultrasonographic examination of the liver, blood tests like serum bilirubin, serum glutamic oxaloacetic transaminase (SGOT), serum glutamic pyruvic transaminase (SGPT), alkaline phosphatase, etc. are also useful in the diagnosis of various liver disorders.

Cancer of the liver, especially when it occurs as a result of primary cancer at some other place, may remain hidden and, therefore, an ultrasonographic examination of the liver is important for its detection. It has also been observed that in many cases of prolonged low-grade fever, the lesion/pathology is seen in the liver. As such, in all these cases of fever, so-called pyrexia of uncertain origin (PUO), i.e. when the cause of fever is not easily detectable, an ultrasonographic examination/computed tomographic (CT) scanning of the abdomen is a must. Alpha-fetoprotein that is a marker for cancer of the liver (hepatocellular carcinoma) is one of the diagnostic tests.

As a special reference, it must be pointed out that the vaccination for hepatitis-B is highly recommended for the prevention of this serious liver disorder. In view of the increasing incidence of this disorder, the WHO has recommended the introduction of this vaccine to cover the entire population. It may be mentioned that a case of hepatitis may lead to liver failure which may not be controlled by usual conventional treatment. Although in such terminal cases, liver dialysis and transplant are required, we still have to wait for such facilities. Tests like serum viral markers for hepatitis A, B, C, D and E may be required to identify the virus inflicting the liver, and to plan the treatment accordingly. Hepatitis A and E are caused by faecal-oral route and hepatitis B, C, and D are caused by percutaneous route. History of unsafe sex is essentially important in cases of hepatitis B, and also in cases of hepatitis D. Information regarding the use of drugs by unsterilized injections/ needles as in the case of addicts is important both in cases of hepatitis B and C. Mother to infant transmission may occur in cases of again hepatitis B and C. History of blood transfusion in the past should also be elicited in cases of viral hepatitis.

After identifying the disorder, treatment of hepatitis should be carried our energetically under the guidance of a specialist. The patients who are carriers i.e. say their HBsAg (hepatitis B surface antigen) serum test is positive but are asymtomatic need to be treated till the disease is totally eradicated.

In the case of HBsAg carriers prescribe antiviral drug like lamivudine 100 mg once daily. It should be continued till Hepatitis B e antigen (HBeAg) that is a marker of viral replication both in acute and chronic infection is negative. This test may be repeated 4-6 monthly and if it becomes positive again, the above drug may be started again. In case the test for antibody to hepatitis B surface antigen (Anti-HBs) that is a marker of recovery and immunity is negative, it indicates that the patient has fully recovered from HBsAg infection and has developed immunity as well.

As regards the role of ultrasonography in other diseases, it has a significant role in detecting the presence of cancer of the kidney, the urinary bladder, including cancer of the prostate and the testis in males, and of the uterus (the most important being the cervix) in females, etc. The warning signals of cancer have already been described in the chapter on cancer (pages 4, 5 and 6).

It is remarkable that ultrasonography helps in discovering very early pleurisy.

Tests like upper gastrointestinal endoscopy, also called oesophagogastro-duodenoscopy (OGD), colonoscopy and sigmoidoscoy are useful in diagnosing early lesions of the gastrointestinal tract. Again, trained medical personnel are required for carrying out endoscopy, colonoscopy and sigmoidoscopy. As in the case of ultrasonography, these tests too are entirely dependent on the skill of the operator. The suspected area/s of the gastrointestinal tract are visualized by the operator with the help of endoscope, colonoscope or sigmoidoscope, and he finally forms his opinion regarding the exact pathology inflicting the specific site. It may be cautioned that an inaccurate diagnosis may have serious consequences, and hence the vital need for a specialist approach. These apparatuses are like a tube with a camera at one end which is used for getting an inside picture of the lesion without resorting to surgery. EGD is done by passing a flexible endoscope through the mouth, into the esophagus, stomach and second part of the deuodenum after local pharyngeal anesthesia. Colonoscope, again a flexible tube, is passed through the anus into the rectum, colon up to the caecum. The procedure of flexible sigmoidoscope is similar to flexible colonoscope but one can visualize only the rectum and some parts of the left colon. For the detection of the lesions of small intestine, small-bowel enteroscopy may be carried out. Endoscope ultrasound (EUS) is also helpful in detecting various lesions of the gastrointestinal tract. Besides the above tests, CT scanning, etc. also helps in diagnosing various lesions of the gastrointestinal tract. (Warning signals relating to cancer/s of the gastrointestinal tract have been mentioned on page 3 and 4).

Some of the common surgical problems of the abdomen also require prompt attention/surgery to avoid fatal complications.

Appendicitis is one of the common surgical emergencies. If immediate steps for its treatment, either medical and/or surgical, are not taken, the inflamed appendix may burst inside the abdomen causing a very serious/fatal complication of the disease, i.e. peritonitis (acute infection inside the whole abdomen), which may lead to generalized septicaemia and death. Hence, whenever an attack of appendicitis occurs one should immediately consult one's physician/surgeon so that the disease is controlled with medicine and the appendix is surgically removed (appendicectomy).

Once an attack of appendicitis occurs, even if the disease/attack has been controlled with medicine, it has to be removed surgically, as a recurrence of the attack is possible at any time/place, later in life, which may prove fatal. Hence, a diseased/infected appendix is like a bomb lodged in the body, which may explode any time, even causing the death of the patient.

Another such problem is hernia (commonly inguinal), which, in fact, is a minor surgical problem of the abdomen. If the operation is delayed for too long, it may get obstructed, causing gangrene/perforation of the intestine, which may prove fatal, if an emergency operation is not performed. Hence all cases of hernia should be operated on well in time.

In the end, it should be emphasized that a careful watch must be kept on the possible occurrence of the various serious diseases of the abdomen, for their timely prevention.

11
DISEASES OF THE KIDNEYS

Prevention, especially of a few diseases of the kidneys, is essential so that the end result of these diseases, which is renal (kidney) failure, can be avoided. Everyday, we hear about cases of renal failures/renal transplants.

Some of the important diseases of the kidneys, which ultimately cause renal failure, remain hidden for a long time, and many a time, kidney failure comes to the notice of the patient suddenly, and by then it is usually very late. Much expense is involved, as in such cases, repeated or regular dialysis of the kidneys is required, and ultimately a transplant of the kidney may be the only solution to save the life of the patient. This may not be within everyone's financial capacity and moreover, the kidney is required either from a relation or a donor, and even then, the transplanted kidney may not always prove successful, as such operations entail very high risks.

The author is reminded of an Indian patient who was operated for kidney transplant through his effort and an agency in London sometime back, where the author had gone to present a paper at a conference. The operation was carried out by a renowned surgeon, who had also earlier done a successful transplant of a kidney in another Indian patient. But unfortunately, this operation did not prove successful, and the patient died abroad. Hence the need for caution at every step.

Diseases of the kidneys sometimes are so silent that even routine kidney tests do not help. By the time the blood urea, serum creatinine, which are the routine tests prescribed by the physician, rise significantly, the kidneys may have already been damaged.

It is, therefore, desirable that we know about such diseases of the kidneys in detail, and follow the various preventive measures.

Apparently this aspect of kidney disease is not fully realized, and a general lack of awareness in this regard can prove fatal. This may be so because diseases of the heart and cancer, etc. attract immediate and anxious attention. Needless to say, that diseases of the kidneys are equally important, and with this in view, the author has tried to present a comprehensive picture of the problem. Some of the most common serious diseases of the kidneys are given below.

1. Chronic/recurrent urinary tract infection (UTI)

UTI is a common disease of the kidneys. Its recurrence is very common, especially in females. A chronic infection of the kidneys may slowly damage them, resulting in kidney failure. However, a sudden acute infection of the kidneys may also cause a failure. Hence the kidneys have to be protected against any possible infection. It is, therefore, essential to know the details of the disease, including the preventive measures, which are simple to follow.

How the urinary tract gets infected

The urinary tract (which consists of the kidneys, the ureters, the urinary bladder and the urethra) is free from any infection/organism/bacteria (Fig. 20).

On the other hand, the intestinal canal usually contains organisms, like Escherichia coli (E. coli), which passes out in large numbers in the faeces. Under normal circumstances, they do not cause any harm in the intestine, but they are extremely harmful to the urinary tract when they enter the urethral orifice from the anal orifice. This happens especially when no proper washing/cleaning is done after each defecation, and the area outside the anal orifice remains contaminated with E. coli. It is, therefore, the urinary tract infection, especially recurrent, is more common in women since the anal as well as the urethral orifice/opening is lying close together, and the bacteria can easily enter from the anal to the urethral opening. Moreover, the urethra is very short in women (only an inch long), so infection reaches the urinary

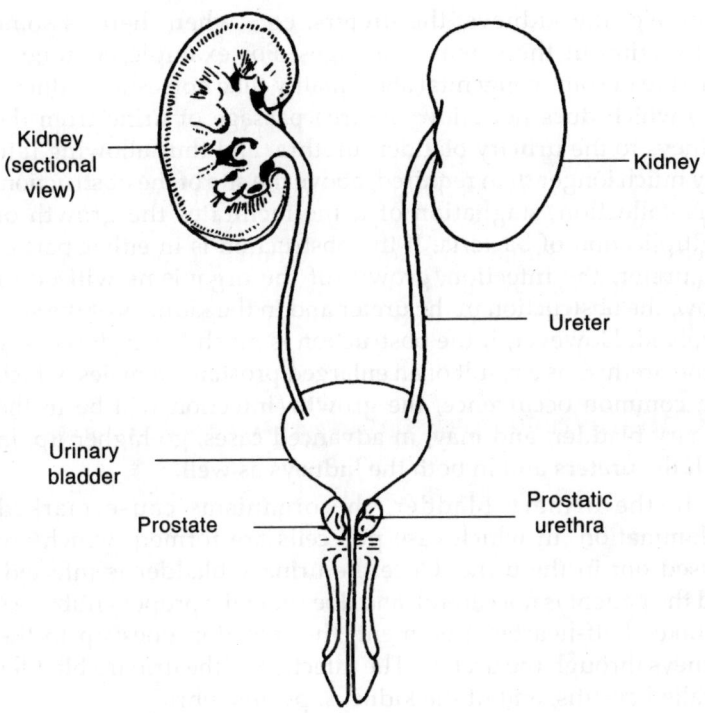

Fig. 20. A diagram of the urinary tract.

bladder in no time. On the other hand, the urethra in males is much longer, and is much farther away from the anus or anal orifice, and thus chances of infection from the anus to the urethra are significantly reduced.

However, infection in the urinary tract may also reach there through the blood, or through lymphatics, and besides E. coli, other bacteria may also damage the urinary tract, especially when the infection is carried by a catheter, directly into the urinary bladder. It may be noted that all strains of E. Coli do not cause UTI. Only those strains that belong to serogroups O, K and H infect the urinary tract.

As soon as the organisms reach the urinary bladder, they start multiplying in the urine present in it, which happens to be an excellent medium for their growth. Chances of the growth of these organisms become much more in any part of the urinary tract, e.g. the kidneys, the ureters, etc., when there is some obstruction in the urinary passages. For example, a stone, a stricture or some congenital abnormality (like horseshoe kidneys, etc.) which does not allow the free passage of urine from the kidneys to the urinary bladder/urethra, and thus allowing it to stay much longer than required, above the site of the obstruction. This collection/stagnation of urine facilitates the growth or multiplication of bacteria. If the obstruction is in either part of the ureter, the infection/growth of the organisms will occur above the obstruction in the ureter and in the kidneys of the side involved. However, if the obstruction is much lower down, say in the urethra, as a result of an enlarged prostate, in males, which is a common occurrence, the growth/infection will be in the urinary bladder, and may, in advanced cases, go higher up, in both the ureters and in both the kidneys as well.

In the urinary bladder, the organisms cause marked inflammation, in which case pus cells are formed, which are passed out in the urine. Once the urinary bladder is infected, and the patient is not careful, and does not take proper antibiotics or takes half-hearted treatment, the infection goes up to the kidneys through the ureters. The infection of the urinary bladder is called cystitis, and of the kidneys, pyelonephritis.

Symptoms and signs of acute UTI (cystitis, pyelonephritis)

A patient of cystitis complains of burning while passing urine, as a result of an inflamed urinary bladder. He/she will have the urge to urinate frequently, both in the morning and during night and, there may be pain in the lower abdomen. As the infection reaches the kidneys and causes their inflammation (i.e. acute pyelonephritis), besides the symptoms of cystitis, just mentioned, there will be associated symptoms relating to the involvement of the kidneys. The patient will complain of pain in the flanks (where the kidneys are located), high fever/chill, nausea, vomiting, etc.

In some cases, when the infection gets located in the kidneys, the symptoms of cystitis may diminish, especially in the case of chronic pyelonephritis. Chronic inflammation of the bladder (cystitis) may also occur in many cases, especially in females,

Diseases of the Kidneys

and it is usually extremely troublesome and, being recurrent the patient may go on showing signs and symptoms of cystitis.

Do all the cases of acute pyelonephritis become chronic?

All the cases of acute pyelonephritis may not become chronic. However, in some cases, after an acute attack, the disease may remain silent/hidden for a short/long time, and later present itself as a case of chronic pyelonephritis. However, there may occur repeated attacks of pyelonephritis in between, before the disease becomes chronic.

Symptoms and signs of chronic pyelonephritis

It is one of the most hidden diseases, and may remain symptomless/undetected for years together, and sometimes comes to light in a routine medical check-up where a routine urine examination shows the presence of albumin or pus cells, which gives a hint in the diagnosis of this disease. Sometimes, there are only vague symptoms like a headache, fatigue, tiredness, etc., and again a casual analysis of urine helps in diagnosing the disease. It is also seen that hypertension may be the only manifestation of the disease. Other patients may directly be diagnosed as cases of chronic renal failure.

Hence a case of chronic pyelonephritis has no definite presentations/signs or symptoms, and, therefore, the disease has to be detected/suspected by periodic urine examination. In all cases of vague symptoms, as well as hypertension, a urine analysis should be an essential feature. The best thing is a complete six-monthly/yearly examination of the urine, or earlier, depending upon the case in question.

As in other hidden/occult diseases, various clinical presentations of both acute and chronic pyelonephritis/cystitis should be recognized by all, especially those who are more prone to UTI, e.g. cases having some congenital abnormality in the kidneys, the cases of enlarged prostate or urinary stones, i.e. stones formed in the urinary passages, causing constant obstruction in the flow of urine, and also in all old recurrent cases of UTI. Patients who have undergone catherization in hospital, at one time or the other, need also to be highly cautious.

How kidneys are damaged and cause 'hidden' kidney failure

Kidneys are one of the most vital organs of the body, and damage to them must be prevented by all means. Survival is threatened when kidneys are badly damaged in a disease, and their function impaired severely. Hence, the infection must be controlled/eradicated immediately with proper antibiotics, otherwise the kidneys will be damaged as a result of a long-standing/recurrent infection, called chronic pyelonephritis.

The situation becomes grim when an attack of acute pyelonephritis/cystitis subsides in about 1-2 weeks, even without treatment. This happens in cases especially where there is no obstructive lesion in the urinary tract. Although the patient feels no symptoms, the infection persists and damages the kidneys in a slow gradual manner. This asymptomatic infection of the kidneys (although the patient goes on passing bacteria/pus cells or albumin in urine), is most dangerous, as ultimately the kidneys may fail silently, and the patient begins to feel helpless, unexpectedly. Such is the treacherous nature of infection of the urinary tract.

As a result of chronic infection, the size of the kidneys goes on reducing. It becomes small, scarred and contracted, with hardly any function it can perform; it fails markedly/completely — this is called renal/kidney failure.

A patient of UTI should never feel that since he has no symptoms, he needs no test or antibiotics. Hence one should realize the value of mass awareness with regard to UTI. It has been aptly said that 'what the mind does not know, the eyes cannot see', and, therefore, chronic UTI can be arrested/controlled soon enough, if there's general awareness in this regard.

Detection of occult / hidden cases of UTI

If a survey is conducted regarding the detection of occult/hidden cases of UTI, one will find a substantial number of cases that have no symptoms of any kind related to cystitis/pyelonephritis. Hence, a periodic examination of urine for albumin, as well as a microscopic examination of the urine collected properly (refer to page 183, last para) for pus cells is the most useful test for the

Diseases of the Kidneys

detection of such cases. A frequent examination of urine is an essential requirement in cases which are more prone to this trouble. All such symptomless cases of UTI must be treated with suitable antibiotics so that infection in the urinary tract is eradicated and the kidneys are saved from damage.

What should be done for UTI?

Under these circumstances, the only way to safeguard against kidney infection/UTI is to strictly follow the preventive guidelines which are mentioned later, and one should be aware of the various clinical signs and symptoms of both cystitis as well as pyelonephritis, so that the patient can report to the physician/specialist concerned at the earliest, for investigations, treatment/eradication of infection from the urinary tract, before the disease subsides on its own, or recurs, causing irreparable damage to the kidneys. Treatment should be taken under a specialist's guidance, and even the maintenance dose of antibiotics for the urinary tract may be required for a long time/even for years in some cases, so as to keep the kidneys free from infective organisms. Treatment should commence at the earliest possible moment. A case of cystitis should not allow pyelonephritis to develop, and cystitis should be treated energetically, so that the infection does not flare and damage the kidneys.

Details of predisposing factors / obstructive lesions in urinary tract responsible for UTI

It is essential to have an idea of such obstructive factors in the urinary tract, as they are likely to cause UTI. Chances of UTI diminish markedly when there is no obstruction in the urinary tract. Any obstruction, however mild it may be, will affect the flow of urine in the urinary tract, and as the stream slows down, chances of the growth of organisms increase, since urine is a favourable medium/source for the growth of organisms, and thus chances of infection in the urinary tract increase substantially. Once the stream of urine is running normally, organisms get fewer chances to stay and grow further. Hence the removal of such obstructive factors is absolutely necessary. In case the obstructive factors are not properly cared for, i.e., investigated as well as treated, irrespective of the amount of antibiotics administered, the UTI can hardly be controlled and the infection is likely to occur again and again. Some examples of obstructive factors are given below:

1. Urinary stones/calculi

The usual stones in the urinary tract consist of calcium oxalate or calcium phosphate (or combined with ammonio-magnesium phosphate), or uric acid, etc. However, the stones may occur as a combination of these constituents, called 'mixed stones'.

What are the symptoms of urinary stones?

Stone/s in the urinary tract may remain symptomless for long, and may be detected by routine X-rays. Stones which are stagnant/motionless in any part of the urinary tract do not show symptoms, although they may cause massive harm, as they grow in size. However, there is very severe pain (renal colic) as the stone starts moving downward.

A renal colic pain usually subsides with the administration of a strong pain-killer injection. Blood may also pass in the urine during an attack of renal colic, as a result of some injury in the urinary tract, caused by stones. Infection will also occur in the urinary tract due to the slowing down of the flow of urine. In which case pus cells will also be seen in the urine, when examined under the microscope.

What should be done for urinary stones?

It is advisable that the treatment of urinary stones is done in the earliest possible time after the acute attack has subsided, so that UTI is prevented. If neglected, besides causing repeated attacks of renal colic, the obstruction in the urinary tract will grow due to the increase in the size of the stone, which may show serious consequences later.

Small and early stones, causing little/no obstruction are usually pushed down and out, when the patient takes plenty of fluids, at least 3 litres of water per day.

In case the stone is not ejected, it must be removed either surgically, or by lithotripsy.

Lithotripsy is a non-surgical method of removing stones from the urinary tract. It is called extracorporeal shock-wave

Diseases of the Kidneys

lithotripsy (ESWL), and in this procedure electrically generated shock-waves are focused on the stone and fragment it. Hence this mode of non-surgical therapy is ideal as it excludes surgery and late complications.

What tests are required in a case of urinary stones?

Tests like plain X-ray as well as ultrasonography of the urinary tract are important in order to detect the exact location of the stone, and to see the extent of damage caused to the urinary tract by the stone/s. However, uric acid stones are not picked up in X-rays. Therefore, an intravenous pyelography may be required in some of the cases, to prove the presence of stones in the urinary tract. Intravenous pyelography is also useful in locating any associated lesion/s of the urinary tract, such as a stricture, horseshoe kidneys etc.

The above tests should not be forgotten in a case of UTI for excluding urinary stones, especially when the patient has no signs/symptoms of renal colic.

It is essential that the stones once passed out or removed must be analysed regarding their constituents, so that appropriate steps can be taken so as to avoid a recurrence of the stones. A restricted diet should be prescribed, depending on the stone analysis report.

2. Benign enlargement of the prostate (BEP)

The prostate is a walnut-sized gland in males, located below the urinary bladder, and it encircles the upper part of the urethra. This part of the urethra is called the prostatic urethra. Urine from the urinary bladder passes out through this urethra (Fig. 20).

Hence it is clear that whenever the prostate becomes enlarged, it is likely to put pressure on this part of the urethra, i.e., the prostatic urethra, causing obstruction when the patient passes urine. In very early cases, there may not be any symptom or there may be negligible/minimal symptoms, since the force of the contraction of the urinary bladder may be able to overcome the small initial obstruction caused by the enlargement of the prostate gland.

As the obstruction increases, urine will stay in the urinary bladder for a longer period, and if obstruction is severe, urine may collect, as a result of back pressure, in the ureters, and finally in both the kidneys. One can imagine that such stagnation of urine in the whole urinary tract will cause an enormous growth of bacteria, leading to inflammation of the entire urinary tract, from the urethra to the kidneys. There will then be inflammation of the urethra (urethritis), the urinary bladder (cystitis), the kidneys (pyelonephritis) and even the prostate may be affected by the infection called prostatitis.

If early steps are not taken, kidney failure may occur as a result of the chronic infection of the kidneys, i.e. chronic pyelonephritis.

Regarding cancer of the prostate, it has already been described in the chapter on cancer (page 5, serial 13). Here we are dealing with the 'benign' enlargement of the prostate, i.e. the condition is non-cancerous in nature. Such an enlargement of the prostate occurs in old people, usually after the age of 50. It has been rightly said that as the hair turn grey, there is, likewise, an enlargement of the prostate gland.

What are the early symptoms and signs of the BEP?

Since an enlarged prostate causes obstruction in the flow of urine in the urethra, the patient experiences varied difficulties while passing urine. There is a narrowing or decrease in the calibre of the urethra, and, therefore, (i) the patient does not pass urine with normal force, and the stream becomes thin, (ii) he experiences difficulty both while starting and stopping urination, (iii) he always feels that he has not passed the whole urine, (iv) urine falls in drops/trickles after he has passed urine, (v) the patient passes urine frequently, especially during the night, (vi) he takes more time in passing urine, (vii) he always feels like passing urine, and it becomes unavoidable most of the time.

The above early symptoms and signs must be known by old people, so that they can report it to their physicians/surgeons for early diagnosis and treatment, and save themselves from the grave complications of UTI.

As the prostate enlarges more, and the calibre of the urethra decreases further, the patient experiences more and more inconvenience while passing urine.

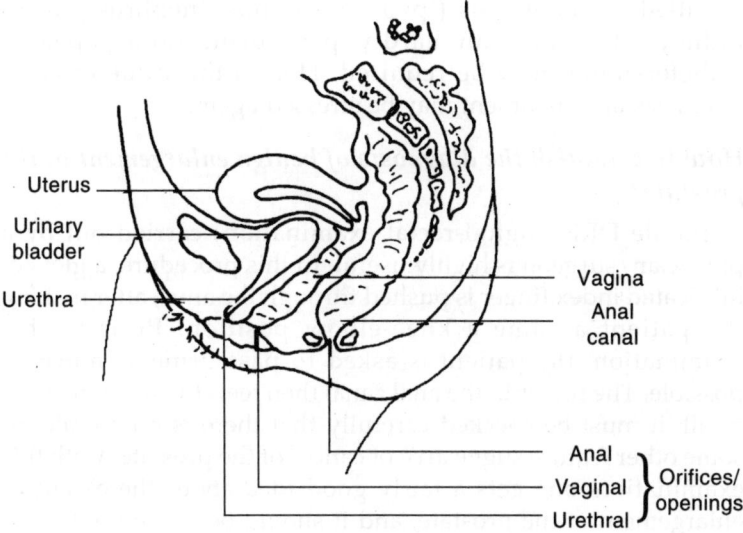

Fig. 21. A diagrammatic representation of the three openings, i.e. of the anus, the vagina and the urethra, lying close together (in females).

One factor is of great importance in such a diagnosis. If the patient is unable to pass urine completely, there is a strong possibility of 'residual urine' in the urinary bladder. This increases as the disease progresses. Residual urine is a valuable guide and indicates the severity of blockage in the urethra. The amount of residual urine is measured with the help of ultrasonography, and the line of action of the treatment is decided. Residual urine, more than 40-50 ml in the urinary bladder, is considered significant, and at this stage, treatment should not be delayed further.

Late symptoms and signs of prostate enlargement

If the disease is neglected, there will be a marked retention of urine, and the back pressure of the urine increases more and more, resulting in dilation of the ureters (called hydroureters), as well as of the kidneys (called hydronephrosis). An enormous growth of bacteria will occur in the entire urinary tract, leading to pus formation, and the kidneys will be grossly infected. This is called pyonephrosis ('pyo' means pus, 'nephros' means kidney). Patients can hardly pass urine, and repeated catheterization may be required. Hence, the value of early diagnosis and treatment may be stressed again.

How to establish the diagnosis of benign enlargement of the prostate?

A simple DRE (digital-rectal examination) carried out by a physician/surgeon is highly useful. In this procedure, a gloved, lubricated index finger is pushed through the anus, after making the patient assume a knee-elbow position. Prior to this examination, the patient is asked to pass urine as much as possible. The finger in the anal canal then feels the prostate. First of all, it must be checked carefully that there is no nodule, or some other feature suggestive of cancer of the prostate. With this examination, one gets a fairly good idea about the extent of enlargement of the prostate, and it should be carried out in all cases systematically.

The above examination should be followed by an ultrasonographic examination of the prostate. It is a very useful as well as accurate test. It gives all the details of the prostate, like its exact size, weight, any nodule suggestive of cancer, or any stone in the prostate, including the exact amount of the residual urine. If need be, a more specialized ultrasonography (trans-rectal prostate sonography), in which a special probe is used, can be carried out to rule out any doubt regarding cancer of the prostate, in selected cases.

If in a case of enlarged prostate, there is an associated infection of the urinary tract/renal failure/renal insufficiency, more tests will be required.

Treatment of a benign enlargement of the prostate

It should be stressed that an enlarged prostate alone is not sufficient indication for an operation. The patient must have symptoms, and, above all, a significant quantity of 'residual urine', for considering medicinal/operative treatment.

In early cases, some of the drugs available may be tried. However, in cases where symptoms are markedly distressing to the patient, and the 'residual urine' is highly significant, the

Diseases of the Kidneys

operation should not be delayed. Above all, what is needed is the quick removal of any obstruction from the passage of the urinary tract, for the prevention of UTI.

As regards the diverticulum of urinary bladder that may be seen in cases of BEP, it may be considered to be removed at the time of operation as it may become a chronic source of UTI threatening the functioning of the kidneys. However, a small diverticulum need not be removed to eliminate possibilities of infection or even development of tumour. In a communication, Dr. Emil A. Tanagho, Professor, Department of Urology, School of Medicine, University of California, San Francisco, U.S.A., author of the book *Smith's General Urology* wrote to the author regarding his opinion about a patient who had 3½ cm posterolateral diverticulum of the urinary bladder that was considered to be left as such at the time of operation, "...relief of the obstruction will minimize the significance of this diverticulum. This is a relatively small one compared to the huge one that we might encounter. The fact that the patient developed one infection after prostatectomy in itself does not really mean that the diverticulum is the source of it. Many patients do develop one or two infections after prostatectomy due to the foreign tubes or catheters, or just the healing process. Such diverticulum needs no particular surgical attention." The follow up of this patient has been satisfactory.

If the patient takes care of his enlarged prostate, he can be easily operated on by a transurethral resection of the prostate (TURP), in which no surgical incision is required. The instrument is simply passed through the penis, of course, under anaesthesia, which cuts the prostate into very small/tiny pieces. These can be easily sucked out, and the obstruction in the urinary tract is removed. The results are highly promising.

3. Other predisposing / obstructive factors of UTI

Stricture/scarring, congenital abnormalities of the kidneys, such as horseshoe kidneys, are some other predisposing factors which can be diagnosed by ultrasonography, and/or by intravenous pyelography. These should be treated accordingly so that UTI could be prevented.

Some other conditions relating to UTI which should also be discussed:

1. UTI and pregnancy

It is routine in a prenatal check-up that the urine of all women is examined for UTI. It is probable that during pregnancy the urinary bladder becomes more susceptible to infection. There may be altered immunity during the course of pregnancy that the urinary bladder becomes weak, and retention of urine increases, giving more time to bacteria to grow, leading to UTI. Early detection and treatment of UTI is, therefore, important in pregnant women, for safe delivery.

2. UTI and sexual activity

Incidence of UTI among school girls is not very common. If detected, one should look for any congenital obstructive lesion in the urinary tract, responsible for UTI.

However, UTI becomes more common in women after marriage. During sexual intercourse, bacteria gain entry into the urinary bladder through the urethra, as in a woman all the three orifices/openings of the urethra, the vagina and anus are closely located (Fig. 21). Thus, infection is frequently introduced in the urinary tract, and reactivated, following sexual intercourse. It should be prevented as explained later. In men who have history of rectal intercourse, UTI is likely to occur.

3. UTI and diabetes

If the kidney has already been affected by a disease, it becomes more susceptible to infection, as in the case of a diabetic kidney, which occurs due to uncontrolled diabetes. Sugar contents in the urine add to infection of the urinary tract. Hence the control of diabetes is important to prevent infection of the kidneys.

4. Hypertension and UTI

Similarly, a hypertensive kidney, i.e. one damaged as a result of prolonged uncontrolled hypertension, may become more prone to infection. On the other hand, chronic infection of kidneys (chronic pyelonephritis) may also cause hypertension called renal hypertension. Hence the control of hypertension as well as

UTI should be considered important to save the kidneys from damage.

5. Catheter and UTI
In case all aseptic precautions are not taken while catheterization of the urinary bladder in an emergency, the infection may enter directly into the urinary bladder through the catheter leading to UTI. Hence, a strict sterilization is required during catherterization.

Genetic factors
UTI is likely to occur if there is family history of this disorder

What tests are necessary for the diagnosis/treatment of UTI?

At the outset, it may be said that in case there is any predisposing/obstructive factor (like urinary stones, benign enlargement of prostate, congenital abnormalities of urinary tract, etc.), it must be investigated and treated according to the lines already described.

The various tests required for the diagnosis/treatment of UTI are as under:

1. Examination of urine
It is one of the most important tests, and it should not be taken casually. It indicates whether the patient is suffering from UTI or not especially, when symptoms of cystitis/pyelonephritis are not marked, or happen to be completely absent.

The urine specimen for test in laboratory should be very carefully collected, keeping the following steps strictly in view:
  (i) The specimen should be from midstream. The patient must pass some urine outside, before passing the urine in a sterilized container.
  (ii) Before giving the sample of urine, wash the whole area properly so that there is no contamination of E. coli, especially in women.
  (iii) The specimen should be given in laboratory as urine sample often gets spoiled, on the way to the laboratory.

(iv) Second morning sample is always preferred. In the first morning sample, some changes are likely to occur due to overnight standing of urine, in the urinary bladder.

2. Urine for culture and sensitivity

If the examination of urine shows the presence of pus cells, the urine should be given in the laboratory for culture and sensitivity. It may be noted that 0-5 pus cells and 0-1 RBC (a little more in females, and markedly if a woman is in menses) per high power field may be normally present in urine, especially when there is no associated/contributing factor to UTI. The report of culture and sensitivity is usually available after 48-72 hours, and it guides the physician regarding the administration of antibiotics in a particular case. The treatment of UTI may not be possible without this test, and the entire course of treatment depends upon the report of this test. Therefore, it should be carried out by an experienced laboratory technician and the urine must be collected under strict aseptic conditions.

Besides the examination of pus cells, as well as of the culture and sensitivity of the urine, a complete detailed routine examination of the urine must be carried out so that any other abnormality, if present, can also be considered while treating the case. Many a time one finds in the urine analysis report, traces of albumin, although there is no apparent cause of passing albumin in urine in the concerned case. Traces of albumin in urine could be due to the contamination of the urine sample by vaginal secretion/semen of the previous night's intercourse. Hence the importance of proper washing of the whole area, especially in women, before giving the sample, is again emphasised. And, if still, in spite of all such precautions, traces of albumin in the urine persist, total protein should be measured in 24-hour urine, and normally it should be less than 150mg/dl (30mg/dl of albumin) per day. However, presence of albumin in urine is an important finding for kidney damage, not only due to pyelonephritis, but also due to other diseases of the kidneys, mentioned later. It tells us that the patient is passing into the chronic stage, although he/she may remain asymptomatic. Hence a periodical examination of urine is an important factor to assess the extent of kidney damage.

3. Blood urea and serum creatinine tests

Normal levels of blood urea range from 15-35 mg/dl with an average of 25 mg/dl. Normal serum creatinine levels range from 0.8 to 1.4 mg/dl, the average being 1.00 mg/dl. Both these tests should be carried out in order to be on the safe side, although blood urea is a simple test and serum creatinine a little more difficult to carry out — serum creatinine is more sensitive than blood urea. If the levels of serum creatinine are 1.5 mg/dl, although the kidneys may be fairly damaged, it is still considered early. When levels of serum creatinine are raised to the extent of 3.5 to 5.5 mg/dl, the kidneys may still be said to be moderately damaged and one should not lose time in initiating the necessary tests and treatment. But if levels of serum creatinine rise above 8 mg/dl, it means that the kidneys are severely affected, leading to renal failure, requiring urgent dialysis.

4. 24-hour creatinine clearance

It is much more reliable than the serum creatinine test. But it is somewhat cumbersome as in this test, a 24-hour collection of urine is required. It may be carried out to diagnose very early cases, wherever facilities exist.

5. Ultrasonographic examination

It must be carried out in each and every case of UTI. It is a non-invasive test and usually gives valuable information regarding occult causes of UTI. For example, there may be an asymptomatic stone lying in the urinary tract, or there may be some congenital abnormality of the kidneys causing obstruction in the urinary tract, or there may be an early enlargement of the prostate, in the case of males.

6. Plain X-ray, CT abdomen, intravenous pyelography

These may be required depending upon the case.

7. Renal / kidney biopsy

It may be indicated to know about the exact nature of pathology causing renal damage.

What is the schedule for taking antibiotics for the treatment of UTI?

The main aim of treatment is to eradicate the bacteria from the urinary tract so that kidney damage/failure can be prevented, under all circumstances.

As already stated, the predisposing/obstructive factors in the causation of UTI, if any, must be looked into and treated accordingly. For example, the removal of urinary stone/s/, enlarged prostate, etc.

The patient should be put on antibiotics according to the culture and sensitivity report of the urine. Repeat culture and sensitivity of the urine after 72 hours. If there's no growth of organisms, it shows that the antibiotic initially started has been effective. Continue with this antibiotic for a total period of 7-10 days.

On the other hand, if the culture indicates sensitivity to another antibiotic/s, stop the antibiotic initially started, and switch over to the antibiotic according to the second culture, and repeat culture and sensitivity of the urine after 72 hours of starting the second antibiotic. If this culture, i.e. the third culture shows no growth, continue with the second antibiotic for a period of 7-10 days. However, if the sensitivity of the drug shown in the third culture is different, change the antibiotic, and so on.

The infection is usually arrested after 7-10 days of continuous administration of antibiotic. Then start with the maintenance dose of the same antibiotic at bedtime for a period of 3-6 months, even much longer, say, years, in some cases. But go on doing culture and sensitivity of the urine, initially, weekly/fortnightly, so as to be sure that the maintenance dose of the required antibiotic is constantly effective.

In case, at any time, culture and sensitivity of the urine shows new organism/antibiotics, it means that the drug prophylaxis, i.e. the administration of antibiotic at bedtime has failed to prevent infection. Then, one has no choice except to start again as usual with the next antibiotic, and repeat culture and sensitivity test of the urine after 72 hours from the start of this antibiotic, and so on.

Norfloxacin, amoxycillin, ciprofloxacin, lomefloxacin, amikacin, ceftriaxone, cefixime, cefepime are some of the common urinary tract antibiotics, to name a few.

It needs emphasizing that drug prophylaxis, i.e. administration of a single dose of antibiotic should never be forgotten, and its effectiveness must be checked periodically by repeating culture and sensitivity of the urine monthly, two-three monthly, or after a longer period, depending on the case, so that no chance is given to the organisms to damage the kidneys/the urinary tract. Hence, constant vigilance, as well as effort, also patience, is required for such a long prophylaxis.

What are the various guidelines for the prevention of UTI

From the foregoing information on UTI, one should realize that the best course is to follow, strictly, the preventive measures, which are very simple, mostly relating to routine hygiene, rather than being on long-term prophylactic antibiotics; or, in neglected cases, developing terminal kidney disease, i.e. kidney failure, which may, as mentioned earlier, require repeated dialysis, or even kidney transplant, depending on the case.

Various guidelines are mentioned below, and all individuals, irrespective of age and sex, are required to carefully follow them in their everyday life.

(i) Perineal hygiene

The perineum is the area where the openings of the anus, the urethra and the vagina are situated (of course, the scrotum and the penis in the male). It is the most dangerous area, especially in females, as all the three openings are lying close together (Fig. 21), and there is always a threat of infection to the urinary tract from anal-faecal organisms, which invade the urinary tract through the urethral opening. Hence if proper hygiene is maintained after each defecation, the infection from the anus to the urethra can be stopped/prevented, since UTI is caused, mostly by E. coli organisms present in the faeces. Of course, the various predisposing/associated factors responsible for UTI, if present, have to be simultaneously investigated and treated.

A simple cleansing with water, and preferably with soap and water after passing stools, and urine in the case of females, is strongly recommended at all ages, more so in children, girls, both married and unmarried women. However, those using toilet-paper, after passing stools, should be more careful, and see that the area has been thoroughly cleaned, especially in the case of females. Hence, it is of the utmost importance to always keep the perineal area clean, and thus it has been rightly said that 'cleanliness is next to godliness.'

(ii) Passing of urine after sexual intercourse (postcoital voiding)

Since during sexual activity, the organisms may gain entry through the urethral opening into the urinary bladder, it is advisable for all women to pass urine after each sexual intercourse, so that the bacteria, in case they have entered the urinary bladder, are washed out. It is safer if urine is also passed before sexual intercourse.

Further, women who are more prone to UTI, or get recurrences of UTI as a result of intercourse, are advised to take a single dose of prophylactic broad-spectrum antibiotic like norfloxacin, ciprofloxacin, lomefloxacin or ofloxacin, etc., after sexual intercourse/coitus. This is an important step in the prevention of UTI in such patients, and has shown promising results.

The above step for the prevention of UTI is very important and calls for an urgent need to impart sex education at the appropriate age. Physicians/obstetricians/gynaecologists/paediatricians can also guide their patients as and when an opportunity arises. Mothers can also advise their children in this matter.

(iii) Passing of urine frequently

All persons, and especially those who are more prone to UTI, should pass urine frequently, say every 3-4 hours, so that the urinary bladder is constantly washed out, and the bacteria, if any, are pushed out in the urine. If the bladder is not evacuated frequently, the bacteria will get more time to increase in number in the urine collected in the urinary bladder. Hence, frequent urination is an essential step towards the prevention of UTI, which should be observed by everyone.

Diseases of the Kidneys

In any case, urination should not be postponed, as this will increase the rise of UTI.

(iv) Passing of urine at bedtime

Similarly, urine must be passed at bedtime, so that the minimum quantity of urine remains in the urinary bladder during the night. Since the duration of the night is long, there should be as little urine as possible in the bladder, and one should pass urine even during the night, if he or she happens to wake up.

(v) Plenty of fluids

It is obvious that the intake of plenty of fluids is required, so that there is frequent urination, and the bladder is constantly kept clean. At least about three litres of water/fluids must be taken daily to achieve the desired results.

Ideally, the habit of frequent urination or bladder training, including cleanliness, should be instilled right from childhood, especially in the case of female children. Above all, once the subject is made clear to the sufferers/others, it becomes routine.

(vi) Immediate treatment of predisposing factors

As soon as some predisposing/obstructive lesions happen to occur, e.g. urinary stones, benign enlargement of prostate, etc., immediate attention should be paid, and surgery, if required, should not be delayed, so that UTI does not develop at all, and there is absolute prevention.

(vii) Control of high blood pressure and diabetes

Control of high blood pressure and diabetes is an essential requirement to prevent the kidneys from contracting an infection, since a damaged kidney, as a result of high blood pressure and/or high blood sugar, is always prone to get infection. The infection in such kidneys can only be avoided/prevented if it is protected from damage by these diseases. That is, a strict control of both high blood pressure and diabetes is required. This aspect has also been emphasized earlier.

(viii) UTI and catheter

As already mentioned, catheterization of the urinary bladder should always be done under aseptic conditions. It should not be taken casually, and the catheter should be used by trained/experienced medical personnel. Catheterization is one of the causes of UTI, as it pushes the bacteria directly into the urinary bladder, if appropriate steps are not taken. It is an important aspect of the prevention of UTI, since in some cases repeated catheterization may be required, while in others, a catheter may have to be left in the urinary bladder for constant drainage, during an emergency period. Hence, all necessary precautions are required during catheterization to safeguard against UTI.

(ix) Periodic examination of urine

Besides the various preventive measures given above, a periodic examination of the urine is also important for at least pus cells and albumin, so that asymptomatic/hidden cases can be detected in time. As mentioned earlier, urine should be examined six-monthly/yearly to check the functioning of the kidneys from time to time. More frequent examinations of urine are required, even monthly, when the patient has suffered from an attack of cystitis and/or pyelonephritis, or has some associated, predisposing/obstructive factor responsible for UTI. A regular check-up of urine, as explained earlier, is essential during the period of pregnancy.

In the end, it should be stated that UTI can be prevented by following everyday personal hygienic measures, and we only need to know their importance, for following them wholeheartedly. It may seem amazing that the simple principle of cleanliness can prevent the most serious/fatal disease of the kidney, i.e. kidney failure, which may necessitate repeated dialysis to keep the patient alive. Even a renal transplant may be required in some cases.

Besides personal hygiene and the other measures already discussed, even if UTI occurs, it should be treated with patience, as long therapy may be required. If there is any factor contributing to UTI, it should also be treated at the same time.

In addition to the above, an active drive to find out hidden cases of UTI, and for creating a mass awareness about each aspect of the disease is urgently required, so that the goal for the prevention of UTI can be effectively achieved. A UTI vaccine will certainly help in solving this problem to a great extent. An E.coli vaccine (one of the organisms inflicting UTI) is now available in some of the developed countries.

2. Glomerulonephritis (GN)

This is one of the diseases of the kidneys, which may remain hidden for years, and the patient may suddenly suffer from kidney failure.

What is the cause of this disease?

Whether one believes it or not, the disease in question is caused as a result of a sore throat. It may be tonsillitis/pharyngitis, or both. However, not all cases of sore throat cause this serious disease of the kidneys. It only occurs when the sore throat takes place due to the invasion of a specific bacteria called group A beta-haemolytc streptococcus (GABHS). It is the same organism that is responsible for the causation of rheumatic fever (RF)/rheumatic heart disease (RHD). As in the case of RF/RHD, this bacteria does not directly involve the kidneys, but it remains confined in the throat, and the disease manifests itself after 1-3 weeks (average 10 days) after the subsiding of the sore throat. It is said to be an allergic manifestation, as a result of streptococcal infection in the throat. Hence the disease may be labelled as post-streptococcal glomerulonephritis (PSGN). The strains of GABHS that are responsible for the causation of acute GN include M types 1, 2, 4, 12, 18, 25, 49, 55, 57 and 60. It may be noted that once the disease occurs, the immunity to these strains is very long lasting. In other words, once acute GN occurs, it does not manifest a second time. Hence prevention of sore throat in such patients (which is a must in cases of RF/RHD) is not required. However albumin in the urine may be checked periodically to watch the chronic phase of the disease. Further, prevention of sore throat will be required among masses so that the disease does not manifest.

What are the symptoms of GN?

The disease may be acute, subacute or chronic. The acute manifestation of the disease is very troublesome. It commonly occurs in children, and is called acute GN. This condition subsides in about 7-10 days, but in some cases, the disease may be so serious that a sudden kidney failure may occur, requiring urgent dialysis. In other cases, after the disease has subsided with treatment, or in some mild cases, even without treatment, being self-limited in nature, it may pass on to the subacute, or directly into the chronic phase, called subacute GN and chronic GN respectively.

Although patients of acute GN report to the physician/hospital immediately, as the symptoms are of an emergency nature, yet the cases of subacute GN remain so concealed that sometimes the patient is diagnosed in a normal medical examination. Chronic GN is the terminal stage of the disease, and it is one of the important causes of chronic renal failure. And, interestingly, the patient may directly/suddenly report to the physician with the symptoms of chronic GN, without passing through either the acute/subacute phase of the disease. Further, most of the time, a previous history of sore throat may also not be available. Therefore, the occult nature of the disease is clear both in the subacute and chronic stages of this ailment.

Acute GN

A child may suddenly report the passing of a large amount of blood in the urine (as the blood leaks into the urine due to the involvement of the blood vessel walls of several glomeruli in the kidneys), which looks a dark-brown/coca-cola colour, and the urine passed is also small in quantity. There may be pain in both the flanks due to the pathology in the kidneys, which get enlarged/swollen. As a result of haemorrhage, the whole surface of the kidneys show tiny haemorrhagic spots, and are hence called 'flea-bitten kidneys'. Such kidneys are only seen in the museums of medical colleges where they are kept/preserved for the study of medical students. Besides blood in urine, there is puffiness/swelling of the face of the child as well. A sudden rise of blood pressure in the child is also noted. Simultaneous manifestation of RF is extremely rare.

A urine examination shows marked red blood cells (RBC), there may be a small amount of albumin in the urine and the blood urea will be slightly raised. There will be no pus cells in the urine, and the urine culture will be sterile as there is no direct invasion of bacteria, and hence no infection/pus formation.

The child should be given bed rest till all signs and symptoms disappear. If RBC or albumin persists in the urine, rest may be prolonged, or the child may be temporarily mobilised, and if RBC or albumin increases, rest should be again advised. Proper follow-up/treatment of all these cases is important so that they may not pass on to the subacute/chronic GN, silently.

In view of sudden hypertension, a salt-restricted diet is also recommended.

With usual supportive therapy and rest, most children recover in about a fortnight. As mentioned in the beginning, the patient, especially when the disease appears in adulthood, may pass on to the subacute/chronic stage, after remaining asymptomatic for a long period. Hence a prolonged follow-up of such a case is required, and a periodic examination of urine, especially for albumin, should be the rule, so that as soon as the patient shows the earliest sign of the disease, it can be treated.

Subacute GN (Nephrotic syndrome - NS)

Surprisingly, the patient may suffer from the subacute stage of the disease, without passing into the acute stage of GN.

The disease is highly dormant, and remains without any symptoms for long periods, even for years, and is diagnosed/ discovered sometimes incidentally when proteinuria (albuminuria) is detected during a routine urine analysis, as a part of a general medical check-up.

At this stage of the disease, the defect in the kidneys, more precisely in various glomeruli of the kidneys, occurs in such a way, that the patient loses only protein in the urine, called proteinuria. Specific proteinuria is the rule of this disease that results from disturbed permeability of glomerular filtration barrier for protein i.e. of glomerular basement membrane (GBM) due to immune process. Other features of nephrotic syndrome (mentioned further) are all secondary to the loss of protein in the urine.

So hidden is the nature of the disease that the patient goes on passing protein in the urine, and the disease is usually discovered when it reaches a fairly advanced stage, i.e. the patient passes significant amount of protein in the urine. As a result of which other complications occur in the body, like that the protein in the blood decreases to less than 3.0 g/dl (hypoproteinaemia), and a swelling (oedema) of the feet occurs initially, and later on, of all the extremities. In due course, entire the body swells.

Another notable feature of the disease is that the level of blood cholesterol markedly increases. This is called hypercholesterolaemia. Hence the disease is known for its triad manifestations, i.e. proteinuria, hypoproteinaemia and hypercholesterolaemia. Besides cholesterol, LDL (low-density lipoproteins) is also increased, and in severe cases TG (triglycerides) and very LDL also tend to rise. Increased levels of lipids probably occur due to increased formation of lipoprotein by the liver following loss of proteins in the urine that regulate lipid levels in the blood. Increased levels of lipids in NS may be responsible for the manifestation of atherosclerosis in such patients.

Besides the above, there occurs hypercoagulability in such cases i.e. there are chances of clot formation in blood vessels. Patients may develop sudden peripheral arterial or venous thrombosis. Renal vein thrombosis may also occur. Further, the thrombus or clot that has formed in the veins may dislodge or break off and travel to lungs leading to pulmonary embolism which is a life-threatening emergency. Hypercoagulability occurs in such cases due to more formation of fibrinogen by the liver, impaired firrinolysis, and there is more collection of platelet.

Several complications may appear e.g. the patients become malnourished due to loss of proteins, and vitamin D deficiency leads to low level of calcium in the blood. The patient becomes anaemic and due to loss of immunity, infections are likely to occur.

Normal total protein in urine is less than 150mg/dl (30mg/dl of albumin) per day, and in this condition, it would be more than 3.5 g, and may rise to even 30 g per day. Of course, initially, the loss of protein is usually minimal when the disease remains silent, and this is the time when it should be diagnosed to prevent the patient from going to the advanced stage of the disease.

It is worth noting that proteinuria and oedema (swelling) feet/whole body are important signs of the disease. It may be mentioned that NS may also occur as a result of diabetes mellitus or amyloidosis.

Another valuable point is that if the disease manifests itself in a middle-aged person, it may be associated with malignancy.

Diseases of the Kidneys

How can the disease be suspected early?

Since the earliest manifestation of the disease is mild/moderate proteinuria (i.e. passing of protein in urine), without producing any symptoms, the only way to detect it would be a frequent check-up of urine, following an attack of acute GN, as well as of all those persons/children who are more prone to sore throats. In normal healthy persons, urine examination for albumin should be carried out six-monthly/yearly. Urine examination for albumin in various medical camps should be made a routine feature, as we have done many a time, with promising results. However, whenever a patient reports to the doctor for any ailment, a complete urine examination should be prescribed and this may prove rewarding in many cases.

Another important feature of the disease is oedema of the feet. It is seen that mild oedema of the feet may persist for a considerable time, and such patients should be alert, and must get a urine examination for albumin done, to exclude the possibility of NS. However, there are other causes for oedema of the feet as well.

Hence, to repeat, albuminuria and oedema/swelling feet are the early guidelines for the diagnosis of this disease.

What is the prognosis and treatment of this disease?

If timely detected, the disease can be arrested. In very early cases i.e. when proteinuria is just > 3.5 G%, angiotensin converting enzyme (ACE) inhibitors will suffice. This drug lowers the levels of proteinuria as it lowers the intraglomerular pressure. As the amount of proteinuria increases from initial to 8 G% corticosteroids like prednisolon need to be added. Other drugs may be needed depending upon the condition of the patient. Anticoagulants may be required if the patient has developed deep venous thrombosis (DVT). Anaemia and deficiency of vitamins need equal attention. Prednisolon has its own side-effects and needs to be tapered. Many a time, as soon as the drug is tapered, a relapse occurs, and again the dosage of the drug has to be increased, and this goes on in many of the cases. However, spontaneous and temporary remission may also occur.

With the control of proteinuria by administering the above drugs, oedema decreases/subsides. A good way to see the prognosis of the disease is a daily check-up of 24-hour urine for total protein, and look for improvement in the swelling of the feet/body of the patient.

As regards high levels of blood cholesterol (hypercholesterolaemia), which is also an important manifestation of this disease, specific measures explained in Chapter 5 on cholesterol should be strictly followed. Besides aggressive use of drugs, dietary modifications and exercise need to be stressed. This aspect of the treatment should be given equal weightage, and one should not concentrate entirely on the aspect of proteinuria/hypoproteinaemia.

In case NS occurs as a result of any other cause like diabetes mellitus/amyloidosis, besides the above line of treatment, the patient should be investigated/treated on the lines of the underlying disease, which may require urgent control.

If prednisolone alone does not work, other drugs are also available, which can be tried along with prednisolone, in selected cases. The patient is also put on diuretics to relieve the swelling/ oedema of the body. A daily record of body weight also gives a fair idea of the reduction in the swelling of the patient's body. The patient may need antibiotics to prevent secondary infection in the urinary tract or elsewhere.

Although there is protein malnutrition as a result of proteinuria, the patient is given balanced diet, as high protein diet may further increase the urinary excretion of protein leading to more renal damage.

The sad part of the disease is that in the absence of specific treatment or cure, especially in late cases, which are difficult to control, it may progress to the chronic stage, i.e. chronic GN, which may result in kidney failure. Hence the value of the awareness of early detection of the disease, i.e. by a simple examination of urine for albumin, is the key to the speedy control of the disease.

Chronic GN

It is one of the important causes of chronic kidney failure. Again, like subacute GN, the disease may remain underground for several years, and the patient may directly come to the physician/nephrologist, with varied signs and symptoms of chronic GN/kidney failure. It is indeed a tragic experience that even after a detailed enquiry of the patients, in about 50% cases, there is no previous history of either acute/subacute GN. However, some of the cases may give a history of acute GN, of a few or several years back, which has not been seriously followed up after the acute attack subsided, and hence the disease has passed on to the chronic stage, unnoticed.

As a result of the chronic nature of the disease, the kidney reduces in size. It gets scarred/contracted, as in cases of chronic pyelonephritis, which is another cause of chronic kidney failure. In this way, there occurs a marked damage to the kidneys, and thus, its functions adversely affected. The patient may pass urine repeatedly, in an attempt on the part of the kidneys to excrete waste products, as far as possible. There may be associated high blood pressure as a result of the kidney involvement, called renal hypertension. Blood urea, serum creatinine and other kidney function tests start deteriorating soon, and as the disease advances, the patient may enter into the terminal stage, i.e., chronic renal failure.

The disease usually comes to notice when (1) routine examination of urine shows the presence of protein and/or blood in the urine (2) routine blood tests show raised levels of blood urea and creatinine (3) imaging of abdomen for any cause reveals small kidneys on both the sides (4) routine tests for high blood pressure give clue of diseases that have given rise to the development of high blood pressure (called secondary hypertension).

Hidden cases of the disease can be detected by periodic (six-monthly/yearly) examination of urine for albumin, and if possible, by determining the levels of serum creatinine of all persons, and more frequently, in cases who have suffered from acute/subacute GN. However, the disease should be suspected in persons who complain of vague symptoms, such as loss of energy, fatigue, headache, excessive urination (polyuria), thirst, etc. The presence of albumin in such cases gives a clue to the diagnosis.

The patient is investigated and treated on the lines of chronic renal failure, described later.

Prophylaxis of GN

Since an attack of acute GN occurs as a result of sore throat, prophylactic steps should be taken to eradicate the infection in the entire family, and ideally in the whole community, where a particular case has occurred, so that further spread of infection can be prevented. The patient, as well as other associated persons, should be treated for sore throat with a suitable antibiotic. If possible, culture and sensitivity should also be carried out after taking throat swabs, and the antibiotic indicated in the culture report should be given. Immediate treatment should be taken in cases where the culture shows the growth of beta-haemolytic streptococcus, responsible for sore throat/an acute attack of GN. Such urgent measures may save various other members of the family/community from an attack of acute GN.

Since a sore throat infection is the main culprit in such acute cases, general measures are required to prevent its incidence in masses. Overcrowding, highly-populated areas, especially like the slums, should be avoided as far as possible. In other words, living conditions have to be improved. A patient with a sore throat should take an antibiotic at the earliest, and keep himself/herself isolated, so that the infection of the throat does not spread to others, while coughing, etc. The patient coughs out droplets of sputum, contaminated with organisms, into the air, which may be inhaled by other persons, and hence the infection spreads in a family/community.

Hence general measures regarding the prevention of sore throat, as well as its prevention in a community/family, who are likely to contract sore throats, are urgently needed, so that the disease can prevented, and its further spread arrested.

At the same time, steps should be taken to detect hidden cases of GN as early as possible, so that the disease can be brought under control, and further progress, including fatal complications, prevented. For this, the only way is to examine the urine for albumin in a population, preferably through various medical camps, periodically, say, six-monthly/yearly, as in the case of UTI, so that if the disease is suspected, it can be diagnosed, and treated.

Further, the public should also be made aware of this disease, so that patients can report to the physician for timely action.

Diseases of the Kidneys

Hence, prevention of sore throat and the early detection of GN are strong measures for the overall control of this disease.

3. Acute renal (kidney) failure — ARF

ARF is a condition when both kidneys almost suddenly fail to perform their functions. The failure occurs within a few hours/days. This may result from an acute disease of the kidneys, as a result of allergic manifestation operating gravely on the kidneys, i.e. acute GN, described earlier. Besides, sometimes blood pressure may be so acutely elevated, that it may knock down both the kidneys, resulting in their sudden/acute failure. Further, an acute infection of the kidneys (pyelonephritis), following some obstructive lesion in the urinary tract, like a urinary stone, or benign enlargement of the prostate, may also cause ARF, if the infection is not controlled promptly. This aspect has already been discussed under the head of UTI — urinary tract infection.

ARF may occur due to other conditions in the body, which cause reduced blood flow to the kidneys, so that the excretion of waste products from the blood is greatly hampered. Such conditions are common enough, and one needs to know about these. The most common is dehydration, due to loss of fluids in severe vomiting, diarrhoea, burns, crush injuries, etc. ARF develops when such conditions are not immediately attended to, and intravenous fluids are not administered in time. Similarly, severe haemorrhage from the body, necessitating immediate blood transfusion, may cause this condition. A similar situation arises when there is a marked fall in blood pressure (hypotension) due to heart attack/failure, shock etc., so that blood supply to the kidneys is adversely affected.

Another important cause of ARF may be the indiscriminate use of drugs, especially those drugs which are toxic for the kidneys. If one studies the causes of renal failure in general, one will find a substantial number — to the extent of 50 per cent in this group. These are called 'iatrogenic' cases, i.e. when the disease has been induced in the body by the person himself, for example, by the unnecessary use of drugs, etc.

How to suspect a case of ARF?

The most important step in the clinical diagnosis of the disease is that, as a result of the acute involvement of the kidneys, both of them become badly affected and their function becomes markedly deranged, to the extent that the kidneys are not able to excrete urine in sufficient/normal quantities. Thus, the patient starts passing less urine, and slowly the excretion of urine becomes so little, that on measuring it in 24 hours, it will be hardly 400 ml, while an individual is expected to pass about 1500-2000 ml of urine per day.

Serum creatinine and blood urea also rise. These are two important tests. ARF may be asymptomatic and detected when in the patients admitted in the hospital, the levels of blood urea and serum creatinine indicate a recent rise. As already mentioned, serum creatinine is a more sensitive index of kidney function than blood urea, which varies with the intake of food by the patient. Both the levels of these tests rise daily, if timely treatment is not initiated. Levels of serum creatinine have already been mentioned, and to repeat, normal levels of serum creatinine are 0.8 mg/dl to 1.4 mg/dl, with an average 1.00 mg/dl. If the levels of serum creatinine rise more than 8.00 mg/dl, urgent dialysis is required to save the kidneys/life of he patient.

Signs and symptoms of ARF

The clinical picture depends upon underlying causes, like acute GN (allergic disorder of kidneys), sudden acute rise in blood pressure (malignant hypertension), or it may be a case of acute infection of the kidneys (pyelonephritis), or an advanced case of dehydration (due to repeated vomiting, diarrhoea, etc.), or due to loss of blood as a result of sudden bleeding, or due to marked hypotension, i.e. fall in blood pressure in a case of heart attack, or acute kidney failure may manifest itself due to the use of toxic drugs, as explained earlier. Hence, the signs and symptoms vary with the basic disease the patient is suffering from.

Immediate treatment should be started whenever any of the above diseases/conditions occur, and a close watch should be kept on the daily output of urine. A general awareness is required on the part of everyone that whenever a kidney patient starts passing less urine, he/she should consider that the function of

Diseases of the Kidneys

the kidneys is markedly threatened, and therefore, it is advisable that the amount of urine passed each day should be collected and measured. It may seem very simple, but since collection of 24-hour urine is somewhat cumbersome and distasteful, people may not like to follow it. As a result, excretion of urine goes on reducing day by day, till it becomes around 400 ml, and at this volume of urine, kidney failure occurs. Even serum creatinine or blood urea does not run parallel to the initial damage to the kidneys. Hence, it is vital to keep a close watch on the volume of the daily output of urine, in the various circumstances mentioned above, which are responsible for sudden kidney damage/failure.

Initially, during the first week of the disease, the signs and symptoms are of the primary disease, i.e. acute GN, dehydration, etc., and the patient starts passing less urine than normal. If the condition remains undetected, i.e. specific attention is not paid, or the patient does not report to his physician about the low output of urine, the vital period for saving the kidneys is wasted, and the volume of urine passed daily goes on decreasing till it becomes less than 400 ml, when an acute kidney failure is said to have been initiated. Due to the retention of water, swelling of the face and other parts of body may develop. The patient will have marked symptoms of nausea/vomiting, drowsiness and convulsions, and even death may occur. Both blood urea and serum creatinine will be raised.

Treatment

The patient should be treated in a hospital. Most of the patients recover fully as the kidney has the unique property of recovering even when its function has been totally impaired. Besides urgent measures, the underlying cause of the ARF should be simultaneously looked into. If blood pressure is markedly elevated, it should be lowered with suitable drugs. If infection is the sole reason, it needs to be treated on the lines of UTI, already discussed. And, if there is some obstruction in the urinary tract, say, as a result of an enlarged prostate, etc., it should be immediately dealt with in the hospital, by a team of doctors, including both physicians and surgeons. In case of loss of fluids/blood, measures should be taken accordingly. If drugs are the causative factors, they ought to be stopped immediately.

What happens during the recovery of ARF?

With suitable therapy, blood flow to the kidneys improves, and the patient starts passing more and more urine, and in about a few days, conditions start normalizing. The general condition of the patient becomes better, and the appetite also increases. Serum creatinine, as well as blood urea, may also start falling, but usually these take much more time to come to normal levels, and, therefore, the biochemist should not be asked to repeat these tests time and again on the same day. Swelling of the face / body also starts decreasing day by day.

But is a word of caution. Sometimes during the phase of recovery, urine may be passed more than normal, in an attempt by the kidneys to excrete accumulated waste products. It may increase considerably, threatening the life of the patient again. Hence, both too low and too high an output of urine are serious in nature. Therefore, during the recovery period in ARF, if the patient passes more than the normal quantity of urine, and even otherwise, treatment must be immediately initiated, and a close watch kept on the blood chemistry of the patient. This is of utmost importance so that the hard-earned improvement in the function of the kidneys is not lost. Great vigilance, particularly on the quantity of urine passed during an attack of renal failure, during treatment, as well as during recovery, is required.

Urgent tests in a case of ARF

Again these depend on the basic lesion. Besides, urine examination, blood urea, serum creatinine, other detailed blood tests, like the estimation of blood sodium, potassium, etc., may be required. A plain X-ray of the abdomen, and ultrasonographic examination is needed in most of the cases. Even magnetic resonance imaging (MRI), which is a more sensitive test (non-invasive), may be indicated in a few patients. Renal biopsy to confirm the clinical diagnosis may be desirable in some of the cases.

When is dialysis required?

When the patient is not improving, i.e. the urinary output goes on decreasing, and, even in some cases, there may be a complete persistent stoppage of the excretion of urine (anuria), the serum creatinine rises more than 8.00 mg/dl, the blood urea, which is a

Diseases of the Kidneys

rough guide, also usually rises correspondingly, and the patient is also entering into a stage of coma, he has to be put on urgent dialysis to save his life. Dialysis is highly valuable in ARF, as repeated dialysis may not be usually required, as in chronic cases, and the cost of a few dialyses can be easily borne by the patient.

Renal transplant

It may be recommended in cases where, in spite of dialysis, the blood chemistry does not improve, i.e. the dialysis is not enough to bring the deranged renal functions back to normal.

Prevention of ARF

1. It is obvious that we should to prevent/control/treat all those factors/diseases which lead to ARF, like acute GN, UTI, urinary stones, enlarged prostate, etc. The preventive steps, including treatment of all these diseases, have been mentioned earlier, under respective heads.
2. Use of drugs indiscriminately should be totally prohibited.
3. Urgent attention is required in routine cases of dehydration/ loss of blood. Such cases are of common occurrence, and if they are quickly handled, kidney failure can be prevented.

Needless to say that awareness regarding the various diseases of the kidneys and other related factors/conditions is the only key to prevent ARF.

4. Chronic renal (kidney) failure - CRF

CRF is a disease which may remain asymptomatic/occult for several years, and may be even ten years in existence before it becomes evident. At that time, it is usually very late. The reason for the hidden nature of the disease may be because even a limited portion of the kidney remains capable of meeting the demands of the body, i.e. excretion of waste products from the body. Even in early cases of the disease, the symptoms (mentioned later) are so vague, that one can hardly suspect the presence of this disease unless one is highly aware of its possibility, with the result that, usually, the patient reports when the disease has gone to a fairly advanced stage. In such a situation, even lifelong dialysis, at varied intervals, may be required, which is an expensive affair. In such cases, if there is no dialysis, it means no life. One can thus clearly imagine the fate of those who cannot afford even a single, or more than a couple of dialyses.

What are the causes of CRF?

There are only 4-5 common causes of CRF, and if one reads them, it may look simple, but the situation is different. The causes relate to common diseases, which the person has not taken note of out of ignorance, neglect or apathy. The causes are:

1. *Undetected/uncontrolled*
   (i) Diabetes mellitus (Diabetic nephropathy)
   (ii) High blood pressure (Hypertensive nephrosclerosis)
   (iii) Glomerulonephritis (GN)
   (iv) Urinary tract infection (UTI)
2. *Indiscriminate use of drugs*

The above-mentioned diseases responsible for CRF are very familiar ones, and we only need to detect and confirm them in time. In other words, one should not allow these diseases to remain concealed in one's body. As already explained in the related topics, these diseases go on progressing very slowly, day by day, for years together, and still remain subclinical, i.e. the patient feels no symptoms whatsoever, and thus, they act like 'silent human killers'.

A patient may suffer from more than 1-2 diseases at a time. It is also possible that one disease may be detected at one time, and some others still may remain in a dormant form, in a particular case. The incidence of these diseases may vary from country to country, and even within different areas/communities of the same country. In some places, chronic GN may be more common, while in others diabetes and/or hypertension may be more prevalent. However, one may not be able to detect any such disease, or any other disease responsible for CRF in a particular patient. In other words, the underlying cause/s of CRF may remain undiagnosed, and this usually happens when the patient reaches hospital in an advanced/terminal stage, when both the kidneys have been fully damaged.

What happens to the kidneys?

As a result of slow or chronic involvement of both the kidneys, the size of the kidneys reduces, i.e. they become small in size. As the disease progresses, they become more and more small. An ultrasonographic examination of the kidneys can give a fair idea of the progress of the disease, by measuring the size of the kidneys. However, in acute renal failure (ARF), discussed in the earlier topic, the size of the kidneys remains almost their normal size, since the condition has developed suddenly. Besides the size of the kidneys, an ultrasonographic examination of the concerned organs may also indicate the underlying pathology causing CRF, e.g. BEP, or urinary stones, or any congenital abnormality of the kidneys, responsible for obstruction in the urinary tract, leading to chronic UTI. As detailed in the topic of UTI, whenever there is an obstruction in the urinary tract, chances of infection in the urinary tract increase considerably.

As a result of small/shrinking kidneys, their functioning becomes markedly deranged and blood urea, serum creatinine start increasing, leading to various signs and symptoms of CRF. This happens when the disease manifests itself in clinical form, after its hidden phase.

As time passes, due to the constant adverse effects of the disease on the kidneys, the size of the kidneys may be so markedly reduced, that their functioning may be adversely affected, and these organs may never attain normalcy, i.e., there may occur an irreversible damage to the kidneys, and the patient may have to live on repeated dialysis. Such is the importance of the kidneys in the body, and these are indeed vital for the life of an individual, like other organs of the body, e.g. heart, lungs, liver, brain, etc. Therefore, the kidneys should also be given due attention and care in maintaining the normal health of an individual.

At what stage can the disease be diagnosed/suspected clinically?

As already mentioned, the disease remains hidden for years together; therefore, it can only be diagnosed through a periodic estimation of serum creatinine and urine for albumin, especially in cases that are more prone to the disease, for example, those with GN, with a history of earlier attacks of acute GN, of hypertension, of diabetes mellitus, of UTI, etc. It is ideal if the above tests like serum creatinine and urine examination are carried out in all normal persons, at least once a year, and more preferably six-monthly, if facilities are readily available. At least a urine examination for albumin should be done regularly.

Even very early cases of the disease can be screened by a strip test called Micral - Test II, which detects microalbuminuria (MAU), i.e. a very small quantity of protein in the urine. More precisely, MAU is characterised by the protein in urine being 80-200 micrograms/minute. In this test, a reagent strip is dipped in the morning sample of urine. The results are available in one minute. The depth of the red colour indicates the intensity of albumin in the urine. Hence it is a quick and simple test, which can be carried out by all concerned. It is a very useful test for the early detection of renal/kidney involvement (nephropathy), as a result of various causes of CRF, in a mass survey/medical camps, etc.

If one fails to detect the disease in its hidden form, it should be suspected if the patient complains of any of the vague symptoms, like loss of appetite, general weakness, nausea, vomiting, more so in the morning, especially when these symptoms cannot be accounted for. Though vague, these are some of the early symptoms of the disease. In such cases, the level of serum creatinine can be determined in the blood, and if it is raised, or even slightly raised, it shows that chronic renal failure should be seriously considered. The raised levels of serum creatinine in the blood shows the extent of derangement of the functions of the kidneys.

What are the various investigations required to establish the diagnosis of CRF?

Besides a complete examination of the urine, serum creatinine, blood urea, ultrasonography, plain X-ray of the abdomen, and intravenous pyelography in some of the cases, are the tests required both for the hidden as well as evident cases of CRF. These tests will also help to detect the underlying pathology operating on the kidneys. Magnetic resonance imaging (MRI)/computed tomographic (CT) scanning, renal biopsy may also be indicated.

Besides various tests, a detailed history and examination of the patient will be required, so as to assess the level of the complications, which the patient may have developed over the years, as a result of kidney failure. Blood pressure readings should be taken, and if elevated, other tests mentioned in the chapter on high blood pressure, should be carried out. Similarly, diabetes should be excluded, and besides confirming a family history of diabetes, various tests for the exclusion of diabetes should be performed. It may be again said that both hypertension and diabetes are 'hidden' in nature, and a thorough probe must be made for the presence of these diseases, so that important underlying causes of CRF may not be missed under any circumstances.

A culture of urine may be required to see the growth of bacteria, if any, which may be acting on both the kidneys, causing their slow/chronic infection/damage.

However, in a complicated case of CRF, more tests will be required both for diagnosing the various complications, and for their treatment. In such cases, the patient suffers from various distressing symptoms which make his life miserable.

Complications / symptomatology of CRF

As the disease advances, various systems/organs of the body start deteriorating due to the collection of poisons/toxins in the body, which the diseased kidneys cannot excrete fully.

As already mentioned, the patient complains of marked loss of appetite, nausea and recurrent vomiting (especially in the morning). These are the early symptoms, and the patient may report only with these vague complaints, and at such a stage, it is only the clinician who can clinch the diagnosis, provided the patient reports to him well in time.

The taste of the mouth gets altered. A marked ulceration may follow in the mouth as well as in the stomach and/or intestine, leading to haemorrhage in both the stomach and the intestine, causing vomiting of blood (haematemesis) or the passing of blood in stools (melaena). There is a marked pain in the abdomen and the patient usually reports as a case of bleeding peptic ulcer. Loss of fluids, as a result of vomiting/haemorrhage, further deteriorates kidney functions as a result of dehydration. Hiccoughs are another symptom as the disease progresses.

In addition, blood pressure rises as a result of the damage to the kidneys, called 'renal hypertension'. Sometimes, the patient may be already suffering from high blood pressure, which may have contributed to the injury to the kidneys. Further, heart failure may occur due to the persistent elevation of blood pressure. In advanced cases, the pericardium, i.e. the membrane covering the heart may also be involved (pericarditis).

Fall in haemoglobin (chronic anaemia) becomes a constant feature of CRF. As the blood urea/serum creatinine rises, haemoglobin falls accordingly, and both are so correlated that even an estimation of haemoglobin, which is a simple test, can indicate the progress of the disease. The fall in haemoglobin occurs due to the toxic effect on the bone marrow, which gets depressed, as well as due to haemorrhages in the stomach/intestine, etc. Renal production of erythropoietin (EPO) is also impaired. Anaemia is difficult to treat as the patient cannot tolerate oral iron due to constant nausea, vomiting and ulceration in the gastrointestinal tract.

Soon the lungs may be affected, and the patient may experience difficulty in breathing (uraemic lungs).

In the same way, the bones may be affected (renal osteodystrophy), and, likewise, the peripheral nerves may be involved (neuropathy), and there may develop a marked weakness in the muscles (myopathy), and a number of other conditions like muscle twitches/tremors etc. may show up.

The brain or the central nervous system may be involved, leading to drowsiness and even coma. CRF or uraemia is one of the important causes of coma.

Sometimes epilepsy/epileptic fits may also manifest itself. Epilepsy may be the only presenting signal of CRF, i.e. the patient can present himself as a case of epilepsy, and if blood urea/serum creatinine estimation is done, his blood urea may be as high as 400 mg/dl, and likewise there will be a higher level of serum creatinine. Although such cases are not common, the estimation of blood urea/serum creatinine in all cases of epilepsy may prove rewarding, in excluding advanced cases of CRF.

One such case of a child (four and-a-half year old) came to the notice of the author, and he wrote to the noted specialist, Dr. H.E. de Wardener, Charing Cross Hospital Medical School,

London (author of the book *The Kidney*), regarding the pathogenesis of uraemia presenting with the clinical manifestation of epilepsy alone. In his communication to the author, Dr. de Wardener pointed out "... I don't know if there is a simple answer to this except to point out that in general children seem to be able to withstand renal failure far better than adults. We have seen boys of 17 and 18 who have been playing Rugby football a week before they come up with a spontaneous nose bleed and are found to have a blood urea of 400 mg%." Hence, it is clear that the whole phenomenon seems to be a complicated one, and that the disease remains hidden for long, and sometimes may present only with a solitary symptom, as a result of the complications of uraemia, like epilepsy or epistaxis (bleeding nose).

There may also occur high levels of blood uric acid (hyperuricaemia), as a result of blood uric acid not being excreted by the kidneys fully. This results in the various complications of high blood uric acid, as mentioned in the chapter on uric acid. Marked itching (pruritus) of the whole body adds to the misery of the patient, and it hardly responds to any treatment.

Hence, as a result of CRF, almost every part of the body gets significantly involved, threatening the life of the patient.

Treatment

A patient of CRF needs a specialist's care. Steps for the treatment are taken depending on the levels of blood urea/serum creatinine, serum potassium, complications/severity of the disease. Factors that aggravate the CRF, like sudden dehydration/loss of blood, or hypotension (fall of blood pressure) due to a heart attack, shock, including indiscriminate use of drugs, should be avoided so that the disease can be prevented from going to an advanced stage.

Underlying diseases, like diabetes, hypertension should be controlled. Those lesions causing obstruction in the urinary passages, like BEP or urinary stones, should be taken care of on a priority basis, because these are some of the causes that can be treated. In other words, a treatable case of CRF must be given immediate consideration, as it will substantially bring back renal functions towards normalcy. A special diet is prescribed in such cases to prevent further rise in blood urea, which is dependent on the food intake. Protein is specifically restricted in such cases.

Dialysis

If the patient is not responding satisfactorily with the above line of treatment, this means that he has gone to an advanced/end/ terminal stage of renal failure. There is, then, no alternative except to put the patient on regular/periodic dialysis to save his life. Besides unresponsive failure to improve with usual treatment, there is a specific criterion for placing the patient on dialysis. This includes raised levels of serum potassium, serum creatinine/creatinine clearance, refractory acidosis, and a bleeding diathesis. The periodicity of dialysis varies from case to case, considering the severity of the disease. But in such an expensive treatment, periodicity of dialysis, as is usually seen, depends more upon the financial means of the patient, since most hospitals cannot afford free dialysis for the whole life of the patient, and usually all patients cannot bear the expenses for several, or even few years that he may be expected to live. In such conditions, i.e., when the life or functions of the kidneys are dependent on dialysis, the life of the patient continues till the hospital/patient can bear its expenses. That is the worst part regarding the treatment of this disease.

Therefore, above all, preventive steps should be taken to completely avoid the occurrence of this disease, or at least, to prevent its further progress, when it is diagnosed at a later stage. However, the prognosis is promising when the disease is detected in time.

Renal transplant

It may be recommended in selected cases of CRF, provided a donor kidney is available, and the patient can afford the cost of the operation (which has its own risks) and the long use of post-operative drugs, so that the donor kidney remains safe in the body of the patient. However, the results of renal transplants are not promising in all patients.

Prevention of CRF

It is the most significant part of our discussion, relating to this malady. Preventive/therapeutic steps have to be discussed

Diseases of the Kidneys 211

under various heads, since the disease manifests itself in its various stages — for example, in its hidden form, early clinical form (when detected early), stable form, i.e. when the remaining healthy portion of the kidney is able to cope with the demands of the body. Therefore, preventive/therapeutic steps are required to deal with the condition at its various stages of manifestation, depending upon the time of the detection of the case. The aim is that the patient should not enter into the end/terminal stage of renal failure.

The awareness of the patient who knows the various steps regarding the manifestation of the disease, and the medical specialist's help in providing at least an easy life for the patient as far as possible, irrespective of the stage at which the disease has been detected, are essential steps. Above all, total prevention of the diseases (CRF being under immediate consideration) is the key aim of writing this book. Which means that such preventive measures should be taken, so that the disease does not show up at all.

The various preventive and/or therapeutic measures regarding CRF, therefore, can be divided into four groups:
1. *Total prevention:* That the disease does not occur at all in an individual.
2. *Detection of hidden cases of CRF:* i.e., if the disease is detected at this stage, it should not be allowed to manifest itself in clinical form, and the abnormal condition is reverted to normal with proper measures.
3. *Detection of early clinical cases of CRF:* If the disease is detected at this stage, preventive/therapeutic steps should be taken so that it may not progress further and damage the kidney, and the condition is reverted back to normal fully, or as far as possible.
4. *Preventive measures for maintaining stable cases of CRF:* This includes various the vital steps for its prevention/ treatment, which keeps the condition stable, and prevents it from progressing to an unstable stage. If preventive steps are not taken, most of these cases may become unstable forever, i.e., irreversible. In other words, they will not revert to normalcy, as the kidneys are damaged badly. In these cases lifelong dialysis is the only answer.

Now let us discuss each of the above heads carefully.

1. Total prevention of CRF

Kidneys can be prevented from any damage, provided one is careful to prevent all those diseases, at least the common ones, which harm the kidneys. Since CRF usually occurs as a result of undetected/uncontrolled diabetes, high blood pressure, GN, UTI, especially the cases where there is an obstruction in the urinary tract, due to an enlarged prostate, urinary stones, etc., all these predisposing factors/diseases have to be avoided/prevented right from the beginning/early age, so as to achieve total protection against damage to the kidneys. Therefore, it would be advisable to look up the preventive measures of each of the above diseases, mentioned under the respective topics/chapters.

Needless to say, that total prevention, through early detection and proper control of the above-mentioned diseases, is the most important key to keep the kidneys safe, for all practical purposes.

Prevention of drug-induced renal/kidney failure: Besides the above, an indiscriminate use of drugs is a serious cause for CRF. If all the above measures are taken care of, and equal attention has not been paid to drug abuse, CRF is bound to hit the person. In other words, no stone should be left unturned for the prevention of CRF.

All drugs should be used cautiously and under strict medical advice. Any of the drugs can cause renal failure. When drugs are administered into the body, they are excreted by the kidneys, directly, or as their end-products. Since the kidneys bear the brunt of handling the various drugs/chemicals, they are likely to be damaged by the various drugs, which are toxic to the kidneys, leading to drug-induced renal damage.

Various antibiotics, like ciprofloxacin, lomefloxacin, gentamicin, etc., pain-killers (analgesics), diuretics, radiographic dyes (used in various radiological tests like intravenous pyelography) are some of the examples that may prove to be toxic for the kidneys (nephrotoxic) and cause renal failure.

It is seen that people take drugs, especially pain-killers, tranquillizers, and even antibiotics, indiscriminately on their own, not once or twice but frequently, and even for long periods. It is not advisable, and today, even the food composition or intake

Diseases of the Kidneys 213

is properly monitored. Further, as mentioned in acute renal failure (ARF), the administration of drugs is an 'iatrogenic' phenomenon, i.e. the disease is induced by the patient, due to sheer ignorance. Hence it should be avoided by all concerned. One only needs to be aware about this and be careful in the use of drugs. If one is already taking these, one must stop all such drugs, and take medical advice for one's ailment and get the drugs prescribed, if they are at all required.

Hence, to prevent drug-induced CRF, the following steps should be taken:

(i) Use only the prescribed drugs, and only for the duration necessary for the treatment of the disease.

(ii) Use drugs with caution, especially in the case of patients who are prone to CRF, e.g. all cases of glomerulonephritis (GN), hypertension, diabetes, etc.

(iii) Besides the above, administration of radiographic dyes, which are used in certain radiological tests like intravenous pyelography, should also be discouraged, and other alternative tests should be done so that their use is avoided. If required essentially, all precautions must be taken, like the intake of fluids before and after the administration of the dye. Only the least toxic dyes, in their minimum dosage, should be used. Estimation of blood urea and serum creatinine must be done before the administration of the required dye. If these tests show higher levels of blood urea and serum creatinine, the dye should be avoided, as it may cause damage to the kidneys.

(iv) While on drugs, take adequate fluids, so that their excretion may become easy through the kidneys.

2. Detection of hidden cases of CRF

These cases must be detected. Since they are hidden, the only way is a periodic examination of urine, at least for pus cells and albumin, and if possible, serum creatinine among the general population, in camps, six-monthly/at least yearly, and more frequently in cases who have suffered from GN, UTI at one stage or the other, or are diabetic, hypertensive, including those who are in the habit of taking drugs indiscriminately.

In such camps, besides the examination of urine and serum creatinine, blood sugar tests, blood pressure measurement should also be carried out so that occult cases of these diseases should also be detected, which are responsible for CRF, and in this way CRF can be prevented. If possible, ultrasonographic examination of the kidneys should also be carried out to see the size of the kidneys. If the size is reduced, it shows that the patient is a hidden case of CRF, and the disease may manifest itself clinically, at any time.

Once albumin and/or pus cells in urine are detected, or serum creatinine is found raised, their exact cause must be determined, and a diagnosis of CRF should be established.

3. Detection of early clinical cases of CRF

In all such early suspected cases, when there are vague symptoms (page 206, second para), one must request one's physician to prescribe tests, like a complete urine examination, serum creatinine, for the timely detection of the disease. When such a patient reports, the physician takes the final decision regarding the various tests that he may order to eliminate CRF, as well as other possibilities that he may be considering.

Once it has been confirmed that the patient is suffering from early CRF, the case should be investigated in detail, and predisposing factors, operating on the kidneys, should be located, like, again, GN, diabetes, hypertension, UTI, etc., and all possible steps should be taken to control such factors, including the treatment of the patient as a whole. With this timely action, the damaged kidneys are likely to revert to normal. However, preventive steps and important lines of treatment may have to be carried out for almost the entire life of the patient. One has to be vigilant on this account forever, so that an early detected case of CRF may not revert to the hidden form, or progress further into an advanced stage of the disease.

4. Preventive measures for maintaining stable cases of CRF

Being on the borderline, this group of cases needs constant care. In this group, there is an irreversible damage done to the kidneys, and only a limited portion of the viable kidney is left to meet the just daily minimum demands of the body. So long as the daily

Diseases of the Kidneys

body requirements are met with, such cases are said to be stable. However, there are certain routine factors which are likely to disturb the normal functioning of the kidneys, which is being delicately maintained by a little portion of the kidney, leading to the worsening of renal functions. The patient then becomes unstable. The prevention of such factors, which shift a stable patient into an unstable one, is the most important aspect of the life of the patient, as once he becomes permanently unstable, i.e. the functions of the kidneys are impaired forever, lifelong dialysis/kidney transplant is required.

Hence, one may say that the condition is like the pendulum of a clock. By strictly adhering to the preventive steps, mentioned later, one can keep the pendulum towards the 'stable' side, and if it goes towards the 'unstable' side, one can quickly bring it to the 'stable' side by attending/treating the causative factors. Utmost vigilance is required to keep the condition stable permanently. Once the condition becomes unstable, serum creatinine rises quickly, but reverts to the original levels as soon as the patient's condition becomes stable again. When permanently unstable, serum creatinine may go on rising, and when it is markedly abnormal, i.e., above 8.00 mg/dl, dialysis will be required. Since after a period of dialysis, depending on the case, serum creatinine again rises, another dialysis is required, and so on. Hence 'unstable' cases will have to live on maintenance dialysis forever.

Various preventive steps to keep the person in a stable state are given below. The same steps should be followed by patients who are on permanent dialysis.

(i) Prevent dehydration

Since vomiting and/or diarrhoea, haemorrhage of the gastrointestinal tract, are some of the features of this disease, together with the use of diuretics in this condition, the patient frequently becomes dehydrated, and his condition may quickly become unstable. This condition is so sensitive, that if dehydration is not attended to immediately, serum creatinine rises in no time, and the patient may even become permanently unstable. Hence, quick oral or intravenous fluids should be given, and if need be, hospitalization of the patient should not be delayed, under any circumstances. If the patient is handled in time and carefully, he will soon revert to a stable state and serum creatinine will also come to its original level.

There are other everyday points to be kept in mind. To avoid the risk of dehydration, fluids should not be stopped in the morning, while taking morning blood samples for various tests or for taking X-rays, etc. Similarly, purgatives are not recommended, which are usually given the night before taking an X-ray of the abdomen, as loose motions may add to dehydration. As far as possible, X-rays etc. should be avoided, and blood samples ought to be collected very early in the morning before the patient wakes up. Further, surgical intervention, even of a minor nature, needs to be carried out with proper hydration with intravenous fluids, both before and after the operation.

Since a patient of CRF passes more urine in an attempt to excrete body waste products, both during the day and night, therefore he feels more thirsty. When more urine is passed during the night (nocturia), he may feel dehydrated/thirsty in the morning, which may bring the patient to an unstable stage. And if nausea/vomiting is also there, this will further add to dehydration, which will make the patient more and more unstable, if the condition is not immediately controlled. This can be prevented to a reasonable extent, if the patient takes a little water after each urination at night, or he takes water when he gets up in the morning.

In view of the above, it may be said that one has to know even the minute details in order to preserve a viable portion of the kidneys, and to prevent further damage to them. However, excessive fluid should not be taken which the damaged kidney may not be able to excrete.

(ii) Prevent infection of kidneys

There should be a regular/periodic check-up of the urine, for any infection/pus cells or growth of any bacteria. A CRF kidney is more prone to infection, and if infection is not prevented/ controlled, there is a danger of further kidney damage/failure. The infection should be treated on the lines explained in the topic on urinary tract infection (UTI). However, a word of caution — if on culture and sensitivity of the urine, various antibiotics are

Diseases of the Kidneys

available for treating the infection, only those should be administered which are least toxic for the kidneys.

(iii) Prevent obstruction in the urinary tract

In case there is an obstruction in the urinary tract, as a result of the benign enlargement of the prostate (BEP), or urinary stones, or some other cause, the obstruction should be removed. Since obstruction in the urinary tract increases the infection in it, it can further damage the kidneys.

(iv) Avoid unnecessary usage of drugs

A case of CRF should not take any drugs on his own unnecessarily. He should take only limited drugs, as prescribed by a specialist. Any indiscriminate use of drugs may immediately shift the patient to an unstable condition. If that happens, stop the drug immediately, so that his condition may revert to the stable state.

(v) Avoid radiographic dyes

As mentioned earlier, radiographic dyes should also be avoided as far as possible, since these dyes are likely to damage the kidneys. Thus, intravenous pyelography, etc. is least recommended in such cases. Now other tests are available. Moreover radiation has its own side-effects.

(vi) Strict control of diabetes and hypertension

Both these conditions, if not strictly controlled, will damage the kidneys further. Hence the prevention of further damage to the kidneys requires a rigid control of both these conditions. Hypertension is usually associated with CRF, and sometimes blood pressure may be markedly elevated, making the condition unstable, which must be brought to normal quickly, so that the condition returns to the stable level.

(vii) Strict control of diet

If this step is not strictly followed, the patient may enter into an unstable stage. And, if taken seriously, an improvement in the condition of the patient may be noticed. The diet of a patient of CRF is prescribed by the specialist. However, broadly speaking, an intake of more protein in the food will elevate the blood urea, which is dependent on protein, and this elevated urea in the blood will further worsen the condition of the patient, which should be avoided. Protein alone makes the condition stable/ unstable. A high-protein diet may make the condition of the patient so unstable so that a dialysis may become necessary. On the other hand, a low-protein diet may make the condition absolutely stable.

(viii) Rigid follow-up

A case of CRF has to be monitored strictly and regularly, even constantly. Depending on the condition of the patient, it may be assessed weekly/fortnightly/monthly. At each visit, serum creatinine should be repeated, besides a detailed check-up of the patient. It is understood that the patient will get his blood pressure and blood sugar, if diabetic, checked up daily. However, any sudden rise in serum creatinine should be noted carefully, and critically examined. It can be a true sign of uncontrolled diabetes/hypertension, infection, dehydration, necessitating immediate attention, and treatment. Otherwise the condition is likely to become unstable, either temporarily or even permanently. In such a situation, the condition of the patient is somewhat alarming and he may need dialysis at any moment. However, constant vigilance and quick response to any complication may keep the patient stable for years together. Maintenance dialysis is expensive, and may not be within the reach of everyone. Therefore, prevention of the disease is the only way to meet the situation.

It would be ideal if there is some national policy/programme for the overall prevention of this disease. At the same time, all hidden cases must be discovered/treated. Summing up, early detection, prevention, including mass realization about the various especially serious aspects of the disease, should be the key to such a national programme.

12
DISEASES OF THE THYROID GLAND

The thyroid gland is one of the vital organs of the body and is situated at the front and lower part of the neck. It consists of two lateral lobes (each lobe is about 5.0 cm in length, 2.5 cm in width and 2.5 cm in thickness) which are fixed on their back surfaces to the sides of the trachea, and are joined by a band (called isthmus), which crosses the front of the trachea, to which it is also firmly attached (Fig. 22). An adult weight of the thyroid gland is 20-25 grams.

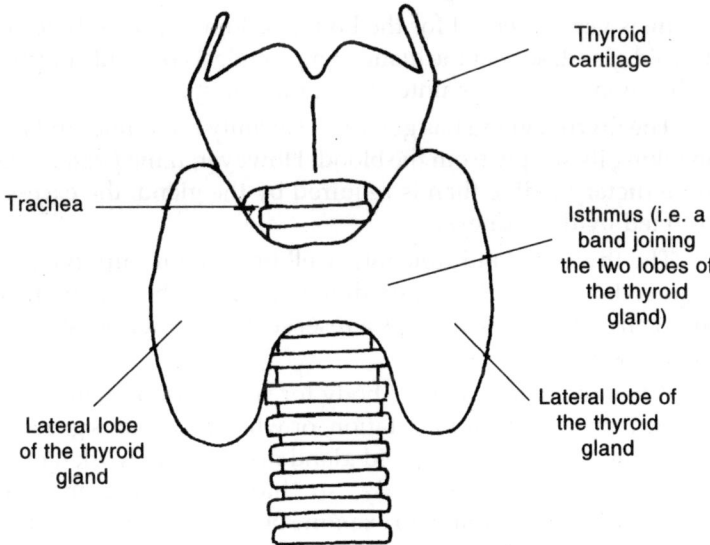

Fig. 22. The thyroid gland.

The thyroid gland secretes essential hormones called thyroxine or tetraiodothyronine (called T_4), and also a small amount of triiodothyronine (called T_3). These hormones are responsible for various functions/activities of the body. They regulate/maintain the metabolism of the body. Overactivity or underactivity of the thyroid gland occurs whenever the thyroid secretion increases or decreases as a result of various disorders of the thyroid gland (mentioned later).

More about T_4 and T_3

Normal life is hardly possible if the levels of these hormones in the blood are disturbed. As stated above, they are produced by the thyroid gland, and for their production, the thyroid gland needs a proper and regular supply of iodine. This supply of iodine to the thyroid gland is met from the food and water we take in our daily life. The iodine in the thyroid gland is converted into T_4, which is the chief hormone of the thyroid gland.

Some vital information about iodine and thyroid hormones

Iodine is very essential for the body, and more precisely for the thyroid gland, so that the gland can provide a constant supply of its hormones for the maintenance of the body.

The thyroid gland has got a great affinity for iodine, and goes on taking its supply from the blood. However, if the person takes more dietary iodine than is required by the gland, the excess is excreted by the kidneys.

The thyroid gland functions well on its own, supplying the required hormones, as per demand of the body. Even for emergency purposes, it keeps a reserve of these hormones in the gland itself.

When the demand of the body for such hormones increases, during a pregnancy or in lactation, or when the child is growing, i.e. during puberty, the thyroid gland may have to work more to meet the needs of the body, so that it may get enlarged temporarily. It is common to examine both boys and girls in their growing years, with enlarged thyroid glands. One only needs to assure them, emphasizing that such an enlargement of the thyroid gland is only physiological — called puberty goitre.

Diseases of the Thyroid Gland

1. What is goitre?

It means an enlargement of the thyroid gland, and in Latin, guttur means throat.

What is iodine deficiency goitre?

It occurs due to a lack of iodine in the diet, in vegetables and/or in the water. It is common among the people living in the hills, where the iodine content of the soil is limited, due perhaps to soil erosion by continued rains, etc. It is thus endemic, i.e. at such a place, one can find several people with swollen necks, as a result of an enlarged thyroid gland. More precisely, the disease is called endemic iodine deficiency goitre.

Hence, when the food/water taken by persons in such areas is deficient of iodine, the supply of iodine to the thyroid gland suffers, and there is a constant pressure on the gland to secrete normal amount of hormones. As a result, the gland goes on increasing in size, and even its shape may get distorted, and it may become nodular, the so-called multinodular goitre. In its initial stages, there may be only a smooth enlargement of both the lobes of the thyroid gland, as in puberty goitre.

Hence it may be said that the thyroid gland is very loyal to the body, so that even if there is a constant inadequate supply of iodine to the gland, it goes on supplying/manufacturing/producing sufficient amount of hormones for the normal activity of the body, although the gland itself increases in size enormously.

One may think that if the thyroid gland is enlarged, there should be a corresponding increase in the production of thyroid hormones. But that is not always so, although in some of the cases, the gland may turn toxic or hyperactive, or underactive, and yet in some other cases, malignancy may develop, as in cases of multinodular goitre. Hence the size of the thyroid gland may not indicate the true pathology developing in the gland.

Practical approach / hints for investigating a case of goitre and/or solitary nodule / s

In any case of goitre and/or solitary nodule/s in the thyroid gland, one needs to look for the following:

(i) Is it malignant?
(ii) Is any treatment required?
(iii) Has it caused hyperactivity or underactivity of the thyroid functions?

All the above points have been explained further, and they are necessary so that nothing remains undetected, and the specific treatment is not delayed.

Although an enlarged thyroid gland (goitre) may not disturb the functioning of the body, yet due to its enlarged weight/size, it may press the underlying trachea (windpipe) or oesophagus (food-pipe), so that the patient may have some difficulty in breathing as well as in swallowing. Cosmetic factors, especially in females, should also be considered. Thus, a portion of the thyroid gland may have to be removed surgically in selected cases.

Prophylaxis for endemic iodine deficiency goitre

As a prophylactic measure, in endemic areas, for all normal persons/children, iodised salts should be used as a matter routine.

Other causes of goitre

An enlargement of the thyroid gland may also occur in persons who are addicted to heavy smoking, and those who are taking PAS (paraaminosalicylic acid) for the treatment of tuberculosis.

2. Cancer of the thyroid gland

Early detection of cancer of the thyroid gland should be given priority while dealing with any problem related to this gland.

There may be a solitary nodule/s in a thyroid gland, or even a nodule/s of a multinodular goitre, which may be malignant. Or, the whole gland may undergo a malignant change.

Hence, nodule/s in a thyroid gland must be given prompt consideration, and if the whole gland is enlarged, one needs to palpate, to check if there is any hard/indurated area of the thyroid gland, which may be of a malignant nature. It may happen, especially when the swelling of the thyroid gland is of recent origin, and has rapidly increased in size. This aspect of malignancy of the thyroid gland has also been mentioned in the chapter on cancer, while mentioning major warning signals for the detection of various cancers (page 5, serial 10).

Tests for detection of thyroid cancer

Ultrasonographic examination of the thyroid gland and/or computed tomographic (CT) scanning/magnetic resonance imagining (MRI), as well as fine needle aspiration cytology (FNAC), help in establishing the diagnosis of the malignancy of the thyroid gland. A radioisotope scanning of the thyroid gland may also be required in some of the cases. It tells precisely about the hyperactive area/s in the thyroid gland.

Prophylaxis for thyroid cancer

Even if the above tests do not prove malignancy in thyroid nodule/s, still such nodule/s must be removed surgically as a preventive measure against cancer. These nodule/s may be responsible for the hyperactivity of the thyroid gland, and hence their removal is a must. Once removed, all such nodule/s must be subjected to histopathology which may prove very helpful in establishing the diagnosis.

3. What is hyperfunction of the thyroid gland (also called hyperthyroidism/thyrotoxicosis/hyperactive/overactive thyroid/toxic goitre)?

In this condition, due to the overactivity of the thyroid gland, there is an increased production of thyroid hormones which are constantly pushed into the blood, so that the whole metabolism of the body gets elevated.

As explained above, solitary nodule/s in a thyroid gland, or nodule/s of a multinodular goitre may become responsible for the overactivity of the thyroid gland.

The whole thyroid gland may become enlarged in many middle-aged or younger persons. The blood supply in such an enlarged gland may be increased markedly, so that on placing a hand on such a thyroid gland, a thrill may be felt. This autoimmune thyroid disease is called Graves' disease — named after Robert Graves.

As a result of the increased metabolism/activity of the body, the patient feels restless, tense or excited, and even emotionally upset. Fine tremors of the fingers/hands are usually noticed when the patient is asked to stretch forward both his arms with fingers opened wide.

Due to the same reason, the heart rate is markedly increased, and palpitation is a normal complaint. The pulse, while sleeping, should be counted to differentiate the condition from nervousness/anxiety, in which case the pulse rate should be normal. On measuring the blood pressure, the upper or systolic blood pressure should be elevated, and the lower or diastolic should show a lower level. The difference between these two readings of blood pressure is called pulse pressure, which increases in such cases.

In some cases, and more so in young patients, other manifestations of the heart, like supraventricular tachycardia, atrial fibrillation, congestive heart failure may occur, and one may think of a basic heart problem rather than a thyroid disease.

Another symptom of an overactive thyroid gland is a loss of weight in spite of an increased appetite. The skin is moist and warm even in cold weather, and one can easily feel this by touching the hands of the patient. Especially in Graves' disease, the eyes may look prominent, or may even bulge out (exophthalmos).

What are the early symptoms/warning signals of a hyperactive thyroid gland? Is it an occult/hidden disease?

In spite of the above symptomatology, the patient is often late in reporting his problem, may be more than a year, in some of the cases. Hence, whenever, one observes symptoms like palpitation, especially when there is an increased pulse rate in sleep, nervousness, loss of weight, one must look for a swelling/nodule/s in the thyroid and/or immediately consult the physician. It is not unusual to see the patient with a reasonably enlarged thyroid gland and he/she is totally unaware of it.

The disease may actually remain hidden for quite a long time, and may be precipitated when the patient feels mentally upset due to unforeseen circumstances. One should be more cautious when there is a positive family history of Graves' disease.

Diseases of the Thyroid Gland

Late cases of hyperactive thyroid gland

However, if the patient has neglected his ailment, all through, weakness of the muscles of the limbs may develop (thyrotoxic myopathy). He may even suffer from a serious disorder/emergency called thyrotoxic crisis.

Tests for a hyperactive thyroid gland

Since the hormones of the thyroid gland, i.e. T_4 and T_3 are increased in the blood, a blood analysis of the patient for estimation of these hormones, will make clear the diagnosis. However, for a screening programme for detecting the occult/hidden cases of hyperthyroidism, estimation of the serum free T_4 is ideal, since T_4 is the major hormone of the thyroid. Thyroid-stimulating hormones (TSH) secreted by the pituitary gland (see later) is a very sensitive marker of thyroid function and its levels in the blood get lowered during increased activity of the thyroid gland. Levels of TSH rise as the activity of the thyroid gland is decreased.

All thyroid function tests, like TSH, T_4 and T_3 must be interpreted with care. The levels of various thyroid function tests may be altered in patients who are on drugs like salicylates, propranolol (one of the antihypertensive drugs), glucocorticoids.

Other conditions in which thyroid function tests may be changed are in the case of patients who are taking nonsteroidal anti-inflammatory drugs. Or, in whom contrast media have been used for imaging studies, or in the cases of severe/recurrent vomiting during the period of pregnancy, although in such conditions, the effect is only transitory.

Further, in cases which are acutely serious, as a result of some disease, or in the case of patients who are suffering from severe mental/psychiatric disorders, thyroid function tests have to be read with caution.

It is important to note that all tests for locating a malignancy in a hyperactive thyroid gland are a must, as detailed on page 223.

Treatment of a hyperactive thyroid gland

Overactivity of the thyroid gland as a result of Graves' disease can be successfully brought down to normal levels by the use of various antithyroid drugs, and the one commonly used is neomercazole (carbimazole). While on antithyroid therapy, one has to regularly watch the activity of the thyroid gland, because it is a disease in which both natural remissions and relapses may occur from time to time. Hence, such patients will need lifelong care.

After initial therapy, the patient may be put on a maintenance dose of antithyroid drugs. As the drug shows its effect, TSH, T_4 and T_3 will return to the normal level, and the size of the thyroid gland may also decrease. However, at any time, thyroid activity may become low (hypothyroidism), even when the patient is on a maintenance dose of the antithyroid drug, as he may get natural remission. Therefore, TSH, T_4 and T_3 may have to be repeated frequently, when the clinical picture so warrants.

Further, the patient may even get a natural relapse of overactivity of the thyroid gland, while still on the maintenance dose of antithyroid drugs, and in such cases T_3 (rather early) and T_4 will rise, and will give the true status of the thyroid gland. Hence it is clear that thyroid function tests must be carried out from time to time so that the function of the thyroid gland is perfectly maintained, and the patient lives a normal, satisfactory life.

Radio-iodine or even surgery may be considered necessary in some of the cases.

In the case of solitary nodule/s responsible for the overactivity of the thyroid gland, after controlling the elevated activity of the gland with an antithyroid drug, these may be removed surgically for a lasting cure of the disease.

4. What is hypofunction of the thyroid gland (also called hypothyroidism/myxoedema/underactive thyroid)?

In hypothyroidism, as the name indicates, there is a decline in the functioning of the thyroid gland. The gland is either damaged as a result of an autoimmune disease of the thyroid gland, or in the case of an overactive thyroid gland, when more than the required amount of antithyroid drug has been administered. Similarly, hypothyroidism may occur following radio-iodine treatment or surgery, in cases of an overactive thyroid gland.

Subclinical hypothyroidism

The most characteristic feature of an underactive thyroid gland is that it remains asymptomatic for a long period, and there are only vague symptoms in the beginning. Sometimes the diagnosis is made when a person is undergoing routine tests for a general medical check-up.

The hidden nature of the disease is clear enough. Such early cases of hypothyroidism are suspected, diagnosed/investigated and labelled under the head 'Subclinical Hypothyroidism'. They may, however, still be in the infancy stage and have only minimal symptoms. This truly highlights the need for early diagnosis and treatment of all cases of hypothyroidism.

When to suspect subclinical hypothyroidism?

The disease may be suspected when the patient feels lethargic, especially in the case of a patient suffering from hyperthyroidism, who is undergoing antithyroid drug treatment, or radio-iodine therapy, or has undergone surgery of the thyroid gland. Or, the condition may occur in cases which have a positive family history of hypothyroidism.

How to diagnose subclinical hypothyroidism?

Once suspected, estimation of the thyroid-stimulating hormone (TSH) in the blood should be carried out. The levels of this test will be elevated significantly, although the levels of T_4 may be just on the lower side of the normal, or just below the normal level. T_3 does not play a significant/diagnostic role in the detection of hypothyroidism, and its level may be found within normal limits.

What is TSH?

It is a hormone secreted by the pituitary gland, lying in the brain, which controls the activity of the thyroid gland. This hormone has got a highly stimulating action on thyroid activity, so that as soon as the activity of the thyroid gland decreases (hypothyroidism), and the quantity of the thyroid hormone, the major being T_4 falls, or even when it touches the lower limit of its normal range, there will be an increase in the secretion of TSH from the pituitary gland.

Hence there is a close relationship between the pituitary and thyroid glands so that a normal level of thyroid hormones may be maintained in the blood as far as possible. (However, it may be said in passing, that if hypothyroidism occurs as a result of the involvement/disease of the pituitary gland, the levels of TSH will not be elevated, although T_4 may be on the lower side. Rarely there may be TSH-secreting pituitary gland tumour leading to high levels of TSH. Hence in a disease of pituitary, TSH levels may not prove useful to assess the functions of the thyroid gland).

Since the raised levels of TSH in the blood is the most sensitive/earliest index for the decreased function of the thyroid gland, this test, along with T_4 must be carried out whenever there is the slightest suspicion regarding the underactivity of the thyroid gland.

Does subclinical hypothyroidism require treatment?

Difficulty does arise in such cases. However, it may be said that in the absence of significant, rather troublesome symptoms, the physician will have to make his own judgement for the initiation of therapy. If no therapy is considered necessary for the time being, the patient must be monitored at least 3-6 monthly, so that the disease does not progress unnoticed. A thyroid peroxidase antibodies (TPOAb) test is useful in this disorder. If it is positive and the patient has symptoms that may be minimal, the treatment may be started. If this test is negative and the patient has no symptoms, annual follow up would be required.

As regards the size of the thyroid gland, in cases of hypothyroidism, it may be noted that the gland may be either enlarged or atrophied, or may remain normal in size. Hence the size of the thyroid does not indicate the activity of the gland, and, therefore, one has to depend on the levels of thyroid function tests in the blood.

What are the signs and symptoms of hypothyroidism?

In the event that an early diagnosis has been missed in a case of hypothyroidism, it is never too late. The disease must be diagnosed as soon as possible when it is in the most treatable condition.

Many of the symptoms of hypothyroidism are opposite to hyperthyroidism, so that it becomes easy to keep the

Diseases of the Thyroid Gland

symptomatology in view, to create mass awareness. Virtually, everyone is required to keep in mind such symptoms for the information of their physicians, so that the disease is diagnosed at the earliest, if not at the subclinical stage.

Since the metabolism of the body will decrease in a case of hypothyroidism, the entire functioning of the body becomes slow. The patient feels as if he has lost energy or vitality. The pulse/heart rate becomes low, and, in advanced cases, pericardial effusion (i.e. fluid in the pericardial cavity around the heart) may appear, which will markedly disturb the proper working of the heart.

In contrast to the overactivity of the thyroid gland, in hypothyroidism, the pulse pressure is reduced, i.e. the difference between the upper (systolic) and lower (diastolic) blood pressure is less, as in this condition, the systolic pressure becomes low, while the diastolic blood pressure is elevated.

The patient will gain weight in spite of a reduced appetite, due to the swelling of the body. The face will show thickened features, and becomes expressionless (in hyperthyroidism, the patient is smart and immediately responds to questions).

In hypothyroidism, the skin is cool (due to the constriction of peripheral blood vessels). It is dry and coarse, as the secretion of both the sweat and sebaceous glands markedly decrease. The skin may look a bit yellowish due to the increase levels of carotene in the blood.

The hair of the body tends to fall and becomes dry and is without any lustre. There is a loss of hair on the outer part of the eyebrows. Even a marked falling of hair of the head may occur.

The voice may become husky or hoarse. The patient may feel constipated (in hyperthyroidism frequency of stools may increase).

Among females, there may be menstrual disturbance leading to irregular excessive bleeding (menorrhagia). Sterility is also an important manifestation of the disease in both the sexes. There may occur failure of ovulation in females, while in males the sperm count may be reduced. There may be lack of libido as well as impotence. Hence thyroid function tests may be advisable in cases of sterility as well as in cases of dysfunctional uterine bleeding, especially when there is no obvious cause to explain these disorders. There are cases where periods become from irregular to regular with the treatment of hypothyroidism. It is most likely that the periods may become irregular again in case the dose has not been monitored regularly through thyroid function tests. In hyperthyroidism, bleeding during the menstrual period may be reduced (oligomenorrhea) and there may even be a stoppage of periods (amenorrhea).

The blood sugar level may fall (hypoglycaemia) in hypothyroidism, while blood sugar levels may increase (hyperglycaemia) during hyperthyroidism.

Hypothyroidism (myxoedema) may lead to psychiatric manifestations (myxoedema madness or mania). The patient's gait may become unsteady (cerebellar ataxia), and he may become unconscious (myxoedema coma).

Investigations for hypothyroidism

As already mentioned, TSH levels are elevated and the T_4 levels lowered. Other tests, like serum cholesterol, triglycerides may also be elevated in cases of hypothyroidism. It needs to be emphasized, that in cases of hypothyroidism, particularly where the thyroid gland is enlarged and/or there is a nodule/s relating to this gland, all tests for detection of cancer of the thyroid gland (page 223) must be carried out, so that a malignant growth/lesion in the thyroid gland may not remain hidden/undetected.

Treatment of hypothyroidism

As hypothyroidism is a treatable condition, therefore, irrespective of the advanced nature of the symptoms, the patient should take drugs with patience, and with a positive hope of recovery.

Since in this condition there is primarily a lack of T_4 in the blood, the patient is put on proper doses of eltroxin, which is a synthetic thyroid hormone manufactured by Glaxo India Ltd. As the level of T_4 in the blood increases, the patient starts showing signs of improvement in respect of various symptoms. The swelling of the body starts decreasing, and he starts showing signs of activity. The voice as well as the skin also becomes better. After about three months of treatment, the patient may appear quite fit, and in another three months, the levels of serum cholesterol and triglycerides and other lipids may also touch normalcy (page 81 — important steps for lowering high blood cholesterol). Usually, the treatment of hypothyroidism may have to be continued lifelong though in maintenance dosages.

A word of strong caution before starting treatment of hypothyroidism. A true cardiac/heart status of the patients must be assessed before the treatment is started, especially in the case of a middle-aged person. If the patient has associated coronary artery disease, the administration of eltroxin will increase the metabolism of the body, so that the output of the heart will also increase, when the heart is already damaged. As a result of this, a heart attack may be precipitated. Hence all tests like electrocardiogram (ECG), treadmill stress test (TMT), if required, should be carried out before starting therapy for hypothyroidism. A proper history of a previous heart attack/angina must be enquired from the patient.

The administration of eltroxin is safe during pregnancy and even breast-feeding.

5. What is cretinism?

In infants, thyroid hormones are essentially required for the proper development of the central nervous system. In case there is a deficient supply of thyroid hormones to the infant, or these are not replaced by proper therapy during this period, the child may develop permanent mental retardation, and the condition is called cretinism. Also, the growth of the child will suffer adversely, resulting in dwarfism. It is a congenital disorder.

A very early diagnosis of a cretin child is of the utmost importance. The condition should be suspected at the right time, by vigilant parents, especially the mother. Such a child is lethargic, sleeps during feeding, is constipated, does not hold up his head, sit, stand and walk at his age like a normal baby. In such a case, the early advice of the paediatrician must be sought, both for a precise diagnosis as well as for treatment. Ideally there should be countrywide screening programme for the timely detection of this disorder. In such programmes, the newborn needs to be examined and blood measured for the levels of TSH and/or T4.

Hence it is clear from the above that hypothyroidism must be suspected both in adults and in infants, at the earliest, both for early diagnosis and treatment, and for this, only mass realization regarding the early symptoms of the disease can help.

Unusual manifestations of hyperthyroidism and hypothyroidism: personal experience

Since both hyperthyroidism and hypothyroidism (thyrotoxicosis and myxoedema) are treatable conditions, any variant from the textbook description of the disease must be kept in mind, and the disease must be identified by carrying out tests, as described above.

The author came across a case of gross tremors in all the four limbs in a 70-year-old male patient. This patient had hardly any of the usual features of thyroid overactivity, as generally tremors of thyroid toxicity are too fine to be visible. These tremors are usually so inconspicuous, that the physician has to put a little piece of paper on the back of the wide open fingers of both hands of the patient, after the arms are stretched forward, to see whether the paper is moving or not. Under the circumstances, it was hard to imagine that the gross tremors the patient was having could be due to the increased activity of the thyroid gland. The general impression was that these could be senile tremors, at his age.

But this patient was in extreme distress. The tremors were so marked that he could hardly walk a few steps, and on standing, both the lower limbs trembled, making the patient sit or lie down, even at odd places. Similarly, the tremors in the hands were so marked that he could hardly write anything.

On careful questioning, the patient gave a history of loss of weight, and on physical examination, the left lobe of the thyroid gland was also found to be a bit enlarged. Since loss of weight is an important symptom of thyroid hyperactivity, therefore, this symptom alone should be enough to suspect hyperfunctioning of the thyroid gland. With this lead, the patient was investigated for thyroid toxicity, and it surprised many when the tests revealed that he was truly suffering from thyroid overactivity, causing gross tremors in all the four limbs. It was very heartening to the patient when he found that all his tremors, from which he had been suffering for a long time, disappeared completely, with proper medication. This brought the overfunctioning of the thyroid gland to the normal level.

Diseases of the Thyroid Gland

While the case was being investigated, the clinical data of the case were sent to Dr. Robert H. Williams, Professor and Head of the Division of Endocrinology, University of Washington, USA, who has also edited the *Textbook of Endocrinology* (W.B. Saunders Company, Philadelphia). In his communication to the author, he commented, "... I have seen patients who definitely did have a toxic goitre with manifestations similar to the ones that you describe. I think it is important, however, to demonstrate that the protein-bound iodine of his plasma is hyper-normal, and, if you have the opportunity to do an I^{131} uptake over the thyroid gland. I think this is worthwhile but not a necessity ... If, on the basis of all information available, it is decided that he does have a toxic goite, my approach would be to treat him with radioactive iodine". Dr. Williams was so pleased with our approach to this case that in his next communication he wrote, "Some day I hope to go to India, ... I will have the opportunity to see you."

Similarly, there was an unusual case of hypothyroidism (myxoedema) which came to the notice of the author. In this case, the brain was involved, and there was a variation from the usual manifestations of the disease.

It may be pointed out that there are several conditions of the central nervous system which are degenerative in nature, and most of the disorders are progressive ones, without any specific treatment. To take out the treatable, especially the unusual problems, out of this lot, is always rewarding, and a handicapped person becomes perfectly normal with medication/treatment.

The case, under reference, was a case of cerebellar ataxia, in which the cerebellum, a part of the brain, was involved, as a result of myxoedema (hypothyroidism). This made the person ataxic, i.e. the patient walked with an unsteady gait. If the cerebellum alone is involved, and there are other features of myxoedema, there may not be much difficulty in diagnosis and treatment.

In this case, the patient had some borderline features of myxoedema, and besides the involvement of the cerebellum the pyramidal tract was also involved. Thus, the diagnosis went more in favour of spino-cerebellar degeneration, which is usually progressive in nature, with no specific treatment.

Since myxoedema is a treatable condition, the patient was investigated and treated satisfactorily on the lines of myxoedema.

This case was also sent abroad for comments, and Lord Walton, then Professor of Neurology, University of Newcastle upon Tyne, UK, who has also authored *Essentials of Neurology*, published by Pitman, and edited the *Brain's Diseases of the Nervous System*, published by Oxford, while expressing his views said, "It would certainly appear that myxoedema is a strong possibility in his case, and cerebellar ataxia has been described as a complication of this endocrine disorder. However, myxoedema does not give rise to extensor plantar responses or other evidence of pyramidal tract disease, ... My reaction would be to suggest that as the only possible treatable disorder in this case would seem to be one of myxoedema, it might be best to try the effect of thyroid treatment upon this case".

In a serious patient of polyserositis i.e. when the patient has fluid in pleural cavity (pleurisy), fluid in peritoneal cavity (ascites), fluid in pericardial cavity (pericardial effusion) and also has developed massive swelling (oedema) of the lower limbs, the last possibility of myxoedema was considered and the patient treated on the lines of myxoedema with promising results. One such case has been reported from Ukraine. Pitting oedema (usually non-pitting oedema) in myxoedema though occurs rarely is well documented. The above case has also pitting oedema of the lower limbs.

Summarizing the above three cases, it may be said that unusual manifestations of both myxoedema and thyrotoxicosis must be considered seriously, and investigated, so as to bring to light such cases which are treatable, with promising results.

Lastly, it needs emphasising that the value of mass realization and early detection of hidden cases of the various disorders of the thyroid should not be underestimated. Somehow this aspect has not picked up the right tempo. Annual check up for the thyroid would be ideal. Thyroid function tests must be done, at least once in childhood, especially in obese children.

13
TROPICAL DISEASES

In tropical and subtropical countries like India, Pakistan, China, Japan, Africa, Australia, America, etc. (Fig. 23), some diseases like snake-bite, rabies, scorpion-sting, tetanus, plague, etc., are more prevalent. These may prove fatal if timely treatment or necessary preventive steps are not taken. In these countries, these diseases occur, in general, due to socio-economic conditions, a relatively hot climate, the inhabitation of insects and animals, overcrowding, etc.

Since most of the tropical diseases are preventable and there is a limited awareness about them in the general public, some important tropical diseases have been described in detail below.

1. Snake-bite

Snake-bite is one of the fatal diseases of the tropics. A clinical epidemiological study shows that Asia occupies the first position in respect of the incidence of snake-bite. In India, studies indicate that about two lac people are bitten by snakes every year, and that out of these, almost 15,000 succumb to the bite.

Which are the common poisonous snakes?

The common poisonous snakes in India are Cobras, Kraits, Russel's Vipers and Saw-scaled Vipers (Fig. 24). Snakes usually come out during summer and the rainy seasons especially during the nights and may bite anybody who happens to come in contact with them.

TROPICAL COUNTRIES OF THE WORLD

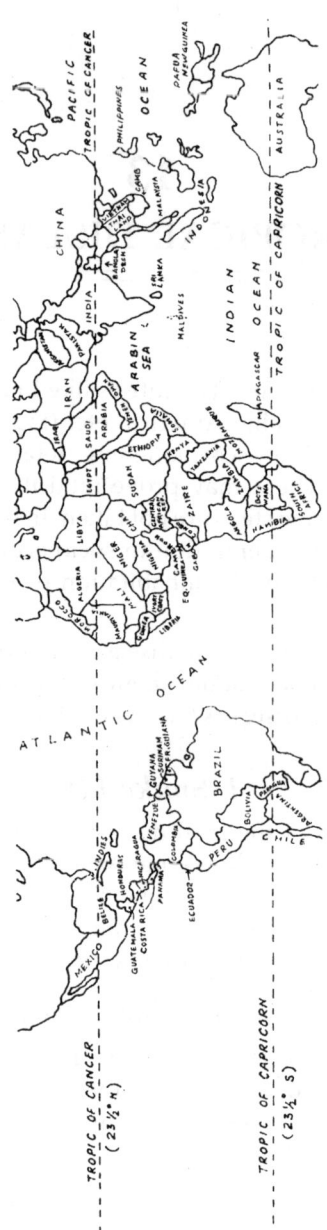

Fig. 23. The tropical countries of the world (situated between the Tropic of Cancer and the Tropic of Capricorn — dotted lines).

What are the symptoms of snake-bite?

Since the snake may be non-poisonous, needless fright or panic may create problems. The person may simply die of shock. However, one should be vigilant as the snake could be poisonous. Vigilance includes the awareness of various symptoms and signs that appear in a person immediately following the bite of a poisonous snake. In case the fang marks are present, it goes in favour of poisonous snake.

In Cobra's and Krait's bite, general manifestations mainly pertain to the nervous system. The patient will feel drowsiness, the eyelids will drop (ptosis), the gait will be staggering and the patient will want to lie down. The patient will feel a marked weakness, especially in the muscles of the limbs. He will have difficulty in speaking (dysarthria) and swallowing (dysphagia), and finally, starting from limbs, a paralytic condition develops.

In the Viper's bite, the symptomatology mainly relates to blood vessels, as the venom acts on the walls of the blood vessels, causing haemorrhage in various parts of the body, like the skin, mouth, stomach, kidneys, etc. Following the bite, the patient soon starts spitting blood, and if you ask him to cough, he may cough out a lot of blood. He may complain of blood in the urine, and may vomit blood. There may be several bleeding spots/areas, both on the skin and in the mouth.

In each of the above groups of poisonous snakes, the symptoms, as described above, start appearing within half an hour, and within the next four hours or so all the symptoms appear.

The severity of the symptoms depends upon whether the amount of poison injected by the snake is small or large (it may be only a dry bite, when in spite of the bite, no venom has been injected by the snake i.e. due to failure of venom gland-fang mechanism), the depth of the bite, interposition of clothing, etc.

In any case, following a snake-bite, whether poisonous or non-poisonous, the attendants or the patient should not be agitated unnecessarily, as in general, nothing will happen until the symptoms, described above, start appearing. As soon as the symptoms start, one should be very alert and vigilant, as there are about four hours for the completion of the symptoms, and this period should be sufficient to transport the patient to the hospital. Needless to say, following the bite, prompt first-aid measures (mentioned under the next heading) must be immediately initiated, irrespective of the type of snake-bite. One should not, ideally, lose time in waiting for the grave symptoms to appear. It is always better if the patient is transported to the hospital soon after first aid has been administered, without waiting for the symptoms of poisoning to develop.

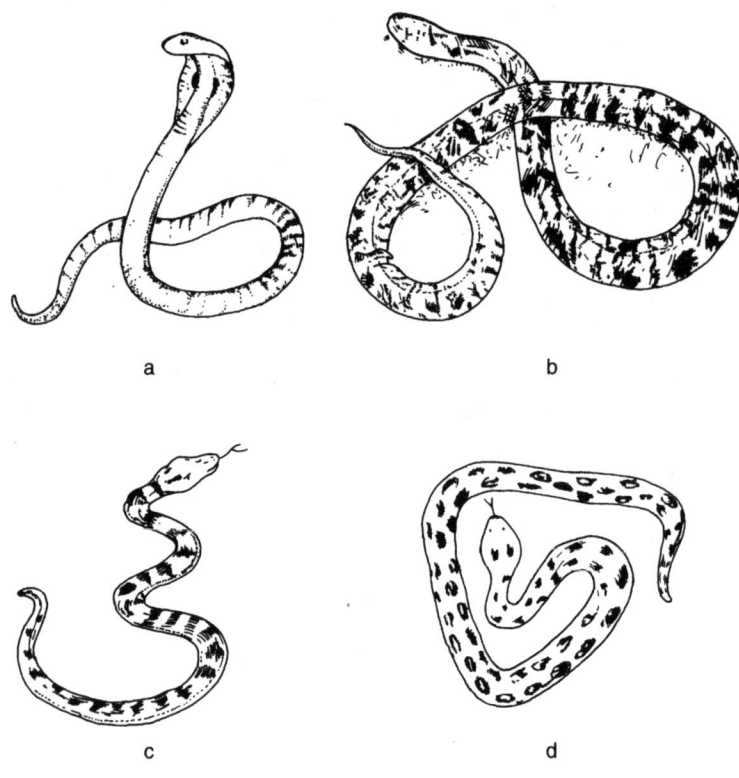

Fig. 24. a. The Cobra
b. The Krait
c. The Russel's Viper
d. The Saw-Scaled Viper.

What should be done immediately after the snake-bite?

Following the snake-bite, immediately tie a tourniquet/string/any cloth available above the bite. The tourniquet etc should be loose so as to allow two fingers underneath it so that venous return is not hampered. Make a small cross cut at the site of the bite, so that some blood comes out, which helps in the slow oozing out of the poison. In case the snake has been killed, it should be handled with caution keeping in mind that the snake can still bite up to one hour after its death due to reflex action.

Ice should be arranged quickly, and the bitten area should be put under an ice-pack, as freezing will detoxify the poison. Here is a word of caution. In case the nerves and blood vessels are exposed, local ice may not be applied to avoid their damage. If possible, and if the patient is collapsing, give an injection of Decdan (dexamethasone sodium phosphate), and if facilities are available, an intravenous 5% dextrose solution may be started immediately. The patient should be given an injection of tetanus toxoid, since the wound created by snake-bite may get infected from outside with tetanus bacilli. Tetanus prophylaxis is a must in all these cases.

However, it should not be forgotten to release the tourniquet after about every half an hour or so, so as to supply blood to the affected limb below the tourniquet. Although with this release of the tourniquet, some poison is likely to travel to the other parts of the body, this release cannot be avoided, and if kept long, the blood supply of the limb below the tourniquet will be markedly affected. This word of caution is very important to keep in mind, as, sometimes, it is seen that people, in their ignorance, keep the string tied for days, and come to the hospital when the whole limb below the string starts deteriorating/showing gangrenous changes due to the stoppage of blood flow. In such cases, there is no alternative left except to remove/amputate the limb, so as to get rid of the gangrenous part. It usually happens when the person is bitten by a non-poisonous snake, and does not seek medical advice. He only reports as a complicated case of a tourniquet which has been tied for several days. If such a person has been bitten by a poisonous snake, he/she will show at least some of the symptoms of poisoning, which will necessitate him/her to seek medical consultation. Such a case of tourniquet complication also came to the notice of the author. Hence, ignorance results in distress and even death.

Administration of anti-snake venom (ASV) and other measures in hospital

On reaching the hospital, the patient is quickly administered polyvalent ASV. Investigations are hardly required in this emergency to initiate treatment. The polyvalent ASV is the antidote of all the above four poisonous snake-bites. Since it is difficult to identify the snake, monovalent ASV is usually not given. Polyvalent ASV covers the risk for the bite of all four poisonous snakes.

ASV should be preferably given in hospital where all facilities like oxygen, etc. are available, so as to treat quickly any adverse reaction of ASV which may prove equally harmful to the patient. Anaphylactic reaction should always be anticipated while administrating ASV, as the skin sensitivity test done earlier may not be proving reliable in a particular case.

As soon as polyvalent ASV is administered, a miraculous improvement is seen in a dying patient within 15-30 minutes, and he opens his eyes and the bleeding stops spontaneously.

Polyvalent ASV should not be given if the patient has no envenomation, i.e., signs of poisonous snake-bite, because, as mentioned above, instances of a dry bite as well as of a bite by non-poisonous snakes are not uncommon. At the same time, family members of the patient should keep a close watch on the patient for the development of any symptoms of poisoning, which may appear even after a few weeks of the bite, say after 3-6 weeks, as in such cases, especially in the case of a Viper's bite, the venom may remain active for a few days or even weeks.

It is important to keep in mind that the tourniquet should be removed after the patient has received ASV.

How is ASV prepared?

It may be of interest to the readers to know about the preparation of ASV. In India, there are snake farms in Calcutta, Madras and Mumbai. The poison of the snakes is collected and given to horses in sub-lethal dosages. Blood from the horses is then collected from the major vein, i.e. the jugular vein and serum is separated from the blood, and the remaining red blood cells (RBC) returned to the horses. This horse serum is used as ASV as a life-saving drug for human beings.

What are the general preventive measures against snake-bite?

Those involved in field service should wear leg guards and have torches while going out at night. They should not walk barefoot, and should preferably use boots which cover the whole foot area. Also, one should avoid sleeping on the ground, especially during the night.

Development of ASV vaccine

Irrespective of the availability of foolproof ASV for the treatment of the bite of poisonous snakes and strictly adhering to some of the preventive measures described above, the role of prevention of snake-bite by vaccination cannot be ignored. Therefore, the development of a vaccine against snake venom is strongly warranted through advanced research and technology. Once the vaccine is made available, it will prove a major breakthrough in the prevention of snake-bite.

2. Rabies

Rabies is a fatal acute viral infection of the central nervous system, and it is one of the most terrifying diseases which afflicts mankind.

Although the disease is more prevalent in tropical countries, it occurs worldwide, and its incidence is ever increasing.

The disease is usually caused by the bite of a rabid dog. The virus of rabies is present in the saliva of the rabid dog, and when such a dog bites a person, the saliva infected with the rabies-virus is transmitted into the body of the victim.

Although the disease commonly occurs through the bite of a rabid dog, it may also manifest itself following the bite of a cat, wolf, jackal, monkey, cow, buffalo, etc. However, rat-bite does not cause rabies.

A bite is the usual mode of transmission of the disease. However, it may also occur if virus-laden saliva comes in contact with broken skin or a wound, or if one is licked by an infected animal. After being bitten by a rabid dog, the rabies virus becomes sequestered, i.e. it remains dormant at the site of the bite, without causing any harm to the patient. From here the virus travels slowly along the nerves of the bitten extremity, and reaches the central nervous system. It is interesting to note that while the virus travels along the nerves, it does not cause any significant damage to these nerves. On the other hand, it causes extensive damage to the central nervous system, making the condition of the patient horrible, as will be explained later. It may, therefore, be said that the rabies virus truly acts like a thief. It gets into the body and climbs to the central nervous system with the help of the nerves, without causing any serious harm either to the nerves or to the site of the bite from where it has entered.

The virus also reaches the salivary glands through the nerves and reaches the saliva either of the man or of the animal whom a rabid animal has bitten. This is how the disease is transmitted through the saliva of a rabid animal. However, transmission from man to man does not occur. But, at the same time, all precautions must be taken by the family members/friends and all others who come in contact with the patient. They should all take preventive measures and, in any case, the saliva of the patient containing virus, should not come in their contact especially with a wound/abrasion/cut, otherwise they are also likely to be infected. Gloves, aprons, face-masks, caps, glasses, etc., should be used. When the patient becomes violent, he may spit saliva on the persons/attendants standing nearby. Moreover, there is also excessive secretion of saliva in these cases.

Following the bite, urgent steps of treatment, i.e., care of the wound, etc., including vaccination (as explained in the next heading) are required to be taken, so that the disease does not manifest itself in clinical form. Once the clinical manifestations appear, the patient dies within seven days. However, the following symptomatology of the disease is required to be known to all so that those who are still ignorant can be helped, and necessary early steps of treatment can be taken, with the hope of saving the life of the afflicted person.

Early symptoms and signs of rabies

The symptoms and signs of rabies start after an incubation period (i.e., the period between the bite and the appearance of clinical manifestations) of, usually, 1-2 months. This long incubation period is a blessing for the patient because, if during this period the patient is immunized, he will be protected against the disease.

As soon as the clinical symptoms appear, the patient starts getting a tingling, numbness, and a dull aching pain, radiating in the affected limb. The wound caused by the bite will become inflamed, causing pain, and there will be abnormal sensations like pricking, irritation, etc. Soon the patient shows signs of restlessness, lack of sleep (insomnia), anxiety, etc., due to the effect of the virus on the central nervous system. The patient also starts complaining of difficulty in swallowing and there is a change in the voice due to the spasm of the muscles of the throat and the larynx respectively.

Late symptoms and signs

As the disease progresses, the patient will start getting convulsions in the whole body, although, in between the convulsions, the patient becomes calm and his mind also becomes clear. The spasm of the throat as well as of the larynx becomes more and more severe. Whenever the patient tries to take water, there is a sudden spasm of the throat causing intense choking. Due to this reason, the patient gets scared at the sight of water. This fear of water is the most characteristic symptom, and hence this disease is commonly called hydrophobia. At the same time, the spasm of the larynx also goes on increasing, the voice becomes hoarse, the patient may make odd sounds (owing to the sudden contraction of the larynx), and the sound may even resemble a 'bark'. The spasm of the larynx may be so intense that the patient may die due to the sudden stoppage of respiration (respiratory failure). The patient may also die during an attack of convulsions, due to heart failure. The patient normally expires within seven days after the onset of the symptoms of rabies. Sometimes there may occur a sudden paralysis of all the four limbs and the trunk, followed by coma and death.

Urgent steps after the bite

Following the bite of the rabid dog, or when the dog has licked a fresh cut or abrasion, or has scratched with its claws, or when the dog has run away after biting the person, unprovoked, follow quickly the undermentioned emergency procedure for prevention of the disease, without waiting for the symptoms of rabies to appear. Once symptoms of rabies appear, death is almost inevitable.

The most effective measure to protect against rabies is to immediately take care of the wound caused by the bite of the rabid dog, or any other animal, and immunization should not be delayed unnecessarily.

Care of the wound

The wound/s should be thoroughly washed with soap and water so as to completely, or as far as possible, remove the infected saliva from the bitten area. As a quick emergency measure, even water alone is sufficient for the purpose. A simple syringe filled with water may be used to clean the full depth of the wound so that the infected saliva is completely washed away.

Immunization

The patient should also be immunized against rabies. Since the disease manifests itself after a period of one to two months following the bite (incubation period), it is possible to prevent the disease by immunization during this period.

However, it must be kept in mind that the disease will start much sooner (i.e., the incubation period will be very short) if the dog has bitten on the neck or face or head, i.e., the area near the brain, since in such a situation the virus takes a very short time to reach the central nervous system. The disease will start a bit later (i.e., the incubation period will be relatively long) when the animal has bitten on the abdomen or the chest. Obviously, the symptoms of the ailment appear much later (i.e., the incubation period will be much longer) if the animal has bitten at a place far away from the brain, i.e., on the extremities.

The incubation period will also depend on the depth of the bite and the number of bites/tooth marks the animal has made. The more severe the injury, i.e., when the bites are deep and larger in number, the shorter will be the incubation period.

The above information is of utmost importance for the initiation of immunization therapy. If the face or head or neck is severely bitten, it requires immediate immunization. In such cases the symptoms of the disease are likely to occur as early as within about 15 days or less.

Schedule of vaccination

The patient should be administered the newly available, less toxic vaccine, i.e., purified chick embryo vaccine or any other available vaccine — like human diploid cell vaccine (HDCV) etc., after giving 1 ml of intramuscular injection in the upper arm (deltoid muscle) on days 0, 3, 7, 14, 28 and 90 after the exposure/bite (0 means first day of the injection of the vaccine). Although this newer vaccine is an expensive one, nothing is more precious than life.

The old nervous tissue (sheep and suckling mouse brain) vaccine is now outdated, as in some of the cases, it causes very serious complications, like paralysis of the extremities, encephalitis, etc., including mortality in a few cases. The author had seen a 25-year-old female patient who developed complete paralysis of all the four limbs on the administration of the eleventh injection of this vaccine, and in one of the communications, the case was discussed with Lord Walton, a noted neurologist in the United Kingdom, and it evoked wide clinical interest there. It is, therefore, advisable that the use of this vaccine should be abandoned, in case it is still being practised at some places, being cheap. Moreover, in the case of this vaccine, 14 subcutaneous injections of 5 ml each are given on both sides of the abdomen.

The above-mentioned newer vaccine has no such side-effects, except a mild reaction like headache, lethargy, fever, etc., and the dose is also small, i.e., only 1 ml.

Tetanus prophylaxis should not be forgotten, as there is every likelihood that tetanus bacilli may infect the wound and, therefore, a dose of 0.5 ml of tetanus toxoid should be given intramuscularly. A booster dose of tetanus toxoid may also be required later.

About the rabid dog and administration of vaccine to the patient

If one is able to catch hold of the dog which has bitten the individual, even if the dog happens to be a pet, should watch it for 10 days. During this period, one should watch the behaviour of the dog daily. If the dog is a rabid one, there will be a change in its behaviour and its appetite will become abnormal. The animal will start swallowing pieces of paper, stones, earth, etc. There will be a change in the tone of the bark of the dog. These are some of the early signs that usually escape the attention of the family unless one is extremely careful in watching the dog, and one has complete/full knowledge regarding such symptoms. After a few days, the animal will become highly excited, agitated, and may bark constantly for a long period. It will try to bite any person whoever goes near it. It will make constant efforts to run away. If the dog runs away, it will run long distances wildly and aimlessly, and may bite person/s, animal/s unprovoked, whoever it encounters. Due to excessive flow of saliva, there will be marked frothing in the mouth. The jaw of the animal will keep dropping and its bark will become high-pitched. In such a situation, it is obvious that the animal is a rabid one. One can imagine the extensive damage such a rabid dog will cause after biting several persons/animals, before it is killed. Hence there is a dictum that any animal that bites persons/animals without provocation must be killed. The animal should not be shot in the head, because its brain will be examined for the diagnosis of rabies. This point has been elaborated in the following paragraphs.

If the dog does not run away and remains chained at home, it will soon develop marked convulsions followed by paralysis. The death of a rabid dog usually occurs within 10 days. In that case, vaccination should be immediately started, if it has not already commenced. It should be started as soon as the condition of the dog deteriorates.

On the other hand, if the dog survives 10 days after the bite, and looks healthy in all respects, further dosages of immunization, mentioned above, may be stopped. However, vigilance over the dog should not be relaxed, at least for some more time, say for about a week, for safety's sake.

In case the dog has been killed immediately after a bite, it becomes difficult to establish whether it was rabid or not, and whether immunization should be administered or not. In such doubtful cases, the only way to establish the diagnosis of rabies in the dead dog, is to examine its brain for the characteristic lesion of rabies called Negri bodies. It is important that the whole head of the dead dog is sent to the laboratory for examination. If some veterinary surgeon is available, the brain may be taken out and sent to the laboratory in glycerine and not in ice. There are places like the Central Research Institute, Kasauli (HP), in India, where round-the-clock-service is available for this test. In case the test report shows that the killed animal was rabid, immunization should be started immediately, if not already commenced. If the result does not show rabies, immunization, if it has started, should be stopped at once.

Treatment

However, if the person unfortunately becomes the victim of rabies, the symptoms of the patient must be relieved by various drugs, and he/she should be kept in a dark quiet place, to avoid convulsions. Strong sedatives/anticonvulsant drugs should be used, and intravenous fluid therapy should be adequately administered. Under no circumstances should the care of the patient be relaxed, as, though the disease is usually fatal, recovery has been reported in a few cases. Moreover, with good therapy, the patient's death will be peaceful.

Prevention

Since the disease is invariably fatal, there is no other way of escaping from this disease than by a foolproof method of prevention. There should be a regular education campaign for the public, emphasizing the various steps for controlling this lethal disease.

At the outset, all stray dogs responsible for rabies should be killed. At the same time, all pet/domestic animals should be vaccinated against rabies. A mass immunization programme to vaccinate all the animals is of the utmost importance.

It is essential to see that domestic/pet animals do not come in contact with stray animals, especially rabid ones, and whenever a rabid dog/animal is reported, there should be a thorough search conducted by the local authorities to trace and kill such an animal.

Truly speaking, a national campaign is needed for the prevention of rabies in animals, and this is an important step which will go a long way in the eradication of this deadly disease. It has already been eradicated in many countries.

It is appropriate that all persons working at places prone to rabies, such as research laboratories or veterinary centres, are vaccinated with at least three doses of one of the newer vaccines, on days 0, 7, 21. If the place of work is highly susceptible to this affliction, booster doses of the vaccination, say after every six months, should be given.

Finally, besides a strict follow-up of the above-said preventive measures, a suitable anti-rabies drug is urgently awaited, so that those afflicted with this disease can be saved.

3. Scorpion-sting

Scorpion-sting poisoning is one of the common life-threatening problems in many tropical countries (Fig. 25).

The period between the scorpion-sting and the death of the person involved may range between a few minutes to about 24 hours. And, therefore, it can be imagined how quickly one has to transport the patient, as following the sting, the patient may collapse almost immediately, and may go into a state of shock, especially when the scorpion happens to be highly poisonous. The difficulty generally arises when the patient has been bitten in a rural area, and the peripheral health centre has no facilities for treating such grave emergencies. Even transportation takes time, and by the time the patient is carried to the main hospital, he is likely to enter into an irreversible deteriorated condition, leading to death. The scorpion venom is also much more toxic/lethal than snake venom, and the amount of venom being minute, it is absorbed into the body in no time.

Are all types of scorpions dangerous?

Not all species of scorpions are dangerous/fatal. There are about 650 species of scorpions. In India, out of these, about 50 are poisonous in nature, and their bite may be fatal. The only difficulty is that following the sting, it is not possible to identify which one is dangerous and will cause almost instantaneous death.

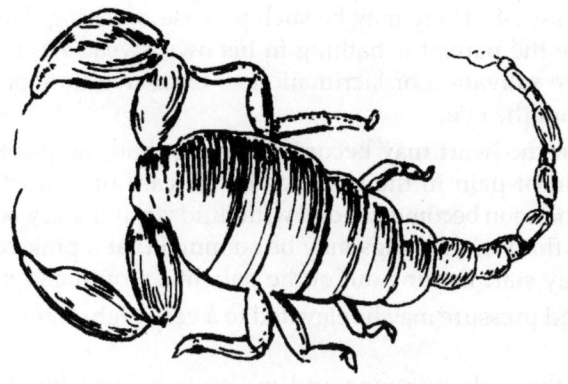

Fig. 25. The scorpion.

On the other hand, some species of scorpions, say about 35 in India, are non-poisonous. The problem again, as mentioned above, is only of identification, and when symptoms of scorpion poisoning start appearing say, even within 2-3 hours, in some of the mild to moderate cases, it may be too late, and death is inevitable, as explained above.

What are the various fatal symptoms and signs of scorpion poisoning?

Following the poisonous sting, within minutes, the patient collapses suddenly, with grave symptoms and signs of poisoning. If he does not collapse at once, beware, he is likely to collapse any time during the next half an hour, depending on the extent of the poison absorbed. The severity of the various symptoms and signs, described below, may vary with the species of the scorpion.

Since scorpion venom is known to cause an injurious effect on the various vital systems of the body, simultaneously, e.g. on the nervous system, cardiovascular/respiratory system, etc., the patient develops many types of serious problems pertaining to several organs of the body. It appears as if the patient is suffering from various lethal diseases at the same time.

The patient becomes markedly restless and shows signs of drowsiness, and may even become unconscious. He may also complain of marked palpitation and difficulty in breathing, or breathlessness. There may be such profuse sweating that it may look like the patient is bathing in his own sweat. Also, there is excessive salivation or lacrimation — excessive flow of water/tears from the eyes.

Soon the heart may become irregular, and the patient may complain of pain in the chest, as in the case of a heart attack. Lungs too soon become flooded with fluids (pulmonary oedema), and the fluid in the lungs may be so much that a pink-coloured froth may start flowing out of the patient's mouth and nostrils.

Blood pressure may be elevated to a very high degree in some cases.

All these fluctuations and multiple system involvement make the condition of the patient not only grave, but also make its management highly difficult and complicated, even in a well-equipped hospital with intensive care unit (ICU) facilities, not to speak of peripheral health centres/hospitals, where facilities are bound to be inadequate.

As time passes, the condition of the patient becomes more serious. Besides these grave deteriorating conditions, other systems may also be involved. Haemorrhage may occur in different parts of the body. The patient may vomit blood, or pass blood in the faeces or in urine. Paralysis of one side of the body (hemiplegia) may occur due to haemorrhage in the brain. Pancreatitis may also occur, causing intense pain in the abdomen. The patient enters into such a deplorable condition, that he even passes urine, stools involuntarily, in a state of delirium.

In such serious cases, death usually occurs instantaneously, or any time within 24 hours. Chances of recovery may brighten when symptoms and signs are not highly fatal from the very beginning, and the patient reaches a suitable hospital at the early stage of the disease. It is all a matter of luck and chance! It is, indeed, a time-bound fatal emergency.

Caution

A word of caution may be mentioned here. All cases of scorpion-sting must be admitted to a hospital, irrespective of age, local or general symptoms and signs. Even when the patient shows no symptoms whatsoever, hospital consultation/detailed investigation and treatment is necessary. Every case of scorpion-sting should be considered highly dangerous, and its severity must be assessed in the hospital.

Treatment in hospital

On reaching the hospital, irrespective of the severity of the disease, all possible efforts must be made to save the life of the patient. Treatment/investigations entirely depend on the condition as well as the system/s of the body that has/have been adversely affected. Complications relating to cardiovascular/respiratory/neurological/haemotological system are taken care of accordingly.

In general, the patient is put on an intravenous drip, oxygen, antibiotics and sedatives, since he may be feeling restless. Urgent drugs are given for the treatment of heart/respiratory/neurological problems, depending on the case. Immediate blood transfusion may be required, especially when haemorrhage has started in the gastrointestinal/urinary tract, etc. Strong antihypertensive drugs ought to be immediately administered, to lower very high blood pressure, as happens in many of the cases.

The patient is constantly monitored, and such cases are always kept in the ICU of the hospital, so that fatal complications, as and when they occur, may be immediately tackled.

How far are early symptoms / signs useful?

Early signs and symptoms or warning signals do help, especially when the scorpion-sting is not highly poisonous, and it does not cause sudden death. We must know these warning signals.

Although following a sting, urgent steps for hospitalization should not be delayed under any circumstances, yet as soon as early symptoms and signs appear, more vigorous steps should be taken for carrying the patient to a well-equipped medical centre/hospital. Aid from the local physician/hospital may also be taken if proper arrangements are available. It should be stressed again that a case of scorpion-sting is never safe till the involved person actually starts receiving aid in a suitable hospital.

About the early signs and symptoms/warning signals, any person who starts vomiting and has excessive perspiration, salivation/lacrimation, and on examination, blood pressure is high or alarmingly raised, one should realize that the grave symptoms and signs (already described) of scorpion-poisoning are imminent, and the life of the patient is threatened. In the beginning following sting, if the patient complains of parasthesias radiating from the site of sting, it should be considered as an important early symptom of poisoning for immediate action.

Does immediate local care of sting help?

If the patient is already in a state of shock, and the symptoms and signs of collapse have already appeared, there is no use wasting time on local therapy. Once manifestations of scorpion-poisoning have developed, or are developing, local therapy will prove to be of little value.

However, if time permits, local first aid may be given at once, provided someone is available on the spot, and he is aware of the procedure of immediate aid in such cases. All steps of first aid for scorpion-sting must be known by all, as it may be said, particularly in the context of this emergency, that the difference between life and death is so small, that only someone who knows what to do in such a difficult situation can be useful. One can never know where 'someone' will be required to give urgent aid to a case of scorpion-sting, and save the precious life of a patient.

Local symptoms include intense pain at the site of the sting, and the patient feels marked uneasiness in the entire limb. There may be itching and a pricking type of sensation in the area of the sting. The site of the sting may become red and swollen.

Various steps of prompt local aid/treatment to the victim are as given below:

Immediately apply a string or a piece of cloth/tourniquet on the part of the body just above the site of the sting. However, it should always be kept in mind to release the tourniquet after every half an hour, so that the blood supply below the tourniquet does not suffer.

At the same time, rub pieces of ice on the site of the sting, or pour ice-cold water over the area. The entire affected portion of the limb may be chilled with iced water.

A local incision/cut is not helpful. However, a strong solution of ammonia may be applied to the sting site and this may neutralise the acid poison of the scorpion. Since the pain at the sting site may be unbearable, a local anaesthesia may be used immediately, if possible, otherwise, any pain-killer injection may be administered.

Any of the above urgent first-aid measures may not help to save the patient. However, these measures must be tried as far as possible, if the situation requires it.

Tetanus prophylaxis should never be forgotten, as tetanus organisms are known to enter even the smallest wound, and scorpion-sting is no exception. Thus, an injection of tetanus toxoid should be administered as soon as possible.

One must be aware of visiting quacks or unqualified persons who claim to treat scorpion-sting cases. Doing so would only delay treatment in a hospital, resulting in dangerous consequences.

What about scorpion antivenin?

Scorpion antivenin is available, and would be certainly useful if administered in very early cases, both locally, i.e., into the site of the sting, and intravenously.

There is a general view that scorpion antivenin does not prove to be effective in many cases of scorpion-sting. One of the important reasons for its ineffectiveness may be that it is usually administered in very serious as well as late cases, when several complications have already occurred. The antivenin may also not be a specific antidote for the species of scorpion that has bitten the person. However, its use should not be overlooked even in advanced cases, as it may prove to be a ray of hope for a dying patient.

Preventive measures

1. A scorpion is a small creature, about 6-10 cm long. It has a segmented body, with two poisonous glands in its tail. It holds its victim with its claws and pushes forward the tail and injects the poison into the body (Fig. 25).

   The scorpion is nocturnal in nature, i.e. it moves around during the night. During the day it remains hidden in various dark places, like in shoes, in clothes/bedding, on the ground, behind the furniture, They are also found in various cracks in the walls, and under rocks, in vegetation/gardens, etc.

They usually move about during the warm season and, therefore, scorpion-stings are likely to occur more in summer, during the night.

Usually they do not jump and sting a person. They bite when someone comes into contact with them, or disturbs them. Children, being ignorant, while catching scorpions, may get bitten.

In view of the above, various prophylactic steps are suggested below:

(i) Shoes should be shaken out before use, especially old ones lying in one place for a long time.

(ii) All clothing, especially towels, bed sheets, blankets, etc., should be closely checked before use.

(iii) The space between the walls and the furniture should be regularly and carefully cleaned.

(iv) All holes/cracks in walls/floors/foundations of the old houses should be plugged and necessary repairs should be undertaken. One should not sleep on the ground.

(v) All rubbish in and around the house should be removed.

(vi) There should be proper maintenance of the lawns of the house.

(vii) Public places, especially gardens, should be carefully inspected, and children should not play there in the dark.

(viii) Persons, especially children, while on tour/trekking/a picnic should not disturb the area beneath the rocks, and should not go near heavy vegetation, or where a lot of debris is lying. One should wear boots in such situations.

(ix) If the particular area is more prone to scorpions, selected pesticides should be used at various places in the house, as well as in the garden/lawns, as a safeguard against scorpions.

2. Scorpion-sting is indeed a public health hazard. Besides abiding by the above preventive measures, which should be meticulously followed, primary health centres, especially in rural areas, where the chances of the presence of scorpions are

Tropical Diseases

greater, should be reasonably equipped, so that cases of scorpion-sting are given proper urgent first-aid measures, while referring the patient to a large hospital, so that the life of the patient is saved.

This information regarding scorpion-sting makes it clear that prevention is the only right way to deal with the problem, which if it is not heeded, has lethal consequences.

4. Tetanus

Why is tetanus still there?

Tetanus is one of the most serious diseases of the tropics and invariably proves fatal, especially when the person is severely affected. In spite of the availability of a highly potent vaccine against tetanus, the dreaded disease is still around. The reason is that a regular schedule of vaccination is not being strictly followed by everyone. The other reason may be poor hygienic conditions at some places. Above all, the main cause is the ignorance of the people. It is seen, even now, at some places, that the dressing of the wound of the umbilical cord of the newborn is done with cow-dung or horse-dung, etc., or with unsterilized powder, which could be infected with tetanus spores, leading to tetanus in the newborn. So much so that, some years back, when various campaigns for the eradication of smallpox were launched, children, of course, unknowingly, used to put earth (which is usually contaminated with tetanus spores) from the ground on the various insertions/wounds created by the rotary lancet, while vaccinating the children for smallpox, with the result that the vaccinated areas used to get infected with the tetanus spores, causing tetanus in the children. The author has also discussed such cases under the head 'Tetanus following smallpox vaccination' in the September 1967 issue of the journal, *Current Medical Practice*.

What are tetanus spores?

Tetanus is caused by an organism called Clostridium tetani (C. tetani). It is a slender bacillus which bears a round terminal spore. The spore gives a drumstick-like appearance. It may be noted that tetanus spores are highly resistant and are ubiquitous, i.e. present everywhere in the soil/dust. They are so resistant that they can survive in the soil/dust even for years.

Since the C. tetani also live in the intestine of horses and other animals (of course without causing any harm to them), these organisms are found in their faeces. As a result, fields which have been subjected to manure containing the faeces of such animals, carry C. tetani in abundance, and, therefore, one should be particularly aware of such a high-risk area, to safeguard against tetanus.

How does a person get a tetanus infection?

Whenever an unimmunized or poorly-immunized person gets an injury, especially on the roadside, he is likely to get the tetanus infection from the soil/dust containing tetanus spores.

The tetanus spores survive better wherever there is a poor oxygen supply. Therefore, these spores will live better wherever the wound/s are severed with deep lacerations, because the oxygen supply is minimal there. If such a wound is not properly cared for immediately, the dirt or foreign bodies, etc. are not surgically removed, and the dressing is done without taking all precautions regarding sterilization, pus/necrotic tissue will develop in the wound, causing further deterioration in the supply of oxygen. Under these circumstances, such a grossly-infected wound will become a safe haven for the germination of tetanus spores into vegetative forms, that will produce the most poisonous toxin in the wound. This toxin reaches the central nervous system, leading to extremely troublesome and distressing manifestations of the disease. However, the C. tetani remain confined to the wound and are harmless themselves. It is only the toxin produced by these organisms which causes various injurious effects on the body, with fatal consequences in many of the cases.

What are the various types of wounds responsible for causing tetanus?

Besides roadside injuries, tetanus may occur from various wounds caused by cuts, especially while working in fields/gardens, or when a deep punctured wound occurs in the case of mechanics engaged in various factories/workshops, etc. Tetanus may also manifest itself in patients with bed sores, or wounds caused by splints, or in cases of burns, skin ulcers or, following tooth extraction. It may be due to gunshot wound as well. A simple pinprick, injury by nail, thorn may also cause this problem. Fishermen may also suffer from it when they get an injury while handling the fish-hook. Frost-bite can also prove dangerous in some cases.

Tetanus may appear when injections or intravenous drips are given without proper sterilization. It is usually seen when drug addicts do not use properly sterilized needles/syringes.

The disease is known to occur when the wound is a tiny one, which can hardly be seen and is completely forgotten/healed. In such cases, the patient did suffer from an injury sometime or the other.

Sometimes tetanus breaks out even in the wards of hospitals. It happens when the various materials used are not adequately sterilized. As already mentioned, tetanus spores are highly resistant in nature, and require very high temperature for sterilization/autoclaving. Boiling for at least 4-5 hours is required to eliminate these spores. In operation cases, tetanus spores get free from the unsterilized material, e.g. cat-gut, gauze, cotton, etc., the wounds caused by the operation serve as the portals of entry for tetanus spores, and their further germination into vegetative forms, which are responsible for the secretion of the toxin.

A pregnant woman may also become the victim of tetanus by a wound caused during labour/child-birth. It usually happens when the woman has not been properly vaccinated against tetanus during her period of pregnancy.

Newborn babies may become infected, as a result of tetanus, when the cut ends of their umbilical cords, or any other injuries, they have suffered during their birth, have not been properly treated, with the result that such wound/s get infected by tetanus spores.

Tetanus may also develop in cases of ear discharge (otitis media), when the tetanus spores which may be present in the discharge of the ear, gain entry into the body through perforation/s in the eardrum of these patients. Such cases are called 'otogenic tetanus'. This is of great importance, because such cases usually remain ignored till they get tetanus. This calls for energetic treatment of the prevailing disease of the ear, as well as urgent vaccination against tetanus. Usually, these cases have not been vaccinated for tetanus earlier. Cases of otogenic tetanus are not uncommon. The author discussed such cases in one of the issues of *Current Medical Practice*. The disease is more common among children, and the parents should have the requisite awareness about this disease.

Warning signals of tetanus

Warning signals of tetanus should be kept in mind, because the disease could occur even when the injury is minor and totally forgotten. In that case, probably, the injury was so minimal that the patient may not have cared to take a booster dose of the vaccination, or may have remained entirely unimmunized. In such cases, the disease appears like a bolt from the blue. However, if the patient is aware of the early symptoms and signs of the disease, he is likely to immediately report to the physician, and the disease can be treated fully with the availability of effective antitetanus serum (ATS). But, if the patient is late and comes with a full-fledged attack of tetanus, survival may not be possible, as firstly, antitetanus serum (ATS) may not prove effective in neutralizing the large amount of tetanus toxin already present in the blood, and secondly, the patient is likely to die of the various fatal complications of the disease in its advanced stage.

Hence, the importance of awareness regarding the warning signals of this disease is vital, so that the patient reaches the doctor quickly, and the treatment is started instantaneously.

The first and the foremost symptom of tetanus is difficulty in opening the mouth (trismus) due to the spasm of the muscles of mastication. Hence, the disease is commonly called 'lockjaw'. It may be noted that this difficulty in opening the mouth is painless, and if one tries to open the mouth, the spasm of the muscles that closes the jaw will increase and, therefore, the patient may not be able to open his mouth widely, howsoever, he may try and, in some cases both the jaws are tightly closed and the teeth clenched.

'Lockjaw' is the earliest characteristic symptom of the disease, and the patient should not delay even if the difficulty in opening the mouth is slight, particularly when there is a history of injury in the recent past.

The incubation period of tetanus, i.e., the period between the injury and the occurrence of lockjaw, is on the average, 1-3 weeks. The disease may manifest itself within 2-3 days in the case of injury of the face (being near to the central nervous system). On the other hand, the incubation period may be much longer, say even months, if the tetanus spores remain dormant in some of the wounds, where the conditions are not favourable for their germination.

However, lockjaw or difficulty in opening the mouth should not frighten the person; it may also occur as a result of acute inflammation/sepsis of the tonsils and its surrounding areas, including dental conditions, especially impacted tooth; but in such cases, the condition is quite painful, and the patient usually points out the area of pain.

Difficulty in opening the mouth may be accompanied with difficulty in swallowing, with or without some change in the voice, due to the spasm of the muscles for swallowing, as well as of the larynx. Soon stiffness of the neck, tightness of the chest and rigidity of the abdominal wall may take place, due to the spasm of the muscles of the neck, chest and abdomen respectively. The warning signals of tetanus may be summarized in its usual order of sequence as follows:

(i) Lockjaw, with or without recent or past history of injury anywhere on the body.

(ii) Difficulty in swallowing and/or change in voice.

(iii) Stiffness of the neck, followed by tightness of the chest and rigidity of the abdominal wall.

Other clinical manifestations of tetanus

As the disease progresses, i.e., when the patient fails to seek medical advice in time, or fails to arrest the disease in infancy, serious signs and symptoms manifest themselves, making the condition of the patient highly miserable.

In such late cases, the stiffness of the neck and the tightness of the chest increase, and the abdominal wall becomes so hard that it may be difficult to push it in. This occurs as a result of the progressive spasm of the muscles of the neck, of the chest and of the abdomen. Difficulty in swallowing increases due to the clenched teeth and also due to the marked spasm of the muscles for swallowing. Breathing too becomes troublesome due to the tightness of the chest, as well as due to the progressive spasm of the muscles of the larynx. Soon all the four limbs turn stiff, as a result of tetanus.

The patient suffers marked restlessness and the rigidity of various parts of the body is soon followed by convulsions.

Many a time, the patient reports to the physician when the tightness of the chest and/or rigidity of the abdominal wall has just commenced. Even at this time, something can be done, but when convulsions of the body have started, treatment becomes very difficult, and chances of survival also decrease markedly.

An advanced case of tetanus is a very painful condition, as a result of repeated convulsions, with marked difficulty in swallowing as well as in breathing. The patient remains conscious, with a clear mind, and this adds to his agony.

Hospitalization

As soon as a patient of tetanus is diagnosed, even in very early cases, when there is only lockjaw, the patient should be immediately admitted to the tetanus unit of the main hospital. Special dark and quiet wards/rooms are kept for the treatment of such cases, as even noise/light may cause marked convulsions in a patient. Early admission is helpful to the patient, so as to arrest the further progress of the disease.

In the hospital, utmost nursing care is required, as in most of the cases, the patient can hardly even drink water, and there is marked difficulty in respiration. Intravenous glucose drip, a ryles tube for feeding, proper oxygenation, and above all, heavy sedatives are required. So heavy a sedation is given that the patient of tetanus is made almost unconscious, so that he is saved from the unbearable pain of repeated convulsions. Muscle relaxants are also administered at the same time, so as to lessen the rigidity of the involved muscles.

Depending upon the severity of the case, a calculated dose of antitetanus serum (ATS) is given intramuscularly, intravenously and also around the infected wound, so that the tetanus poison present in the blood can be neutralized and its further formation within the wound can be stopped. The wound is also surgically cleaned.

In very late and serious cases, when convulsions have occurred, and that too of a very severe nature, in spite of the best nursing care, including administration of high doses of ATS, the patient may collapse and die immediately, as a result of the sudden stoppage of respiration due to the instant spasm of the larynx during the period of an intensive convulsion. Or, the food and other secretions may be aspirated into the respiratory passages, and may cause both infection and obstruction in the airways, leading to the death of the patient. Mortality is greater among children and newborn babies.

There is another factor to be considered. The tetanus toxin, on reaching the central nervous system, gets firmly attached to the nerve cells, so much so that the ATS administered may not be able to break it away or neutralize it completely, although the tetanus toxin circulating in the blood can easily be neutralized. Hence, the patient should report as early as possible, before too much of the tetanus toxin gets fixed in the central nervous system.

What are the various preventive measures?

1. Vaccination is the key for the prevention of this disease. Therefore, a strict vaccination schedule must be followed. Tetanus usually occurs among those persons who are either not vaccinated at all, or to whom proper dosages have not been given.

Therefore, all children should be immunized and this immunization should be maintained throughout life by administering booster dosages of tetanus vaccine at regular intervals. Also, all pregnant mothers should get a cover of vaccination. If the mother is already vaccinated, booster dosages must be administered.

In addition to the above, in all cases of injury or wounds, vaccination must be done as a preventive measure, even if the injury is small. Besides injuries, tetanus vaccination is also indicated in the case of ear discharge (otitis media), as these cases are likely to get tetanus through perforations in their eardrums.

Tetanus vaccination is essential as a preventive measure before minor/major operations. At the same time, a precise regimen of sterilization must be practised so as to avoid the incidence of tetanus in operated cases, as is noticed occasionally.

Since an attack of tetanus does not give immunity to the patient against tetanus, therefore, those cases of tetanus that recover from the disease need to be administered tetanus vaccine for future prevention.

2. The second most important step in the prevention of tetanus is immediate care of the wound. Roadside injuries should be given very careful attention as accidental wounds are almost always contaminated with tetanus spores and are likely to cause tetanus. Apart from a thorough cleaning of the wound, all foreign bodies, debris, etc. must be carefully removed, and if need be, even the whole wound may be surgically excised under anaesthesia so that the wound becomes thoroughly sterile. This is especially required when the wound is mutilated one. If this little step, though of very high importance, regarding treatment of the wound is kept in mind, it will serve as a very helpful measure in the prevention of tetanus.

3. Hygienic conditions must be maintained both at home and outside. One should not walk barefoot even in one's house. All types of injury have to be avoided as far as possible, especially in the case of children.

4. Early warning signals of tetanus (already described) must always be kept in mind, especially 'lockjaw', so that even if tetanus occurs, early urgent preventive/therapeutic steps can be taken, so that the disease is prevented from proceeding to an advanced stage, and the life of the patient is saved.

It may be concluded that it is only by following the above preventive measures religiously that one can succeed in overcoming this deadly disease in all respects. And for that a prophylactic strategy is the urgent need at the national level.

5. Plague Epidemic

Urgent measures are needed to check the outbreak of plague, which takes a heavy toll of life in a very short time. In India, there was an epidemic of plague in 1994 which caused widespread panic throughout the country and abroad.

Although the disease is less commonly seen in daily life, yet in view of the large number of fatalities, as a result of various outbreaks in different parts of the world, important guidelines are required to be strictly followed so that the occurrence of epidemics of this nature can be prevented. This disease may kill the patient/s in about 48 to 72 hours, if immediate treatment is not initiated. Chaos prevails in situations where several people die all at once, and the disease spreads like a wildfire. This way, plague epidemics have been responsible for millions of deaths in human history.

Plague is an acutely infectious disease caused by the bacteria yersinia pestis, which is commonly called plague bacillus. Rats are the main source of infection.

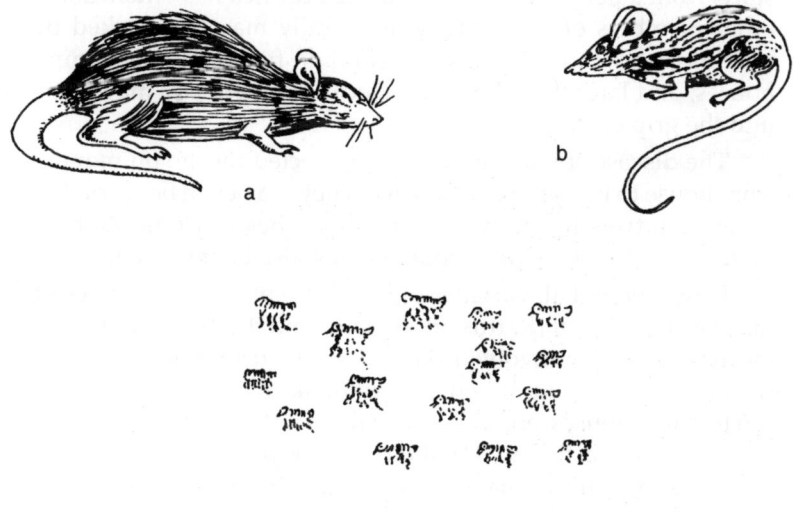

Fig. 26. a. The grey rat (Rattus norvegicus); b. The black rat (Rattus rattus); c. The rat-fleas (Xenopsylla cheopis).

How rats transmit the disease to man?

The disease is transmitted from rats to man by small insects, (about 2-4 mm) i.e. rat-fleas (Xenopsylla cheopis — in India) (Fig. 26c), which act as vector, i.e. they only transmit the disease, but do not suffer from it. Rather, they derive their blood meals from the plague-infected rats till the rats die. While sucking blood from the infected rats, a large number of plague bacilli enter the stomach of rat-fleas where they multiply further. When such fleas bite a rat or man for getting their nourishment, they inject their stomach contents containing large number of plague bacilli into the bite-wound, causing plague in rats or in persons.

Rat-fleas stick to one rat at a time for their food, and they leave the rat only when the rat dies as a result of plague and its body becomes cold. After leaving the dead rat, the rat-fleas become free, and attack more rats in their vicinity for their blood meals. This is how the disease spreads from rat to rat. When many rats die at a time/place, there occurs a scarcity of rats, and therefore, these rat-fleas bite men for their food/survival. This is how the disease is carried from rats to man. Usually, the outbreak starts from a person whom the infected rat-flea has bitten. Soon, other members of the same home/family may be attacked by rat-fleas, and thus the disease spreads further, in adjoining houses, and later the whole area/locality/town/city may come into the grip of plague.

The disease spreads because the infected rats go on moving from house to house/place to place. They may even be carried to other countries in grain-bags by ships. Besides rats, rabbits, monkeys, mice i.e. various rodents may also be involved.

However, not all varieties of rats cause plague. Two types of rats, i.e. the grey rat (Rattus norvegicus) and the black rat (Rattus rattus) are mainly involved (Fig. 26 a, b). Further, usually only wild rats are affected. When an earthquake etc. occurs, wild rats run towards houses, and carry with them infected rat-fleas which attack the domestic rats for their food. When all the domestic rats die as a result of plague, the rat-fleas become free to attack human beings.

Although the rat-flea is the chief insect/agent for carrying the disease, sometimes lice, ticks and even bedbugs may also prove harmful. A moderate and humid climate is favourable for rat-fleas, as they do not survive in dry and hot weather. Hence, chances of the plague epidemic may be less in the hot season and in places with a hot climate.

Can we forecast a plague epidemic?

Yes, we can predict a plague epidemic, but it is a work of great expertise. An epidemic in man is preceded by an epidemic in rats. And, since the rat-induced epidemic is bound to cause the death of large colonies of rats, the matter should come to the notice of the press and the people. Thus, the trouble can be located and localized and treated before it begins to cause widespread panic and havoc. In other words, such an event, when isolated, would serve as a clear warning and as a danger signal. More vigilance is required following earthquakes etc., as plague-infected wild rats, while deserting their habitat, will inflict the disease among urban/domestic rats, causing their sudden deaths, i.e., a rat epidemic would occur, which leads to the human epidemic in about 2-3 weeks.

Hence an outbreak of plague in the human population can be safely foretold about 2-3 weeks earlier from the fall in the rat population as a result of plague.

A regular team/unit/department is supposed to work for such an event. In India, one such surveillance unit is located at Bangalore. It is a survey work. Wild rats are trapped and examined for the infection of plague. Likewise, a careful watch is also kept on urban rats and if a sudden death of urban rats is observed, a plague in rats is immediately suspected, and necessary tests are carried out to confirm the diagnosis.

In doubtful areas, rats should be trapped and examined for plague. They should not be killed straightway. A diagnosis of plague in rats is a useful guide for the prevention of the plague epidemic in human beings.

What are the early clinical symptoms/warning signals of the plague epidemic?

In case an epidemic does occur, the early signs and symptoms/warning signals must be borne in mind so that the patient/s can report at the earliest to their physicians. And if the disease is diagnosed in time and immediately antibiotic treatment started, all early patients will be fully cured, thus preventing the disease from assuming an epidemic form. Also the level of general awareness will rise, to keep the situation under control. Some of these measures will be discussed later.

In an epidemic of plague, people complain of sudden high fever/even up to 105°F, with marked shivering/chills, and soon, within hours or at the most the following day, glandular swellings of the size of an egg appear in the groin, and these are so painful and tender that the patient keeps the limb in touch with the abdomen to reduce the tension in the swellings. As soon as the limb is stretched, there is a marked increase in pain in the groin.

Since the bite of rat-fleas is usually on the legs, the glands of the groin are mostly involved; hence the disease is called *bubo*, which means groin, or it is also called bubonic plague. The infection in the glands of the groin reaches from the area of the bite, i.e. the feet/legs, by the lymphatics which drain these glands. However, if the flea-bite is on the arms, the glands of the armpit will become swollen, painful and tender, like the glands in the groin.

Since the disease spreads rapidly and has a limited span (hardly 48-72 hours in untreated cases), there is a possibility of people ignoring its onset in the initial stage. And when that initial life-saving period of a few hours is usually ignored by the patient, this could prove fatal.

All this happens when the public is not aware of the early signals/symptoms of the disease, and the epidemic strikes suddenly and initiates panic.

Therefore, from the above, it can be concluded that the early signals/symptoms of plague must be made known to all, and these must be vigilantly kept in mind so that one is saved from the tragedy of plague, as and when an epidemic occurs.

The earliest warning signals/symptoms of plague may be described as follows:

Sudden high-grade fever with marked shivering, pain and tenderness in the groin/armpit, followed within hours by the appearance of markedly painful/tender glandular swellings in the groin/armpit — suspect the onset of plague epidemic.

As regards the bite of the flea on the feet/legs/arms, it is so minute that it can hardly be seen or felt. Hence this does not help in suspecting the disease early. The symptoms of plague appear after an incubation period of about a week, or in severe cases, 3 - 4 days following the flea-bite.

Marked septicaemia of plague

The infection/plague bacilli do not remain confined to the glands of groin/armpit only. They also enter the blood stream, reach all parts of the body/internal organs and cause severe septicaemia leading to the death of the patient. Probably, there is no other infection of the body which causes such a marked toxaemia/septicaemia in a very short period of a few hours, as does this infection.

In some cases, septicaemia becomes so marked from the very beginning that the patient dies without passing through the bubonic/glandular stage of the disease, i.e., without the development of glandular swellings either in the groin or in the armpit.

In such serious cases, the bacteria may even damage the walls of the blood vessels, leading to haemorrhage in the skin, mouth, urinary/gastrointestinal tract, lungs, etc. The patient passes blood in the stools, urine, sputum, etc. Bleeding areas are seen in the mouth, and on the skin, haemorrhagic spots/rashes may appear; hence the old name of the disease 'black death'.

The most contagious pneumonic plague

Following the symptoms of bubonic plague, in some of the cases, the plague bacilli, after entering the blood stream, cause marked infection in both the lungs called 'pneumonic plague'. Besides sudden high fever and chills, there is severe cough and expectoration. The sputum is thin and watery and may contain blood, and if examined, shows a large number of plague bacilli. Chest X-rays show pictures suggestive of pneumonia. Initial cases of pneumonic plague occur as a complication of bubonic plague, and it adds to the misery of the patient, and chances of mortality increase, if immediate treatment is not started.

Soon the pneumonic plague spreads quickly from man to man by droplet infection i.e. the plague bacilli, in tiny droplets of sputum are coughed out into the air by the patients, and these contaminated droplets are subsequently inhaled by normal persons leading to an epidemic of pneumonic plague. Such cases of pneumonic plague, which get the infection directly from other patients of pneumonic plague, carry a very high mortality rate, and the patient dies when the administration of antibiotic is delayed even for a day. However, if such cases are taken up well in time and treated immediately, they do respond to antibiotics, and there is every possibility of survival. It is obvious in such cases that there will be no signs of bubonic plague, since it is an airborne infection from patient to patient (no flea-bite in such cases). The 1994 epidemic of plague that occurred in India also included the cases of pneumonic plague. Hence, important warning signal for the early detection of pneumonic plague is:

Any person who develops high fever, chill, cough, breathlessness, passes a large amount of expectoration during a plague epidemic, and more so when cases of pneumonic plague have also been reported, should immediately consult the doctor for diagnosis and treatment of pneumonic plague.

Needless to say, such cases need strict isolation till completely treated.

What are the various tests urgently required for the diagnosis of plague in an epidemic?

At the outset, it may be said that even a few minutes are precious to save the life of the patient. In an epidemic, no tests need to be carried out, and the patient should be straightway put on suitable antibiotics. Tests may be carried out after the drugs have been administered. There is no second opinion on bubonic plague. Glandular enlargement may occur in the groin/armpit in some other diseases, but in plague the swelling of the glands occurs in no time, and these become highly painful and tender, accompanied with fever and chill. And, moreover, many people suffer/die en masse, i.e. it usually comes in an epidemic form.

However, diagnosis can be confirmed quickly and the plague bacilli can be examined in a laboratory, either in the fluid, aspirated from the swollen glands, or in the sputum, in the case of pneumonic plague, or in the blood when there is marked septicaemia. Even these specimens, i.e. the aspirate of glands, sputum and blood can be used for culture of the plague bacilli.

Management of patients suffering from the plague epidemic

Undoubtedly, very early cases of plague can be treated at home with suitable antibiotics like tetracyclines. Even if the disease has gone to an advanced stage, one should not lose heart, since these antibiotics do work to a great extent even in severe/grave cases, and there is always the possibility of recovery. However, mortality is much less in patients who take treatment sooner or later, although recovery will be faster and complete for those who are able to receive therapy at the earliest possible opportunity.

In all moderate to severe cases, urgent hospitalization is essentially required for proper management and nursing care. The patients, besides antibiotics, usually need an intravenous drip of glucose saline, cold sponging to lower temperature, sedatives and antiemetic drugs, etc. Blood transfusion may be required in those cases where haemorrhage has started.

In case there is no proper arrangement for isolation in houses, even early cases should be hospitalised so that the patient is isolated immediately, to avoid the spread of the disease.

Swollen lymph glands, either in the groin (bubo) or in the armpit, should not be incised and drained, so as to avoid the spread of infection in the blood. However, glandular swellings usually subside with antibiotics without local treatment/ drainage.

Prevention of the plague epidemic

A long-term and active anti-plague drive is required at the national level, covering the entire country/population of both rats and man. Preventive steps are required even in normal times, but more vigorously when a plague epidemic is predicted. Specific measures must be undertaken when such a situation arises.

1. Prediction of the plague epidemic

Surveillance units can play a great role. As already mentioned, incidence of plague in wild/urban rats, and/or a fall in the wild/ urban rat population should be regularly monitored.

An epidemic of plague in rats is an indication that an epidemic of plague in the human population is going to occur in about 2-3 weeks. Hence, we have 2-3 weeks to take necessary steps, so that the plague epidemic does not occur in man at all.

Since the plague epidemic in rats usually occurs after an earthquake, such an occurrence is itself a warning signal.

2. What should be done when an epidemic of plague in man has been predicted?

The following measures should be immediately taken:
1. All plague-infected wild/urban rats should be trapped and killed. In case, the rats have already died as a result of plague, they should be carefully disposed off, and the surroundings properly disinfected by spraying insecticides, so that rat-fleas which leave the dead rats are also killed. Those attending/doing this cleansing operation are instructed to wear boots with knee-high socks, gloves, aprons, caps, goggles, masks, so as to protect themselves from being bitten by the rat-fleas.
2. All possible measures need to be taken so that rats from outside do not enter the houses. Grain stores/godowns, ideally the whole building/house, should be rat-proof. Rats harbouring in grain stores are a great nuisance. They may be even responsible for spreading the disease to other countries when infected rats are carried in grain bags by ships. All such rats must be trapped and examined for plague-infection. All grain stores must be free from rats. A close watch is also required to see that ships have no rats.
3. Proper sanitation in and around houses, as well as in the concerned cities is of utmost importance. There should be proper and regular disposal of garbage. This avoids an unnecessary increase in the number of rats/rat-fleas.
4. One should not walk barefoot and with bare legs, so as to avoid being bitten by rat-fleas. Sleeping on the floor may prove dangerous.
5. In case there is sudden death of several rats, authorities must be immediately informed so that all necessary steps can be taken in that area, besides disposing off the dead rats.
6. 'Pest repeller' devices should be used at various places like restaurants, hotels, bars, kitchens, stores, bedrooms, etc. to keep rats away from human beings. These are electronic devices that emit ultrasonic sounds which are highly

disturbing to rats and even snakes, etc., so that rats do not come near the appliance or into the room/hall where the device has been installed. Of course, the sound of the device is not audible to human beings and is harmless.

7. Likewise, insect repellent oils/creams may be used, especially on the exposed parts of the body, to avoid being bitten by rat-fleas.

8. People of the area where plague has been suspected/predicted, should to be immediately vaccinated with anti-plague vaccine, like Haffkine's vaccine, which is available in India. If sufficient quantities cannot be made available for mass immunization, the vaccine should be procured from some other countries, as it is only useful when given in time.

9. Whenever the occurrence of a plague epidemic is predicted, people should be properly cautioned regarding its consequences, and necessary steps of prevention (as detailed above), should be explained through various media, like newspapers, magazines, TV, radio, public announcements, etc. At the same time, detailed instructions must be supplied to all health personnel, including those at the rural level. A requisite number of beds should be kept reserved in the various hospitals of the region/city, and an adequate store of drugs is needed. At the same time, it is necessary to pass on the word to all drug-manufacturers to keep an eye on the production of drugs essentially required for the treatment of plague. There has to be sufficient production of drugs so as to meet the urgent demands of hospitals/chemists.

In conclusion, it may be said that if all the above steps of prevention are strictly followed, an epidemic of plague can be prevented, which will save mankind from mass mortality.

14
LEPROSY

Although leprosy as a disease is known to be of ancient origin, it continues to be prevalent even today. Mass realization regarding the important details of the disease is vital for controlling its spread.

It is crucial to detect leprosy at the earliest possible opportunity before the irreversible deformities and other visible lesions appear. In early cases, the administration of effective treatment will revert the condition to the normal.

World Health Organisation (WHO) has been taking initiative to eliminate leprosy as a public health hazard and also launched a landmark campaign but the target is yet to be achieved. Various voluntary organizations and national health agencies are also working in this behalf.

There are mainly two types of leprosy. In the tuberculoid type, the earliest manifestation is the loss of sensation, and hair on a patch of skin. It is a good warning signal, and should alert those affected by it. The disease should be immediately suspected when one is in contact with a leper. However, in the other type of leprosy, called lepromatous leprosy, there is marked damage to the skin, leading to characteristic thickened facial features. Perforation of the nasal septum may occur in advanced cases. If leprosy is suspected, the diagnosis should be immediately confirmed by taking a biopsy or smear of the skin lesion/s for demonstrating Mycobacterium leprae (causative bacteria of leprosy). Other tests, like nerve biopsy, lepromin skin test, M. leprae PGL-1 (phenolic glycolipid I) etc., may also be required.

There should be no panic when a case of leprosy is diagnosed in a family. It is a curable condition, when the disease is diagnosed in its initial stages. Moreover, long contact with a patient of leprosy is required for the transmission of the disease.

15
AIDS AND OTHER SEXUALLY-TRANSMITTED DISEASES

AIDS

"Natural forces within us are the true healers of the disease" wrote Hippocrates. Hence a natural defence mechanism of the body is essential both for the prevention and the cure of the disease.

In AIDS (acquired immune deficiency syndrome), which is currently rampant in the world, as a result of infection by the virus called human immunodeficiency virus (HIV), (Fig. 27), the body's defence mechanism/resistance becomes so low that the disease eventually proves fatal.

The infection of AIDS travels from the semen to the blood, and so injury is important for the transmission of virus. Therefore, it is more common in heterosexual cases, where the chances of injuries are more. The disease also occurs due to infected blood transfusion and with contaminated needles and syringes. It can also be contracted if an infected shaving blade/razor is used by barbers. The cracked nipple of an infected mother too should be watched. The disease can also be transmitted from an infected mother during pregnancy. It may also manifest itself as a result of deep kissing, when both partners have bleeding gums or mouth sores/ulcers, and one of them is suffering from AIDS.

It is interesting to note that a patient of AIDS may have a longer incubation period (i.e., the interval between exposure to the infection of AIDS and appearance of the first symptom of the disease) of about eight years. This long incubation period is very

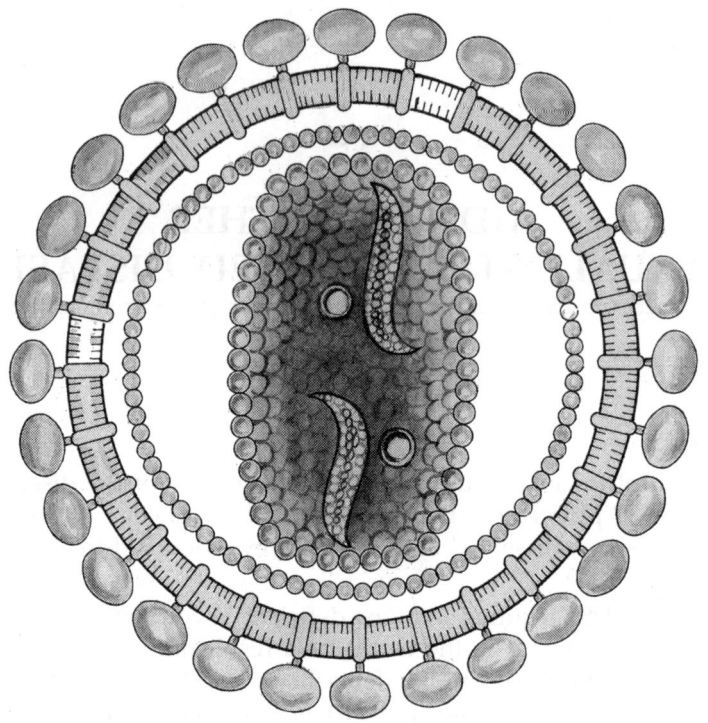

Fig. 27. The human immunodeficiency virus (HIV).

dangerous and results in the spread of the disease. This happens when the patient remains unaware of his ailment throughout the long incubation period, i.e. such a person has no knowledge/awareness about AIDS. Sometimes, even the mode of infection may be forgotten by the patient during this long span.

As soon as the disease manifests itself, i.e. after the incubation period, it has no specific early symptoms/signs. The symptoms are due to the low resistance of the patient, which may be listed as:

(i) Fever, fatigue, loss of appetite and weight, night sweat, and diarrhoea;

(ii) Swollen lymph nodes in the neck, armpit and groin;

(iii) Cough, with breathlessness.

It may be added that AIDS can involve any system of the body. It may be associated with tuberculosis/malignancy. The most tragic part is that once the disease starts showing its effect, the patient may die as disease advances. A patient of AIDS should not be subjected to hatred. The symptoms of the patient must be relieved through proper medication, so that he can live comfortably during the remaining years of his life.

The diagnosis of AIDS should be confirmed by the enzyme-linked immunosorbent assay (ELISA) blood test, and if this test is found to be positive, it must be further confirmed by the Western blot test, since the ELISA test can be false positive in 1% of cases.

The best way to avoid the disease is to prevent it by the measures given below which should be followed rigidly worldwide irrespective of the incidence of the disease in a particular area. Mass awareness is urgently required particularly in younger generation.
1. Avoid sex with suspected persons. Use condoms regularly.
2. Use sterilized needles and syringes.
3. Blood should be tested for HIV before transfusion.
4. When detected, it would be wise on the part of such patients not to spread the disease during the remaining part of the incubation period. Being symptomless, they should be very cautious on this account. If they spread the disease knowingly, they should be liable to be prosecuted. This aspect also needs mass realization.
5. All health-care workers (HCWs) should take all necessary precautions while dealing with patients of AIDS, so that they do not contract the disease. Hands should be properly washed, gloves should be worn, all waste products should be carefully disposed off, and used-needles should be twisted before discarding them. Hands should be washed with some antiseptic liquid like Dettol (chloroxylenol 4.8%), which may be used in 1:20 dilution, and they should be thoroughly rinsed or immersed for at least one minute in this solution. HCWs suffering from skin diseases, like dermatitis, should refrain from working with patients of AIDS.
6. All pregnant mothers are required to be tested for AIDS.

Other sexually-transmitted diseases (STDs)

Although other STDs, like syphilis, gonorrhea, urethritis / cystitis, etc. can now be controlled with various available antibiotics, yet their early detection as well as prevention is more important, so that one is saved from the misery/complications of such is diseases. Hence, it is advisable to have safe sex, and condoms should be used.

Early / warning signals of the above-mentioned STDs may be summarized as follows:

Whenever one gets a painless hard nodule on the penis, and on the vulva in a female (in the case of syphilis), a burning sensation while passing urine in either sex (in case of gonorrhea, urethritis/cystitis), after unsafe sex, he/she should immediately report to the physician for early diagnosis and immediate treatment so as to avoid the very serious complications of these STDs.

It may be emphasized that mass education is a must to prevent various STDs. Parents/teachers can play a vital role in educating their children/students at the appropriate time/age.

And STDs, particularly AIDS, which is rapidly spreading as an epidemic in various parts of the world, must be recognized as a national problem. Priority must be accorded to AIDS prevention measures/programmes. Efforts for the development of cheap and effective drugs, as well as a potent vaccine, should be speeded up.

16
DISEASES OF OLD AGE

Old people suffer more than all other age groups, since there is a general lack of health education/awareness regarding the various diseases and other related aspects of old age.

It should be clearly stated at the very outset that old people constitute an important part of our society. They can work satisfactorily even up to 80 years of age or more, with intelligence, sound memory, provided they are properly cared for. According to the WHO, old age starts at the age of 65. The myth that an old man does not remain useful to society should at once be discouraged. It is a misconception and needs to be removed.

There is no doubt that awareness about the various steps required for proper health as well as the longevity of old people is increasing day by day, and that is the reason that still much more is required to be done in this sphere. It may be appreciated that there is a great heterogeneity in the older population. A 70 year old may run, or on the other hand, may only be able to walk slowly. Globally, the percentage of people of 60 and above is increasing with a rapid pace.

What is geriatrics?

The science dealing with the study and treatment of the diseases of old age is called Geriatrics. Like paediatrics (concerning children), geriatrics (derived from the Greek word 'Geraios', meaning old age) is itself a speciality. The British Geriatric Society has defined it thus: 'Geriatrics is the branch of general medicine concerned with the clinical, preventive, medical and social aspects of illness in the elderly'.

It is worth noting that the presentation or clinical manifestations of various serious diseases are different in advanced age as compared to those among young/middle-aged patients. Unless the public, which includes both the old people and their family members/attendants, is educated/made aware of the symptoms/warning signals of such diseases, the diagnosis of a grave problem in an old person is likely to be missed, and the disease may even prove fatal. Advanced age is in fact a risk factor by itself in the development of several diseases especially vascular. The goal of geriatric care is focused on detection and managing diseases timely.

Is clinical manifestation of various common serious diseases different in old people as compared to that in young / middle-aged patients?

It is true, and there are several serious diseases (mentioned later) which may not appear with classical manifestations in an old man, as compared to their presence in young/middle-aged persons. It is, therefore, necessary to keep in mind these diseases so that they do not remain undetected/undiagnosed.

There is a word of caution both for old people and for their family members, so that whenever an old person makes any complaint, however minor, it should not be ignored. Old people themselves are required to be vigilant in reporting to their physicians any untoward symptom/s. They are advised to actively come forward with their problems, and should not attribute everything to problems of age.

It is for the above reasons that a consulting physician notes down a detailed history of an old person, and is required to spend a lot of time in asking questions, both from the old person as well as his family members, so that a hidden problem may not remain untraced. Truly speaking, the symptoms are coaxed out both from the old man and his/her attendants.

Out of the various serious diseases, some may be mentioned here with atypical symptoms. An old man may suffer from a heart attack and the classical symptom/s of severe pain in the chest, etc. may be missing. There may be only mild chest discomfort, giddiness, breathlessness, etc. Hence an urgent electrocardiogram (ECG) may be required in such cases. (See details of coronary artery disease, page 21)

Old people are more prone to respiratory infection, which may remain undetected until it reaches an advanced stage. Hence, a physician always auscultates the chest of an old person carefully, so that infection may not remain hidden in the lungs. Even tuberculosis of the lungs may remain undetected and the patient may feel all right. There may be hardly any cough or fever, etc. Therefore, at least whenever there is blood in the sputum (haemoptysis), which is an important symptom/warning signal of tuberculosis, urgent steps should be taken to exclude tuberculosis of the lungs, including malignancy. For details, refer to the chapter on tuberculosis.

Indigestion/change in bowel habits (i.e. when there is alternating constipation and diarrhoea) may not be taken seriously by an old person, whereas these may be important warning signals of cancer of the stomach/colon respectively. Similarly, a gastric/duodenal ulcer may be missed until it has become malignant, or has caused perforation leading to haemorrhage in the stomach/intestine of the patient in question. Signals of various types of cancer have been dealt with in the chapter on cancer.

Similarly, diseases like appendicitis may remain hidden in old people. It is a common emergency which causes acute pain in the abdomen, but in an old person there may not be much pain or any symptoms. It is only through an intelligent guess and investigation by the physician that a diagnosis can be reached. If timely proper care is not taken, the appendix is likely to rupture in the abdomen, which may prove fatal.

In the same way, a toxic thyroid gland (hyperthyroidism) may remain neglected due to the lack of classical symptoms in old people. The symptomatology of a hyperactive thyroid gland has been described in the chapter on the thyroid gland. One has to actually enquire about the various symptoms regarding the toxicity of the thyroid gland from the old person, as he/she may not come forward with any of the complaints.

Since the classical symptoms of the diseases are missing in old persons, the physician has to examine these cases in detail during each visit, and routine blood tests, ECG and chest X-ray, etc. should be carried out even on slight suspicion. The detailed previous medical record, including the surgical, is also viewed by the physician. An up-to-date record must be kept ready by the patient or his attendants for the quick attention of the visiting physician/surgeon. The idea is that the society should not lose the old person prematurely, and for this the triad has to work in co-operation, i.e. old person/patient, family members/ attendants and the physician.

The frequency of diseases is also higher in old persons, due to the low defence mechanism of the body, and for the same reason, healing/recovery is also late. The difficulty arises when many of the systems get involved at the same time, which make both the diagnosis and the treatment difficult.

Other diseases in old persons

Diseases of the heart

(i) The rhythm of the heart may get markedly disturbed (arrhythmias). The heart beat may become irregular, or the heart rate may become very slow or even fast. The patient complains of varied symptoms, especially vertigo/ dizziness and in advanced cases, even syncope i.e. transitory unconsciousness/fainting may occur.

(ii) The hardening of coronary arteries may lead to angina or heart attack.

(iii) There may be thickening/hardening or even calcification of the various valves of the heart, like the aortic or mitral valve leading to the aortic or mitral stenosis/regurgitation respectively. Auscultation of the heart will show various murmurs, and the lesion can be confirmed by echocardiography.

Due to the above changes in the heart as a result of old age, its normal functioning may be disturbed, and a physician/ cardiologist may have to be consulted.

Diseases of the brain

(i) Due to atherosclerosis/hardening of the blood vessels of the brain, there may be deterioration of mental functions, like disturbance in memory. The memory of recent events is usually impaired, while past events may be remembered well.

(ii) Similarly, there may occur emotional instability, irritability, rigidity, etc.
(iii) Likewise, the power of judgement/reasoning may suffer.
(iv) Due to the same pathology, i.e. atherosclerosis, the blood supply of a part of brain may be affected, leading to a stroke or paralysis.

It should be made clear that there is no uniform distribution of pathology in an old person. For example, atherosclerosis/ hardening of blood vessels in an old person does not occur equally throughout the blood vessels of the body. In some of the patients, only the coronary arteries may be involved, while in others, the blood vessels of the brain or of any other organ may be affected. Even when one organ, say the heart or brain is involved, the pathology is not the same throughout in the blood vessels of the organ, say in the coronary arteries in the case of the heart, or in the blood vessels supplying the brain. In other words, there may be different degrees of pathology/involvement in different portions of the coronaries/blood vessels of the brain, etc. Hence, if an old man is suffering from angina/heart attack, he may not necessarily suffer from a stroke at the same time.

Systolic hypertension

Elevated blood pressure usually occurs in old persons, and in some only the upper level of blood pressure (systolic) may be raised. Precisely, isolated systolic hypertension (ISH) is said to occur when the upper (systolic) blood pressure is more than 160 mm Hg, but the lower (diastolic) is lower than 95 mm Hg. The patient is required to be investigated on the lines of hypertension (refer to the chapter on high blood pressure).

Care should be taken while administering antihypertensive drugs. An elevated blood pressure should not be lowered suddenly, as chances of thrombosis in a vessel increase, and the patient may suffer from heart attack or stroke. Further, in many old persons, blood pressure is highly labile, i.e., there is a marked fluctuation from a very high level to an equally low level, when the person is taking no drugs. Hence, if drugs are administered for a high level of blood pressure, periodic monitoring is required for adjusting the dosages or stopping the treatment, well in time.

Diabetes

Due to the lack of secretion of insulin, diabetes may be precipitated in old age. It should be investigated and treated as mentioned in Chapter 3 on diabetes.

Osteoarthritis

It is a common disease in old people. The knee joints may be particularly involved, and the patient may have difficulty in walking or climbing stairs. Both the knee joints may be involved at the same time. As a preventive measure, exercise is required at an early age, and those who are prone to suffer from it, must consult their physicians, well in time. Overweight is one of the main factors that damages the knees. Besides knees, the spine, especially the neck (where cervical spondylosis usually occurs), and the back may also be involved. In both these cases, suitable treatment/prevention is required at a very early stage, before the disease reaches an advanced stage, causing considerable damage. Maintaining of proper postures is the hallmark for the care of the neck and the lower spine.

Anaemia/lack of nutrition

It may occur, especially in old persons who are living alone, as they may not be taking a proper nutritious diet, which is essentially required in old age. In India, the joint family system still exists, and thus the diet of an old person can be properly monitored. Besides a balanced diet, a small quantity of iron including vitamins supplements, may also be required in the daily routine of elderly persons.

Osteoporosis

Weakness of bones occurs in old age due to depletion of calcium, more precisely bone tissue/mass. Normally bone mass decreases with age. It may occur in a woman following menopause (i.e. when the menses stop) called 'postmenopausal osteoporosis'. However, as mentioned above, osteoporosis occurs with age, later in life, in both the sexes, called 'senile osteoporosis'. Since the bones are weak, they become more liable to fracture. Even a little fall may cause fracture of the bones, making the life of the old person miserable, as he/she may be permanently disabled.

Diseases of Old Age

Once osteoporosis occurs in certain bones, it is difficult to treat. However, further osteoporosis, i.e., osteoporosis in other bones can be prevented. For an early diagnosis, bone densitometry must be carried out. Sadly, it usually develops silently over many years, without any symptom, until a fracture occurs with minimal trauma. Even the routine day-to-day activities may cause a fracture of the bone and the most debilitating fracture is of the hip.

Old age, family history of osteoporosis, poor diet including low intake of calcium, sedentary lifestyle, use of steroids and other drugs are the major factors in the causation of osteoporosis. Both drugs and a proper diet are required for the prevention of this disorder. Old people should remain active as far as possible, as it helps in preventing osteoporosis.

Causes of falls in the elderly

It would be worthwhile to discuss here the various causes of falls in the elderly. This aspect needs special attention.

Due to the limitation in the treatment of osteoporosis, great care is required in this regard. The old person may fall due to various reasons, like muscular weakness, especially in the lower limbs, syncope i.e. when there is a transitory unconsciousness due to several causes (read the details on page 105), giddiness, etc.

Sudden fall of blood pressure, especially postural hypotension, i.e., when the blood pressure falls almost suddenly when the patient stands after lying down for a long time, say, at midnight or in the early morning, must be kept in mind. Those elderly persons whose systolic blood pressure falls 20 mm Hg or more, and the diastolic to 10 mm Hg or more, within three minutes of standing up from the lying/sitting posture, are suffering from postural/orthostatic hypotension, and should take care that they do not fall when they stand up from a sitting/lying posture. In such a situation, the physician, after taking the blood pressure of the patient in a lying down position, asks the patient to stand by the side of the bed, for at least three minutes, and then takes the final reading of the blood pressure to establish the diagnosis.

It would be appropriate to mention here that during the treatment of fracture as a result of a fall (or during any other illness), an old person should not be put on unnecessary rest. Even if the patient cannot walk, all the joints (except the ones in plaster, or as directed by the physician/surgeon) must be moved by the patient, or by some attendant/physiotherapist, so that contractures do not develop. The principle is either use them or lose them. Once contractures appear, the treatment is difficult and a prolonged one. Even a few days of immobilization of the joints may cause contractures. It is more likely to happen when a person gets paralysis, say of one half of the body in the case of a stroke, and cannot move his limbs. Early physiotherapy is the rule in such cases.

It may be further pointed out that sores/ulcers on the skin may also occur on the back part of the body when the patient remains lying in one particular position on the bed, following paralysis of a part of the body. Hence such a patient must be moved from side to side, or made to sit frequently, so that skin sores/ulcers do not develop due to the constant pressure on various parts of the skin. Needless to say that such ulcers may cause grave complications in an old man, and, therefore, in case these appear, they should be treated immediately.

Benign / senile enlargement of the prostate (BEP/SEP)

It may occur in some old persons, causing various urinary complaints and even retention of urine, if early care has not been taken of the problem. The details of this disease have been given on page 177.

Besides, an old person may suffer from urinary incontinence, i.e. the patient does not have full control on urination. It may be due to some urinary tract infection (UTI), or when there is diminished nervous control on the muscular tone of the urinary bladder.

BEP/SEP, and urinary incontinence should be investigated and treated. BEP/SEP may need surgical intervention.

Functional problems of the elderly

An old person may suffer from various functional problems like difficulty in vision, hearing, sleep, etc. There may be loss of vigour/sexual function, muscular strength, or there may occur a generalized weakness. Menopause may create problems in an old female, and urgent medical advice may have to be sought. Besides, there may be various psychological problems in an elderly person as a result of loneliness, loss of work, identity, etc., and a psychiatrist may have to be consulted, especially when these become troublesome to the old person or to members of his/her family. Depression is also seen in some elderly persons, which may need specific/specialist treatment.

Body temperature

In ageing people, the normal body temperature may become low due to the impaired temperature regulatory mechanism of the body. Hence, the elderly may not be able to cope with adverse weather, heat or cold. If proper care is not taken, an old person may even die as a result of a heat stroke, or hypothermia, i.e. due to excessive cold.

It should be stressed again that all the problems of the elderly must be carefully looked into/listened to for a precise diagnosis. There is great variation regarding the occurrence of various diseases in an elderly person. He may suffer from one or two ailments, or none perhaps. Every illness does not afflict an old person.

Tests in the case of elderly persons

Although routine tests are usually carried out in the case of elderly patients, yet advanced tests, especially invasive ones, may not be carried out, particularly if the patient is not going to get any benefit out of them. However, investigations must be conducted if the condition/disease is treatable, and the life of an old person is going to be comfortable. A careful decision is required in all such cases, depending on the age of the patient, severity of the disease, etc.

Treatment in old age

It should be known to all that adverse drug reactions/toxicity of drugs, drug interactions are common in the aged, or the elderly. Hence drugs prescribed to old persons must be carefully selected, and their dosages also adjusted accordingly.

At the same time, it should be ensured that old people do not take unnecessary medicines, without prescription. On each visit, all the drugs that the old person has been taking should be shown to the physician, so that undue medication is discouraged.

As regards surgical treatment/intervention, any surgery can be carried out on an old person, with due precautions. The old person should not be, in any way, deprived of a surgery when it is essentially required, simply because the patient is too old for it.

In the end, it may be said that there is a dire need for a national policy/programme for the overall care of the old people. Epidemiological surveys should be conducted for the identification/prevalence of various diseases of the old. Camps should be organized for spot tests/treatment of old people. Mass awareness is a must for early diagnosis, as well as for various preventive/therapeutic measures which should be followed by old persons. Old peoples' homes should be opened, especially for elderly persons who are left alone. And a separate department/unit is essential in each medical centre/college/hospital for the specialized treatment of the elderly and for the development of this speciality.

All the above aspects are various challenges which must be faced for the prosperity of the elderly population, which is fast increasing throughout the world. Multidimensional approach is essentially required.

When grace is joined with wrinkles, it is adorable.
There is an unspeakable dawn in happy old age.
- Victor Hugo

Appendix I
SMOKING AND TOBACCO CHEWING-RELATED DISEASES

Since smoking and chewing of tobacco causes serious/fatal diseases, it is important to curb this evil and educate people to avoid its use.

Since the nicotine (toxic substance) present in tobacco products gives a temporary feeling of well-being and facilitates memory, users soon get addicted to it, and the consumption of tobacco increases day by day. It can lead to various dangerous diseases, like cancer of the lung, mouth, pharynx, food-pipe (oesophagus), gallbladder and pancreas. It also causes coronary artery disease, high blood pressure and tends to increase the levels of serum cholesterol (hypercholesterolaemia). A stroke may also be precipitated as a result of excessive smoking and / or tobacco chewing. (The details of these disorders have already been elaborated under respective topics). A smoker is always at a risk of dying early in life as a result of cancer, lung and/or heart disease.

Cancers occurring in the mouth are preventable to a large extent. The risk is aggravated in people who tend to keep/chew tobacco in any of its forms at one particular spot in the mouth. The practice of 'reverse smoking' whereby the lighted cigarette is put in the mouth adds to the problem. It is usually seen in people from Kashmir and south India.

There may also occur gastric/duodenal peptic ulcer (i.e. ulcer in the stomach/duodenum). The patient may get tremors of the hands and muscular weakness. With its use, a woman may become sterile, and if tobacco is consumed during pregnancy, there may be damage to the foetus.

It is, therefore, advisable that smoking or chewing of tobacco should not be indulged in, under any circumstances, and those who are already smoking/chewing tobacco must try to give up this habit at once, or slowly, by reducing the number of cigarettes and the amount of tobacco.

Also, one should not sit in the company of a smoker, as one is likely to inhale the smoke of the cigarette being exhaled by the smoker. It is called 'passive smoking', and if the person constantly is in the close company of a smoker, it may prove as harmful as smoking.

Hence, not smoking, tobacco chewing or sharing the company of a smoker, will certainly help prevent the occurrence of many lethal diseases.

It is very important to educate and create an awareness among school children/youth about the ill effects of tobacco. The main aim is to catch them young, so that they do not become victims of tobacco in their innocence. At this tender age these children can get addicted forever.

Above all, the government should implement a long-term plan to weed-out at least some/all tobacco products in a phased manner and educate people on a mass scale against the ill effects of tobacco consumption. There should be strict prohibition for the younger generation and it is one of the important issues of tobacco prevention.

Appendix II
ALCOHOL AND DISEASES

Alcohol is an important cause of cancer of the liver, oral cavity, food-pipe (oesophagus), stomach, rectum and pancreas. Risk of breast cancer increases if the woman drinks.

When a person starts drinking, he feels relaxed and elated for sometime, as a result of the presence of ethanol in the alcohol. Soon, the person becomes dependent/addicted to alcohol due to its daily consumption in higher quantities, and the side-effects begin to appear.

In the beginning, there may occur only inflammation of the affected organs like the food-pipe, or of the stomach, or of both. Later, ulceration may occur at these sites.

Likewise in the liver, in early cases, there may be only a fatty change of the liver, which is completely reversible, provided the consumption of alcohol is stopped, or markedly reduced. But if the patient continues drinking, the liver may be further damaged, leading to alcoholic hepatitis, which is also reversible. And, if the person is still not careful, the liver may become damaged, and there may occur irreversible alcoholic cirrhosis of the liver, which is the most debilitating disease. Or, lastly, liver cancer may develop.

Heredity and immunity play a great role in the development of alcoholic liver disorders. Besides total abstinence from alcohol, drugs like glucocorticoids do help in recovery of alcoholic hepatitis. Good nutrition is also required.

Sometimes, as a result of taking alcohol, the patient may get an acute attack of pancreatitis, which may prove to be a serious medical emergency. It also carries a high risk of mortality. In some cases, there may be only chronic inflammation of the pancreas, called chronic pancreatitis, which causes severe and repeated pain in the abdomen.

The heart may also be damaged (cardiomyopathy), and the heartbeat may become irregular (arrhythmias) with a constant high intake of alcohol. In such cases, the levels of blood uric acid also rise, leading to further complications. Likewise, the blood pressure may rise, and similarly, an alcoholic may suffer from an attack of stroke. Even an attack of syncope (transitory unconsciousness) may be precipitated due to the excessive intake of alcohol.

An alcoholic may suffer from impairment in recent/remote memory, impairment in judgement, sleep disturbances, hallucinations or any other psychiatric disorder. Also, blood sugar may be markedly lowered for a while in some of the cases adding to the misery of the patient. A careful history from the relation of the patient is all the more important for the information of the physician for treating/motivating such cases.

Alcohol may cause a congenital lesion in the heart of the foetus. Hence, if the pregnant woman drinks, it must be stopped, especially in the first three months of pregnancy, when the development of the heart of the foetus takes place. Even the general development of the foetus, especially of the brain, may be affected as a result of continuous intake of alcohol by the pregnant woman during the period of pregnancy.

A chronic alcoholic may look like a very weak and debilitated person, with alcoholic tremors/gait, and there may be a marked difficulty in walking, as a result of weakness of both the lower limbs (neuropathy/myopathy). He may suffer from cerebellar degeneration as well. Also, the incidence of epilepsy is more in alcoholics as compared to non-alcoholics.

Since alcohol interferes with the absorption of vitamins from the gut and limits their storage in the liver, there may be deficiency of Vitamin B6, B3, Vitamin A and folic acid. There may be disturbance of calcium metabolism reducing the density of the bones, increasing the risk of fractures including necrosis of the head of the femur that is not uncommon and the alcoholic has to face this serious problem. Red and white blood cells including platelets in the blood may be affected by chronic heavy intake of alcohol requiring due attention of the physician.

Further, there may occur testicular atrophy and decrease in sperm count. A limited dose may enhance sexual desire with low

Alcohol and Diseases

penile erection. A woman who drinks may suffer from decrease in ovarian size, infertility, abortions and amenorrhoea. Functions of the thyroid gland may be decreased in chronic cases and thyroid tests may be required in suspected cases.

However, there are considerable individual variations, probably as a result of some genetic factors. Some people do not develop significant side-effects for year, even by consuming large amounts of alcohol daily and go on working at high places, while others develop problems with only a small quantity of alcohol.

It should be stated that low to moderate consumption of alcohol is beneficial in the prevention of coronary artery disease, decrease in the occurrence of heart attack, and it also raises the HDL (high density lipoprotein cholesterol or good cholesterol), which is useful for the heart. Likewise low dose of alcohol helps in preventing/decreasing in the incidence of stroke and gallstones. A low dose of alcohol may not prove useful if the individual is already suffering from a specific disease. The pregnant women are not advised to take even low dose of alcohol to safeguard the foetus from the deleterious effects of alcohol.

If the prescribed limits are ignored, side-effects appear in due course. However, if one takes alcoholic beverages, the prescribed limit is only 1-2 small drinks daily, of 30 ml each, and all concerned should be well aware of this admissible quantity/dose of alcohol. It is the only way one can prevent the above-mentioned serious diseases resulting from an indiscreet consumption of alcohol.

All the more, it is important to detect alcohol dependent/abuse cases who may be suffering from various disorders due to excessive consumption of alcohol, and to treat them on scientific lines, so as to prevent the malady of alcohol dependence. Many of the disorders may yet be reversible only by abstaining from alcohol. It is the need of the hour to create public awareness regarding such cases, so that the sufferers volunteer to have treatment or are brought to the centre by some members of the family. The public must be saved from this 'killer drink' — alcohol. It may cut short the life span by about a decade in cases of alcohol abuse and dependence.

To sum up, it may be said that the above-mentioned information is vital to keep oneself away from the injurious effects of alcohol.

Appendix III
OBESITY AND DISEASES

An obese or overweight individual is always prone to suffer from serious diseases. It has already been mentioned that control of weight prevents coronary artery disease, congestive heart failure, stroke, diabetes, high blood pressure, high blood cholesterol, gallstones. It is obvious that if one is overweight, he/she is likely to suffer from the above-mentioned disorders. There are separate chapters relating to most of these conditions, which may be referred to.

Besides the above, an obese person is likely to suffer from joint problems (osteoarthritis), especially of the knee joints or of the lower back. The incidence of gout may also go up. There may be serious respiratory disorders, like temporary stoppage of respiration during sleep, called 'sleep apnea'. The patient will feel miserable during this period.

Incidence of cancer is more in obese people e.g. cancer of liver, pancreas, oesophagus, rectum, colon and prostate. In obese females, the prevalence of cancer of breasts, uterus (cervix, endometrium), ovaries, gallbladder is higher. Further, in males there may occur hypogonadism and in females disturbances of menses like oligomenorrhoea.

It may be mentioned that risk of complications in obese people vary from person to person. Genetic factors play the predominant role in such cases. The risk of complications can be determined in a particular case by testing the body mass index (BMI) and the ratio between the waist and hip. Normal BMI is 19-26 Kgm/m2 and waist/hip ratio is < 1.0 in males and < 0.9 in females. Person with higher levels of BMR or waist/hip ratio are more likely to suffer from the complications of obesity. The risk is more if a patient is less than 40 years of age and higher in case of children.

Diet and exercise have a great role to play in the treatment of obesity, and if the weight is not controlled by these measures, drugs should be taken. Diet and exercise are mentioned in Appendix VII and VIII respectively. The advice of the physician must be taken, as obesity may not be always related to diet or lack of exercise; it may be a manifestation of a serious disorder (Cushing's syndrome), or the result of taking a high dosage of drugs like corticoids.

Adequate control of diabetes and hypertension does help. In selected cases operative treatment for obesity is also available.

Hence, obese/overweight people must try to reduce/control their weight without fail. At the same time, consulting the physician should not be ignored, so that the disease, if there is any, can be detected and treated in time. If some drug is responsible for obesity, it should be stopped/reduced immediately.

Further, obesity needs to be detected at a very young age and the parents can help their children avert obesity if he/she has a tendency to put on weight easily. Childhood is the habit-forming period and the parents are required to see that the child is eating a healthy food and is developing good eating habits. Outdoor activities and an active lifestyle should be encouraged, and the food intake should be balanced with regular physical activities so as to avoid gain in weight. If required, weight should be lost slowly and crash dieting should be avoided. Urgent tests in childhood should be carried out (see page 89, last para).

Needless to say that awareness of the above factors is of utmost importance for the overall health of those who are overweight.

Appendix IV
SUDDEN CARDIAC DEATH
(SCD)

Prevention of sudden cardiac death is one of the greatest challenges which causes a significant number of mortalities. In the western parts of Europe alone about 1,50,000 people die every year under this category, i.e. SCD. And in the USA, about 4 lac people suffer from this malady annually.

Sudden death can be due to old age. But it may occur earlier, around the age of 45 or later (peak incidence over the age of 30 years ranges from 45 to 75 years), in the case of a person who has been well, and does not apparently show any symptoms. Death occurs rapidly, say within an hour. It occurs usually as a result of diseased/neglected coronary arteries due to the factors already described in the related chapters/appendices — high blood cholesterol/uric acid, uncontrolled diabetes or hypertension, addiction to smoking/tobacco-chewing, etc.

Presence of several risk factors in a patient markedly increases the incidence. Identifying and treating risk factors among patients would go a long way in preventing SCD. This is called primary prevention.

The patient may be revived if immediate proper medical aid (mentioned on page 302, under the head *Technique for Reviving the Heart*) is available before the patient is shifted to the intensive care unit (ICU) of a hospital.

However, if the patient survives, he should be thoroughly investigated, so that the responsible factor/s can be corrected without delay and recurrence of cardiac arrest or death could be prevented. This is called secondary prevention. He may require

Sudden Cardiac Death (SCD)

regular medication under the guidance of a specialist. In most of the above cases, there is a marked occlusion of the coronary arteries/its branches, as a result of atherosclerosis, as shown in various autopsy (post-mortem) reports. (Refer to page 21 for details of coronary artery disease — CAD)

It would be in the public interest/safety that in high-risk cases where chances of recurrence of cardiac arrest are expected, the patients might not be allowed to drive especially the buses, trains and aircrafts etc. for a period of about 8 months following the attack. A specialist's judgment and patient's co-operation are the essential requisite in such cases. Above all, control of the various risk factors responsible for the development of coronary artery disease is vital.

Appendix V

URGENT TESTS FOR THE DETECTION OF VARIOUS COMMON SERIOUS DISEASES

Sr. No	Name of the Test	Name of the Disease
1.	Haemoglobin (Hb), total leucocyte count (TLC), differential leucocyte count (DLC), peripheral blood film (PBF), bone marrow examination.	- Early leukaemias (blood cancers).
2.	Urine examination for:	
	(i) red blood cells (RBC)/ occult blood.	- Disorders of the urinary tract and prostate, like cancer, urinary stones/infection—including tuberculosis, acute glomerulonephritis (GN), etc.
	(ii) sugar (fasting and/or postprandial).	- Diabetes.
	(iii) pus cells, culture and sensitivity.	- Urinary tract infection (UTI).
	(iv) albumin.	- Kidney diseases.
	(v) bile salts and pigments.	- Liver disorders.
3.	Stool examination for red blood cells (RBC)/occult blood.	- Cancer of the gastrointestinal tract.
4.	*Sputum for malignant cells, and for acid-fast bacilli/tubercle bacilli.	- Lung cancer and tuberculosis.

Table contd...

Sr. No	Name of the Test	Name of the Disease
5.	(i) Fasting blood sugar. (ii) 2-hour postprandial glucose test. (iii) Glucose tolerance test (GTT) or 2-hour postchallenge glucose test.	- Diabetes.
6.	** Fasting serum cholesterol/lipidogram.	- High blood cholesterol and other lipids.
7.	** Fasting serum uric acid.	- High blood uric acid.
8.	Creatinine phosphokinase - CPK (MB).	- Heart attack (myocardial infarction).
9.	Serum creatinine, blood urea.	- Kidney diseases.
10.	Liver function tests (i) serum bilirubin, (ii) serum alkaline phosphatase, (iii) serum glutamic oxa-loacetic transaminase (SGOT), serum glutamic pyruvic transaminase (SGPT). (iv) Serum markers for hepatitis A, B, C, D & E	- Liver disorders.
11.	Prostate-specific antigen (PSA). ***Prostatic acid phosphatase.	- Prostate cancer.

Table contd...

* Sputum should be obtained early in the morning after coughing, and if the sputum is blood-streaked, it should be used for examination.
** Patient should not consume alcohol for 48 hours before these tests.
*** Fasting blood sample is preferred, since diet influences the secretion of this enzyme from the prostate gland. The test should be carried out at least two days after the digital-rectal examination (DRE), since palpation of the prostate during this procedure is likely to cause more secretion of this enzyme from the prostate into the blood.

Sr. No	Name of the Test	Name of the Disease
12.	Chest X-ray.	- Lung cancer/metastasis, tuberculosis, etc. - Heart diseases.
13.	Ultrasonography.	- Diseases of the liver, pancreas, gallbladder, urinary tract, prostate in males, uterus, ovaries, tubes, vagina in females. - Disorders of the thyroid gland, etc. - Early pleurisy can also be detected.
14.	Electrocardiogram (ECG), echocardiography and Doppler imaging	- Heart diseases like ischaemic heart disease (IHD), rheumatic heart disease (RHD), congenital heart disease (CHD), etc.
15.	TMT (treadmill stress test) or exercise ECG test, Holter test, thallium stress test, coronary angiography, computed tomographic (CT) coronary angiogram	- Ischaemic heart disease (IHD).
16.	X-ray of the skull, CT scan (head), magnetic resonance imaging (MRI), electroencephalogram (EEG)	- Brain tumours/tuber-culo-sis, stroke, epilepsy, head injury. The CT scan and the MRI are also helpful in detecting various other lesions.
17.	Pap smear.	- Early cancer of the uterus (the most important being the cervix).
18.	FNAC (fine needle aspiration cytology).	- For detecting malignant cells in a growth/lump.
19.	Upper gastrointestinal endoscopy.	- Cancer/ulcer of the oesophagus, stomach and duodenum.

Table contd...

Urgent Tests

Sr. No	Name of the Test	Name of the Disease
20.	Serum free T_4 (thyroxine i.e. tetraiodothyronine), serum free T_3 (triiodothyronine) and TSH (thyroid-stimulating hormone).	- Thyroid gland disorders (myxoedema, thyrotoxicosis, etc.)
21.	Bronchoscopy.	- Lung cancer (more precisely relating to the airways).
22.	Pleural fluid analysis.	- Malignant or tuberculous pleural effusion (pleurisy).
23.	ELISA test for AIDS and Western blot test.	- AIDS.
24.	Pleural biopsy.	- Malignancy of pleura (outer covering of the lung).
25.	ELISA test for tuberculosis.	- Tuberculosis, anywhere in the body.
26.	Troponin T (TnT) and/or Troponin I (TnI) strip tests.	- For urgent and immediate diagnosis of a heart attack.
27.	Micral-test II (strip test).	- Early diagnosis of nephropathies.
28.	Histopathology.	- Malignant growth/nodule and other disorders relating to various organs.
29.	Colonoscopy/sigmoidoscopy.	- Cancer and other disorders of the colon.
30.	Proctoscopy.	- Cancer/other disorders of the rectum and anal canal.
31.	Cystoscopy.	- Urinary bladder disorders.
32.	Laryngoscopy.	- Laryngeal carcinoma, tuberculosis, etc.
33.	Hysteroscopy.	- To examine the inside of the uterus for various disorders.
34.	Bone densitometry	- Osteoporosis.
35.	Mammography.	- Breast cancer.
36.	Radioisotope scanning.	- Various lesions / metastasis, e.g. a bone scan is a must for the detection of the spread of prostate cancer.

Appendix VI

URGENT TIPS: FIRST AID FOR PREVENTION/IMMEDIATE CONTROL OF SOME COMMON SERIOUS DISEASES

Emergency medical treatment is of paramount importance and needs to be carried out in cases of emergencies, contingencies and crises.

The guidelines, given below, regarding the emergencies of various serious diseases, though not exhaustive, will be highly useful in most of the cases. If applied properly and seriously, a life may be saved, or at least further deterioration of the patient may be altogether stopped, till he/she gets proper medical aid.

1. Heart attack

Any pain-killer, especially an injection like norphin/tidigesic or the like, should be administered immediately. These medicines are also available in the form of tablets. There is no harm caused by these drugs even if later investigations do not reveal a heart problem. Half a tablet of Disprin is also valuable in such cases. A tablet of glyceryl trinitrate may be kept under the tongue of the patient with the advice of the physician. The patient should be shifted to hospital immediately. The above therapy will go a long way in preventing damage to the heart to a variable extent, and also later in the recovery of the patient. Sometimes the above therapy is so rewarding that the patient recovers from the heart attack speedily.

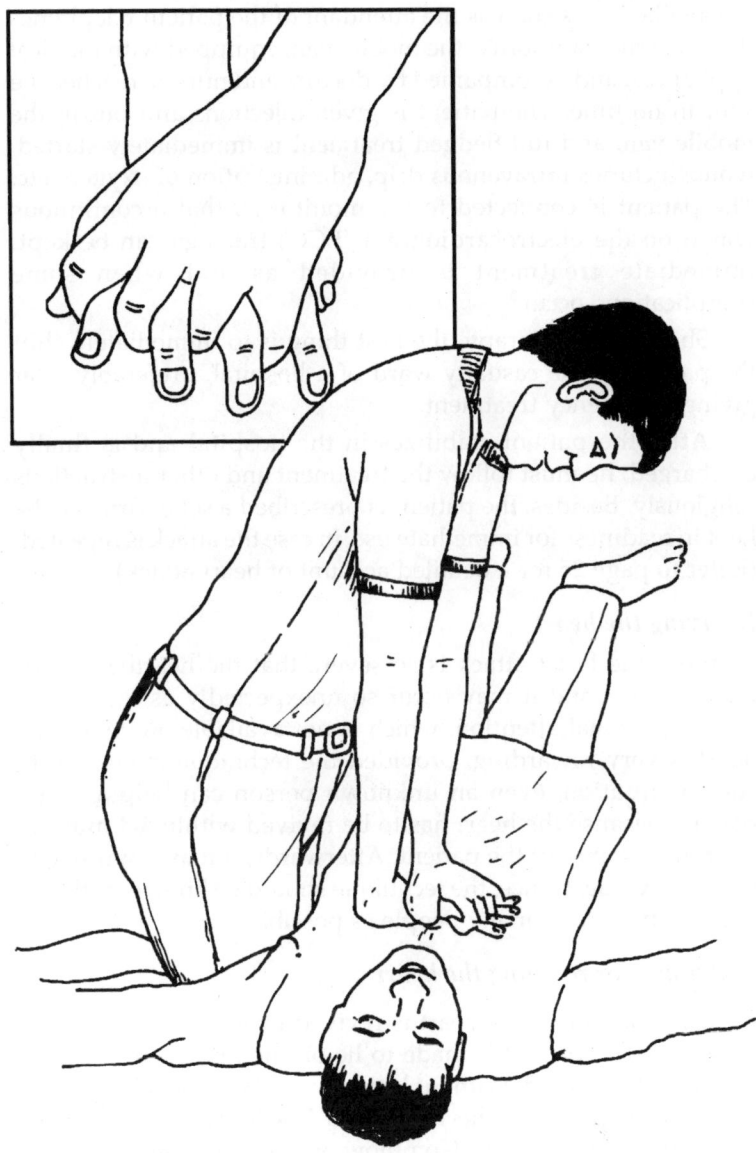

Fig. 28. Reviving the heart with the aid of external cardiac massage.

In some places the facilities of a 'mobile cardiac care unit' are available. As soon as the attendant of the patient telephones the concerned authority, the mobile van, equipped with medical appliances, and accompanied by doctors and nurses, reaches the spot in no time. The patient is given injections and put in the mobile van, and full-fledged treatment is immediately started, which includes intravenous drip, administration of oxygen, etc. The patient is connected to the monitor so that a continuous watch on the electrocardiogram (ECG) tracings can be kept. Immediate treatment is provided as and when some complications occur.

Short of this therapy, the best thing is to immediately shift the patient to the casualty ward of a hospital, preferably after giving emergency treatment.

After the patient stabilizes in the hospital and is finally discharged, he must follow the treatment and other instructions religiously. Besides, the patient is prescribed a set of drugs to be kept in readiness for immediate use, in case the attack is repeated. (Refer to page 25 for a detailed account of heart attack)

Reviving the heart

At times the heart attack is so severe that the heartbeat stops immediately, and it may occur so unexpectedly as to warrant instant personal attention, which is not available. Reviving the heart is very rewarding, provided the technique is known. In such a situation, even an unknown person can help a dying patient, because the heart has to be revived within 3-4 minutes after the collapse of the patient. Afterwards, it may not prove to be of any value. Hence, the technique should be known to almost everybody or to as many people as possible.

Technique for reviving the heart

In such a situation, the heart is revived by an 'external cardiac massage'. The patient is made to lie on the floor with the back touching the ground. Without losing time, the neck of the patient is pulled backward and his legs raised. The legs are kept elevated till the procedure is over. No pillow or anything else is required to be kept under the head. One person places his palm on the lower part of the sternum (i.e. the bone located in front of the centre of the chest), and immediately puts the other palm upon

Urgent Tips

the palm already placed on the sternum, and keeps the fingers extended or interlocked, as shown in Fig. 28. Now, with the help of the two palms, the sternum bone is pressed 80 times a minute, and this pressure should not be more than 4-5 cm. To avoid fatigue, the best course is for the person to kneel against the side of the patient, bending over his chest. He should keep both his arms straight while putting his palms on the chest for the massage/pressure.

If some other person is available, he should start mouth-to-mouth breathing. In this process, he forces his expiration into the mouth of the patient. During this time, the nose of the patient should be closed, otherwise the air forced into the mouth of the patient will come out through the nose. One breath after every five times of the cardiac massage is required. If no other person is available, two breaths should be given after every 15 times of the cardiac massage, by the same person doing cardiac massage.

2. Diabetic coma

This has been discussed in the chapter on diabetes at page 69 and 70.

3. Epilepsy

Marked convulsions may be observed in a patient of epilepsy at odd hours/place. The attacks may come one after another. In such a situation, an injection of lorazepam, slowly and intravenously, is highly useful, and the attack is likely to subside instantaneously, especially in mild to moderate cases. Since the patient will be almost unconscious, it should be ensured that his neck is straight. At the same time it should be seen that the patient does not bite his tongue. This can be prevented by placing the handle of a spoon wrapped in a cloth between the back teeth of the patient. Shifting the patient to hospital should be done after first aid has been administered. The details of the disease are available on page 93.

4. Injury to the head, spine, chest, abdomen, fractures and burn injuries

It would be worthwhile to discuss in this chapter various urgent tips regarding first aid in the case of accidental injuries to the head, spine, chest and abdomen, as well as various fractures, so that immediate steps for treatment are taken, providing some relief, especially to a dying patient.

Injury to the head, spine, chest and abdomen requires immediate attention. The injury may cause a wound, or it may be a blunt one, both are equally serious. There may be a fracture of the skull, or of the ribs, or of the spine.

If there is a wound, emergency measures should immediately be adopted before the patient is taken to the hospital. A sharp wound usually bleeds profusely. Clean the wound, cut the surrounding hair, apply any antiseptic lotion and quickly put the pressure bandage. An injection of tetanus toxoid should be given for the prophylaxis of tetanus.

Head injury

Injury to the head, however minor, must be attended to, as in some of the cases, symptoms of the head injury start appearing after 48-72 hours, and in some even later. The reason is that following the head injury, a small amount of blood goes on collecting in the brain, and when a sufficient amount of blood collects in the brain, say in about one, two or three days, the symptoms become apparent. In view of this, the dictum is that the patient of a head injury must be kept under observation in a hospital, even though the injury may be minor and the patient feels normal. A computed tomographic (CT) scanning of the head must be taken to rule out any pathology in the skull or brain.

In the case of a driver, the author suspected haemorrhage in the brain, following a minor head injury about which the patient did not bother. As a result of it, he developed persistent headache. The patient was strongly advised to undergo scanning of the head immediately, and it astonished many when he went into coma just after the scanning of the head. The scan showed a marked haemorrhage in the brain that could be cleared out by an operation after opening up the skull (craniotomy). Within the next 5-6 hours, the patient regained consciousness, and after being discharged from the hospital, he resumed his normal activities.

The fate of such a case can be well imagined had no early diagnosis or investigation been made available in time. Generally, in such cases, following unconsciousness, a lot of time is wasted in diagnosis/investigations and an immediate operation is delayed, causing several neurological problems, like paralysis of a part of the body, etc. The disease could even be fatal.

The author also had the opportunity to discuss personally a different case of head injury at General Medical Council, London, with the President, Lord Walton, a famous neurologist, regarding the case of a young adult. The detailed records and relevant investigations of this case were taken to London. This patient had a fall from a height of about 15 feet in his early childhood at the age of one year, and he got a head injury. This was not appropriately attended to, and it may be of interest to note that after a long period of ten years after the head injury, the patient developed attacks of convulsions. The conclusion arrived at was that it was clearly a case of post-traumatic epilepsy following head injury in infancy. The injured part of the brain developed scarring which was responsible for epilepsy in this case. At that stage, even surgery had not been considered fruitful.

Lord Walton summarizing this case, commented "In the case of ..., aged 21 years, it does seem to me that the evidence clearly suggests that this boy developed a post-traumatic porencephaly (*cavity in the brain*), involving the parieto-occipital regions of the brain on the right side. Clearly that porencephaly was surrounded by an area of scarring and gliosis which has been responsible for the subsequent picture of focal post-traumatic epilepsy in this case ... My own view is that ..., there is little, if any, prospect that surgery would be of benefit in this case ..."

A word of caution! In some mild cases of head injury, the patient may lose consciousness only for a while (concussion). In this case, the injury is truly a mild one. The brain function which was disturbed for a while reverses to the normal, and the patient regains mental clarity.

But in some cases, if the injury is a little more than mild, the patient may lose consciousness twice. First due to concussion, and later, due to the damage to the brain, as a result of the collection of blood inside the brain tissue. This second episode of unconsciousness is more severe in nature and the patient requires urgent transportation to the hospital for immediate tests like CT scan, and immediate surgery may be required. The period between these two attacks of unconsciousness is called the lucid interval.

The possibility of the occurrence of the lucid interval must be kept in mind, and, following the concussion, one should not relax, as the patient may again lose consciousness, if bleeding in the brain continues, which is a very severe emergency, and any delay in the treatment of such cases may cause more damage to the vital centres/tracts inside the brain, causing neurological deficits, like paralysis, etc.

However, when the injury is severe from the beginning, or the injury to the brain is so much marked, that bleeding in the brain starts immediately following such an injury, there will be no lucid interval, and the patient will lose consciousness right from the beginning of the head injury, and will remain in coma for quite sometime, till the patient gets proper treatment.

There is another important aspect of a lucid interval worth mentioning. In this context, it is stated that besides urgent care in the treatment of such cases, the lucid interval may gain importance in some medicolegal cases. In such cases, the successors/beneficiaries of the diseased may say that following unconsciousness as a result of head injury, the patient did regain consciousness for a while, and gave his dying declaration before he went into coma again. It is a valuable piece of evidence. But it can be questioned regarding its authenticity in a court of law.

The only way to establish the truth of a lucid interval is to study the extent of the injury to the brain of the deceased person. As stated above, the lucid interval is unlikely to occur when the injury is severe, as in the case of a fracture of the skull with marked contusion and laceration/tearing of the brain tissue. The post-mortem report does help in such cases which show marked damage to the brain tissue, like contusion and laceration of the brain, with blood filled cavities.

This aspect of a lucid interval was also discussed with Lord Walton, who commented, "The lucid interval does not occur in severe head injuries causing fracture of the skull, contusion and laceration of the brain. The only circumstance under which the lucid interval occurs is when a blow on the head, perhaps causing fracture and transient concussion, is followed by recovery of consciousness within a short period usually not exceeding a few minutes, but is then succeeded by progressive impairment of consciousness due to rupture of the middle meningeal artery causing extradural haemorrhage. There is no evidence to suggest that such a lucid interval occurs in any cases without such a mechanism being operative."

Needless to say that awareness of the lucid interval is important for the urgent treatment of a case of head injury, as well as in a medicolegal case, if such a situation warrants.

Spinal Injuries

These are mostly either accidental or due to fall from a height. Such cases need urgent attention in specialized injuries centers. These centers need to be increased in different parts of the country so that minimum time is lost in starting the right treatment. Also, awareness needs to be created so that patients reach at the earliest possible and chances of recovery increases. Creation of trauma centers on highways helps in starting the treatment in no time in accidental cases.

Injury to chest and abdomen

In all cases of chest injuries, chest X-rays must be taken and urgent treatment should be given in a hospital, if there is any fracture of the ribs and/or injury to the lungs.

However, cases of injuries to the abdomen require very careful attention. If the intestines have come out, put sterilized gauze or cotton over the protruded viscera and apply loose bandage across the abdomen. Outside the operation theatre, never try to force the viscera into the abdominal cavity as an emergency measure.

Fractures

Fractures may be simple, where there is no wound or compound, which are accompanied by wound/wounds. Sometimes there may be even multiple fractures. In case there is a wound, it should be treated as described earlier on page 304, para 2. In case there is profuse bleeding, a string/tourniquet should be tied on the limb above the bleeding area, so that the patient may not die due to profuse bleeding and shock. A pain-killer injection, whichever is available, should be given promptly, if possible. The tourniquet must be released every half an hour, so that circulation in the part of the limb below the tourniquet may not suffer. The patient should be rushed to hospital after giving immediate support to the fractured area, as described below:

In the case of the fracture of the upper arm (humerus), tie the upper arm to the trunk with a piece of cloth or bandage. Do not forget to keep the other arm free, and the best would be to ask the patient to place the hand of the unaffected side over his head, before tying the fractured arm to the trunk. Use a sling for the fractured arm. For the fracture of the forearm, apply wooden splints (after applying cotton and bandage over these splints) over the two surfaces (anterior and posterior) of the forearm, and then tie with the help of bandage. A sling, of course, will have to be used. For any fracture of the lower limb, tie the fractured limb to the normal limb. For example, if there is a fracture of the femur (thigh), tie the fractured thigh to the other thigh with the help of any bandage, and so on.

Burn injuries

Mass awareness about burns injuries is very important. Adults/elderly should keep in mind that children are likely to get burn injuries from bursting crackers during festivals or special occasions. All precautions ought to be taken so that minors are not inflicted with burn injuries due to any reason. In case accident does occur, pour water on the burnt area of the skin for at least 15-20 minutes depending upon the severity of the burn. With this measure, raised temperature of the burnt area shall be lowered and cells of the skin shall be saved from dying as a result of heat. Cover the burnt area with a clean cloth/towel, as burnt injuries are usually sterile in the beginning. Antiseptic ointments can be applied including the administration of antibiotics and pain-killers etc. In severe cases, the patient should be immediately taken to the hospital. Fire, chemicals, air-raids are some other causes of burns.

Remember that whenever any injury or fracture occurs, the patient should not be given anything to eat or drink, since some sort of immediate operation may be required on reaching the hospital, which may not be possible if the patient has a full stomach. The reason is that administering general anaesthesia, which may be required, will not then be possible immediately. Introduction of post graduation courses like M.D. in emergency medicine (already available in selected developed countries) would help in dealing with all sorts of emergencies more effectively.

To conclude, it should be stressed that the only way to prevent immediate as well as late/serious complications of fatal diseases/accidental cases is that mass awareness should be created for learning and practising various first-aid measures, so that the life of the affected/injured person can be saved. Undoubtedly, this is the need of the hour, considering the fast-increasing incidence of mortalities in such situations.

Appendix VII

URGENT DIETARY MEASURES FOR THE PREVENTION OF COMMON SERIOUS DISEASES

Recommended diet for prevention and treatment of coronary artery disease, brain vessel disease (stroke), high blood pressure, diabetes, overweight, high blood cholesterol / uric acid, and for those above 40. A diet especially advised for prevention of cancer has also been indicated.

Tea and coffee	: To be taken in moderation. Tea should be light, moderately brewed and not boiled. To be avoided in high blood uric acid cases. Longer the brewing time of the tea, more the caffeine extracted. The common practice of wayside stalls and even homes of keeping tea brewing in vessels is not advisable.
Milk	: Skimmed milk preferred.
Sugar	: Low consumption of sugar advisable. None/very restricted for diabetics.
Egg	: Only white portion of the egg to be taken.
Bread	: Brown bread preferred.
Salt	: Should be used sparingly, 2-4 g per day.

Condiments and spices	: Permissible in moderation. Their excessive use causes stimulation of the appetite, and may cause overeating.
High fibre food	: Strongly recommended including for prevention of cancer. It includes: a) Whole wheat, gram, maize or similar flour (bran to be taken along with it). b) Whole pulses. c) Unpolished rice. d) Plenty of green vegetables — cooked or salad. e) Porridge (*dalia*), corn flakes, oats, preferably with skimmed milk. f) Roasted grams. g) Sprouted beans, grams, peas, *moong*, etc. All edible as well as sproutable legumes, grains and seeds may be used.
Cheese	: Cheddar cheese commonly available in tins to be avoided.
Cottage cheese	: May be taken since it is prepared from skimmed milk.
Curds and yoghurt	: Prepared from skimmed milk permissible.
Oils	: To be used in minimal necessary quantities for cooking. Polyunsaturated oils, like safflower, corn, sunflower, soybean, cotton seed oils, etc. are recommended. Oil once used for deep frying should not be reused. A low-fat diet is also useful in the prevention of cancer.
Butter / ghee	: 20% permissible.

Onion and garlic	: May be taken, particularly while using butter/ghee. They tend to lower serum cholesterol and other lipids.
Pickles	: May be taken sparingly as they contain excessive salt.
Meats	: Fish and chicken, i.e., white meats are permissible, but refrain from red meats. In high blood uric acid cases, all meats, including fish, are forbidden.
Soft drinks	: May be taken occasionally. Cola drinks are harmful in high blood uric acid cases. A squeeze of lime-juice added to a glass of water can be taken.
Alcoholic drinks	: Avoid, for prevention of cancer. However, if one drinks, one may consume alcohol only in moderation (see page 291, para 2). High blood uric acid cases should abstain from alcoholic drinks.
Smoking / tobacco chewing	: Strictly prohibited, particularly for the prevention of cancer.
Vegetable soups	: Permissible
Fruit	: Only low-calorie fruits can be taken, e.g. apple, orange, watermelon, guava, papaya, muskmelon, etc.
Sweets	: To be generally avoided. Not advisable in cases of diabetes.
Dry fruit	: To be generally avoided, especially cashew nuts.
Chocolate	: Not recommended in high blood uric acid cases. Can be taken occasionally.
Icecream	: Icecream prepared from skimmed milk with a little sugar or artificial sweetener may be taken.
Cakes and pastries	: May be taken occasionally.

Urgent Dietary Measures

Party / fast / junk food : Better to be sparingly taken, as we do not know what oil, etc. is used. Home-cooked food is ideal. Green diet is preferred. It includes fruits, green vegetables and fresh salad. Use of chips, salty and high fat snacks, pizza, burgers, patties, instant nodules should be minimized.

Water : Two to three litres of water should be taken every day. Take water either before or after meals, only if you are thirsty. Plenty of water may be taken between major meals. More water is required during the summer season.

Some other important instructions

1. It is ideal to have a low/moderate calorie diet. Do consult a calorie reckoner while planning your diet.
2. Take light meals frequently rather than heavy meals at one time.
3. Overeating should be avoided. It is rightly said that we eat to live, not live to eat.
4. Old people require a good balanced diet, as it increases their immunity and prevents serious diseases. Light tonics may be added under the advice of the physician. People with undernourished organs may suffer on account of a poor diet. A diet for old people, therefore, needs to be properly planned.

From the above given details, it is clear that a proper diet is essential for keeping the body healthy and protecting it from various diseases.

"Eating greasy and indigestible food, overeating, excessive sleep, ignoring one's ailment at the beginning, and lack of exercise, are the causes of diseases of the heart related to 'kapha' ".

Charaka-Samhita,
Sutrasthana 17.34

We are what we eat
LUDWIG FEUERBACH

Appendix VIII

EXERCISE — FOR THE PREVENTION/ TREATMENT OF COMMON SERIOUS DISEASES

Exercise plays a significant role not only in maintaining normal health, but also for the prevention and treatment of diseases like coronary artery disease, hypertension, diabetes, obesity, high blood cholesterol, stroke, cancers, etc. (refer to the related chapters and the appendix on obesity for details).

This is not all. There are other several benefits of exercise. It improves bone density and hence helps to prevent osteoporosis that may occur particularly in postmenopausal women. It adds to one's sense of well-being, confers tranquility to the mind, reduces the chances of depression, constipation and improves lung functions. The most important added advantage of increased physical activity is that it prevents premature death.

However, it should be undertaken with care, especially while initiating an exercise programme in the case of a middle-aged person. At this age, it should be carried out after consulting a physician. Only limited activity may be permissible when the heart is involved.

Exercise is useful both in cases of type 1 and 2 diabetes mellitus (DM). It controls blood sugar levels in both the types of DM. Caution is needed in cases of type 1 DM as in this type of disorder while undergoing exercise programme, the patient is likely to suffer from low or high blood sugar levels. Therefore in such cases, estimation of blood sugar would be essential before and after exercise. If need be the test may also be carried out during the period of exercise. Since cardiovascular complications occur more at an earlier age, say around 35 years of age in cases of DM, urgent tests would be required before commencing exercise regime so as to watch the cardiovascular status of the individual patient, more so, if the diabetes is of long duration (say for the last 10-15 years) and/or there is involvement of kidneys (nephropathy), eyes (retinopathy), peripheral nerves (neuropathy) and/or the patient is suffering from other various risk factors relating to coronary artery disease.

In cases of osteoarthritis of weight-bearing joints, regular exercise reduces pain and disability of the joints. It improves the gait and speed in walking. If the patient is not careful, lack of exercise in such cases results in pain in joints and other complications of the disease and the patient passes a sedentary life that invites serious ailments like coronary artery disease, hypertension, DM etc. As time passes, muscular weakness/ atrophy may occur and the patients may become fully disabled. Hence there is an urgent need of exercise programme in cases of osteoarthritis, both for its treatment and prevention

In elderly persons, besides the beneficial effects of exercise on blood sugar, blood pressure, cardiovascular system etc., it helps in maintaining the strength of muscles, coordination, flexibility, balance of body and thereby prevents falls and subsequent fracture of bones that are likely to occur if the old person is not reasonably active. The added advantage is the mental alertness, besides all other uses/benefits of other age groups.

A simple brisk walk is highly beneficial as it improves and energises the whole system. Jogging, cycling, running, etc. are a few common exercises which can be done. The old saying, "I have two doctors — my right leg and my left leg" certainly conveys the most valuable piece of advice. Although all these exercises are good, walking seems to be the ideal one. It can be done conveniently at any place, in any weather and does not need any sports gears. It can be done at any age even by the old persons. 30-40 minutes per day for at least five days in a week is the recommended duration of exercise. There should be no break in exercise programme. It is better if it can be done daily.

Before starting on a brisk walk, it is essential that you warm yourself by walking initially at an exceptionally slow pace, which should be slowly increased to a more brisk walk till you achieve the peak, which too should be comfortable. Cooling down your walk is also important. When you wish to cool down, slow your pace while walking and continue reducing the pace till your heart rate is almost normal or you feel satisfied. Good sports shoes and loose comfortable clothes suited to the weather are recommended.

There is a word of caution. Unaccustomed sudden vigorous/ very heavy physical exercise (or even physical exertion of routine work) may be associated with sudden death, especially in a middle aged person. Regular moderate exercise always helps and also tends to prevent the possible risk of sudden death. Keeping this in view, to begin with, always start your walking exercise programme for lesser duration, which is, for 10-15 minutes or even less and you can always achieve the desired results in due course.

Irrespective of your age, if you are not yet involved in exercise programme, start it immediately. It is never too late but to postpone it day after day is not good for the maintenance of good health. Even elderly persons who remained inactive in their younger age may start their exercise programme for the up keep of their health to avoid both physical disability and premature death. It may be pointed out that physical inactivity is one of the leading causes of disease and disability. Many diseases can be prevented by regular physical activity alone, thereby, reducing the health care costs as well.

Needless to say, both diet and exercise play a vital role in controlling many of the diseases. It is never advisable to straightway take drugs without first resorting to the discipline of diet and exercise, more so in early / borderline cases of diabetes, high blood cholesterol, overweight, hypertension etc. Drugs should be added only when required.

Hence, the value of diet and exercise should always be kept in mind for the treatment as well as prevention of various diseases.

"Any physical activity which suits the liking or taste of an individual and brings strength and stability to the body is called 'physical exercise'. This should be carried out, keeping in view one's own state of health".

Charaka-Samhita,
Sutrasthana 7. 31

INDEX

Abortion 7
Aches and pains 84
Acid fast bacilli (AFB) 126
Acquired immune deficiency syndrome (AIDS) 130, 145, 274, 299
- diagnosis 275
- incubation period 274
- prevention 275
- symptoms and signs 274
- tests 275
Active tuberculosis/
- active cases of tuberculosis 131, 144
Acute anterior poliomyelitis 121
Acute cholicystitis 4
Acute glomerulonephritis (GN) 192, 200, 206, 296
Acute leukaemia 9
Acute nephritis
- high blood uric acid 87
Acute renal (kidney) failure (ARF) 199-203
- dialysis 202
- during recovery 202
- prevention 203
- renal transplant 203
- signs and symptoms 200
- tests 202
- treatment 201
Albumin-urine 173, 174, 192, 194, 197, 208, 214
Alcohol 78, 117
- high blood pressure 76
- high blood uric acid 84, 88
- prevention of congenital heart disease (CHD) 59
Alcohol and diseases 289

Alcoholic/s 130, 165
Alcoholic beverages 19, 37
Alkaline phosphatase 165
Allergens 152, 157, 158, 163
Allergy and bronchial asthma 151-163
- allergic factors 153
- allergy, attack of asthma 152
- asthma in elderly 157
- breathing exercises 161
- complications of asthma 156
- diagnosis 152
- drug treatment 160
- epidemiological survey 163
- general prophylactic measures 158
- immunotherapy 162
- outgrowing asthma 163
- peak flow meter (PFM) 161
- prophylaxis of asthma 157
- tests in a case of asthma 157
- treatment of refractory asthma 163
- warning signals of asthma 151
Alternating constipation and diarrhoea 1, 4
Ambulatory blood pressure recorder 7
Ambulatory ECG (Holter) monitoring 32
Amenorrhoea 230
Amyloidosis 194, 196
Anaemia
- chronic renal failure (CRF) 208
Anal canal-cancer 14
Angina 231, 280, 281
Angina pectoris 23
- diabetes 65

- drug treatment 36
- treadmill stress test (TMT) 33
Anginal pain 24
- awareness/knowledge 24
Angioplasty (ballooning) 25, 35
- rheumatic heart disease – RHD (chronic) 49
Anosmia 8
Anthracosis 130
Anticoagulants 36
Anti-plague vaccine 271
Anti-snake venom (ASV) 240
Anti-tetanus serum (ATS) 260
Antivenin-scorpion sting 253
Anuria 202
Aortic stenosis 47, 56, 280
Aortic stenosis/regurgitation (AS/AR) 56
Apoplexy 90
Appendicitis 167, 279
Appetite
- loss (unexplained) 2
Arrhythmias 47, 106, 110, 280, 290
Asbestosis 130
Aspirin
- high blood uric acid 88
- primary prevention of coronary artery disease (CAD) 39
Asthma
- *See under* allergy and bronchial asthma 151
Asymptomatic
- coronary artery disease (CAD) 21
- detection of CAD 28, 33
- detection of congenital heart disease (CHD) 56
- high blood pressure 74
- subclinical hypothyroidism 227
Atelectasis 157
Atherosclerosis 23, 26, 27, 108, 295
Atrial extrasystolae, flutter or fibrillation
- rheumatic heart disease (RHD) 47
Atrial fibrillation 106, 224
Atrial septal defect (ASD) 52
Aura 94, 96, 99, 104

Backaches
- high blood uric acid 84, 86
Ballooning
- coarctation of aorta and other congenital lesions of the heart 55
- coronary artery disease (CAD) 25, 35
- rheumatic heart disease (RHD) 49
Barrett's oesophagus 3
BCG vaccination 133, 136, 143
Beer
- high blood uric acid 84
Behaviour
- sudden change 8
Benign/senile enlargement of the prostate (BEP/SEP) 5, 177, 183, 189, 199, 284
Beverages
- alcoholic 19
Bile duct
- malignancy 9
Bile salts and pigments
- urine 296
Birth injury 100
Birthmark 2, 8
Black death 267
Black rat (Rattus rattus)-plague 263, 264
Bladder
- habits 1, 5
Bleeding
- contact (vaginal) 2, 6
- following/after intercourse 2, 6
- following tooth extraction 9
- from the nose 9
- in early pregnancy 7
- in hydatiform mole 7
- irregular through vagina 6
- nipple 1, 4, 13
- post menopausal/intermenstrual 6
Blood
- cancers 11, 296
- coagulability 17, 28
- in faeces 250
- in sputum 1, 2, 134, 279

Index

- in stool 1, 4, 207
- in urine 2, 5, 237, 250
- in vomit 237, 250
- occult 14
- oozing from gums 9
- stained froth 96
- through rectum 4

Blood cholesterol
- high 29, 33, 36, 79-83

Blood glucose meter 69, 162

Blood lipids 17, 28, 297 (serum cholesterol/lipidogram)

Blood pressure 17, 199, 201, 224, 250, 290
- apparatus 75, 162
- high 27, 29, 33, 36, 38, 74-78
- in children 75
- low 75
- recorder (ambulatory) 75
- systolic 75, 281 (systolic hypertension), 283

Blood sugar 28, 32, 230, 297
- high 17, 29, 36 see diabetes 60-73

Blood urea 141, 169, 185, 192, 197, 200, 202, 205, 206, 208, 209, 210, 297

Blood uric acid
- high 27, 36, 84-89
- test 297

Blue/cyanosed
- CHD (congenital heart disease) 53

Boils-diabetes 65

Bone densitometry 283

Bone marrow examination 10, 296

Bone scan
- prostate cancer 6

Bones 129, 137

Bowel habits 1, 4

Brain 44, 59, 74, 94, 97, 98, 105, 108, 121, 129, 137, 205, 208, 290
- damage 114
- haemorrhage 91, 250
- high blood pressure 74
- injury 116
- tumours 2, 7, 99, 110, 112

Breasts
- cancer 4, 11, 18, 299

- enlarged in males – gynacomastia 17
- feeding 231
- female 15
- male 17
- self examination 13
- small in females 15
- thickening/lump 1, 4, 13, 17

Breathing exercises
- asthma 161

Breath-holding spells 104

Breathlessness 26, 53, 151

Brisk walk - exercise 315

Bronchial asthma
- *See under* allergy and bronchial asthma

Bronchiectasis 157

Bronchodilator inhalers 161

Bronchogenic carcinoma 2, 18

Bronchoscopy 157

Bubo 266

Bubonic plague 266

Burning sensation 94, 141

Butter
- high blood cholesterol 79

Caffeine
- high blood uric acid 84, 86

Calcium 282

Calcium oxalate stone 176

Calcium phosphate stone 176

Calculi
- urinary 176

Cancer
- anal canal 14, 299
- awareness campaign/programme 11
- blood 11
- brain (tumour) 99
- breasts 4, 13, 292, 299
- cancers and their prevention 1-20
- cervix 6, 14
- colon 4, 14, 279, 299
- dietary preventive measures 310
- duodenum 298

- food-pipe 287, 289
- gallbladder 4, 87, 164
- gastrointestinal tract 296
- general measures for prevention of cancer 19
- kidney 167
- liver 165, 289
- lung 2, 15, 287, 296, 298, 299
- male breast 18
- malignancy and use of female hormones 16
- mouth 287
- oesophagus 287, 289, 298
- pharynx 3, 287
- prevention (general measures) 19
- prostate 6, 14, 167, 178, 296
- prostate-bone scan 6
- prostate-family history 6
- prostate-MRI (magnetic resonance imaging) 6
- rectum 4, 14, 299
- self examination of breasts and testes 11
- stomach 289, 298
- testes 4, 11
- tests (urgent)/regular check-up 13
- thyroid gland 222
- urinary bladder 167
- urinary tract 14, 296
- uterus 6, 17, 167, 292, 298
- warning signals 1

Carbuncle
- diabetes 65

Carotid sinus syncope 107
Carotid syncope 106
Cataract
- diabetes 65

Cerebellar ataxia (hypothyroidism) 230, 233, 234
Cerebellar degeneration (alcohol) 290
Cerebral infarction 110
Cerebral vascular accident (CVA) 90
Cervical spondylosis 30, 282
Cervix

- cancer/malignancy 6, 14, 17
- ultrasonography (USG) 7

Change in bladder habits 1, 5
Change in bowel habits 1, 4, 279
Chest
- injury 307
- pain 23, 26, 30, 250, 278
- pain, tightness or pressure/weight-like 24
- tetanus 259

Chest X-ray 15, 131, 135, 136, 139, 157, 267, 279, 298, 307
Chewing of tobacco 287
Childhood epilepsy 102
Cholecystitis 1, 30, 164
- acute 4
- chronic 4
- High blood uric acid 87

Cholellithiasis 1, 30, 164
- high blood uric acid 87

Cholesterol 79
Chorionepithelioma 7
Chronic renal (Kidney) failure (CRF) 203-218
- causes 204
- complications/symptomatology 207
- diagnosis 205
- dialysis 210
- investigations 206
- prevention 210
- renal transplant 210
- treatment 209

Chronic/recurrent urinary tract infection (UTI) 170-191
- antibiotics 186
- infection 170
- Kidney damage 174
- occult/hidden 174
- other conditions relating to UTI 182
- predisposing factors/obstructive lesions 175
- prevention 187
- symptoms and signs 172, 173
- tests 183
- treatment 175

Index

321

Clostridium tetani 255
Coarctation of aorta 55
Cobras 235, 238
Coca
- high blood uric acid 85, 88
Coffee
- high blood uric acid 85, 88
Coital death 41
Colon
- cancer 4, 14
- colonoscopy, sigmoidoscopy 7, 14, 299
Colonoscope 167
Colonoscopy 7, 14, 167, 299
Coma
- diabetic 65, 70, 303
- head injury (unconsciousness) 305
- myxoedema 230
- renal failure 203, 208
Computed tomographic (CT) coronary angiogram (64 slice CT) 34
Computed tomographic (CT) scanning 8, 92, 95, 110, 138, 167, 206, 223, 298, 304
Concussion 305, 306
Congenital heart disease (CHD) 51-59
- areas of the heart where congenital defects occur 53
- detection of occult/hidden cases 56
- early symptoms/warning signals - tetralogy/pentalogy of Fallot 53
- 'late cyanotic (blue)' congenital heart disease 54
- other congenital lesions 55
- prevention of CHD 58
- prevention of subacute bacterial endocarditis 57
Constipation 1, 4, 279
Contact bleeding 2, 6
Continuous ambulatory recording of
- electroencephalogram - EEG (24-hour) 110

Contraceptives (oral) 16, 29, 76
Convulsions 93, 96, 103, 112, 113, 114, 119, 260, 261, 305
Corn oil
- blood cholesterol 79
Coronary arteries 21, 22
- angiography 25, 29, 33, 34, 298
- atherosclerosis 27
- blockage 35
- cold weather 39
- complete blockage of the flow of blood 25
- hardening 27
- narrowing 26
- sudden cardiac death (SCD) 294
- walls of coronary arteries 36
Coronary artery bypass graft (CABG) 35
Coronary artery bypass surgery 35
Coronary artery dilators 36
Coronary artery disease (CAD) 21-42
- angina pectoris 24
- cause 23
- coronary arteries 22
- heart attack 25
- investigations 32
- occult/asymptomatic/hidden 21, 28
- pain in chest 30
- prevention 37
- primary prevention 37
- rehabilitation after heart attack 41
- risk factors 27
- secondary prevention 40
- See also pages 84, 86, 231, 280 (heart attack in old age), 295, 300 (heart attack - first aid), 311
Coronary occlusion 25
Coronary prone personality/behaviour (CPP/CPB) 27, 38
Corticoids 293
- diabetes 64
- glucose tolerance test (GTT) 63
Corticosteroids 195
Cotton seed oil
- blood cholesterol 79

Cough 134, 151, 267, 279
- persistently troublesome 1
C-reactive protein (CRP)
- rheumatic fever 45
Creatine clearance (24-hour) 185
Creatinine phosphokinase-CPK (MB) 32, 157, 297
Cretinism 231
Cushing's syndrome 293
Cystercercosis 100, 110
Cystitis 172, 174, 178, 183, 190, 276
Cystoscopy 299
Cysts of cysticerci 111

Dandruff from the skin of animals
- asthma 155
Deafness
- unilateral 8
Densitometry 283
Depersonalisation 94
Depression 8, 285
- asthma 154
- rehabilitation after heart attack 42
Detection of various common serious diseases
- urgent tests 89, 296
Diabetes 60-73
- control 66
- general instructions
- glycosylated haemoglobin (HbAIC) 65
- warning signals 65, 69
- *See also* pages 27, 37, 38, 91, 117, 119, 130, 182, 189, 194, 196, 204, 206, 207, 209, 212, 213, 217, 282, 292, 294, 296, 297, 310, 314
Diabetic ambulatory care service (DACS) 73
Diabetic emergency kit 73
Diabetic coma 65, 70, 303
Diabetic kidney 182
Dialysis 169, 190, 192, 200, 202, 204, 205, 210, 211
Diet
- chronic renal failure (CRF) 209

- coronary artery disease (CAD) 27
- epilepsy (infected pork) 116
- high-fiber diet (for diabetics) 66
- low fat, calorie, sugar-free/restricted (for diabetics) 66
- non-vegetarian - high blood uric acid 79
- obesity (good eating habits) 293
- stroke 91
- tuberculosis (good nutrition) 142
- urgent dietary measures for prevention 310-313 (appendix VII)
- urinary stones 177
Differential leucocyte count (DLC) 10, 141, 296
Digital rectal examination (DRE) 14
Diplopia 8
Discharge
- nipple 1, 4, 13
- Vaginal 2
Diseases of abdomen and ultrasonography 164-168
Diseases of the heart 21-59
- congenital heart disease (CHD) 51
- coronary artery disease (CAD) 21
- in old persons 280
- rheumatic heart disease (RHD) 42
Diseases of the kidneys 169-218
- acute renal (kidney) failure (ARF) 19
- Chronic/recurrent urinary tract infection (UTI) 170
- chronic renal (kidney) failure (CRF) 203
- glomerulonephritis (GN) 191
Diseases of old age 277- 286
- anaemia/lack of nutrition 282
- benign/senile enlargement of the prostate (BEP/SEP) 284
- body temperature 285
- clinical manifestation, different in old 278

Index

- diabetes 282
- diseases of the brain 280
- diseases of the heart 280
- geriatrics 277
- osteoarthritis 282
- osteoporosis 282
  - tests in the case of elderly persons 285
- systolic hypertension 281
- treatment in old age 285

Diseases of the thyroid gland 219-234
- cancer of thyroid gland 222
- cretinism 231
- goiter 221
- hyperfunction of thyroid gland 223
  - early symptoms/warning signals 224
  - late cases 225
  - tests 225
  - treatment 225
- hypofunction of thyroid gland 226
- hypothyroidism
  - investigations 230
  - signs and symptoms 228
  - treatment 230
- iodine and thyroid hormones 220
- subclinical hypothyroidism 227
  - diagnosis 227
  - treatment 228
  - when to suspect 227
- TSH (thyroid stimulating hormone) 227
- unusual manifestations of hyperthyroidism and hypothyroidism: personal experience 232

Dizziness 27
Domestic rats 264
Double vision 8
Drug prophylaxis
- penicillin 50
- rheumatic fever (RF)/rheumatic heart disease (RHD) 49
- subacute bacterial endocarditis 57

Drugs
- abuse 117
- abusers 130
- anticoagulants 36
- antiepileptic 8, 113
- causing gynecomastia 18
- causing high blood uric acid 88
- coronary dilator 26, 40
- diabetes 67
- for high blood pressure 77
- for high blood uric acid 89
- glyceryl trinitrate 26, 40
- interactions 285
- reactions 285
- resistance 147
- used for tuberculosis 140

Duodenum
- cancer/ulcer 298
- carcinoma 3
- inflammation/ulceration 30
- peptic ulcer 3, 287
- upper gastrointestinal (GI) endoscopy 7

Dwarfism 231
Dysfunctional uterine bleeding 229
Dyspepsia 3
Dysphagia 3, 8

Ear discharge (otitis media) 257
Ears
- ringing 8
Earthquakes 264
Echocardiography
- cardiac syncope 106
- detection of occult/hidden cases of congenital heart disease (CHD) 56, 57
- Foetal (prevention of CHD) 58, 59
- in heart diseases – congenital heart disease (CHD), ischaemic heart disease (IHD), rheumatic heart disease (RHD) 298
- rheumatic fever 46
- stress echocardiography 35

Egg-yolk
- blood cholesterol 79

Electrocardiogram (ECG) 32, 106, 231, 278, 279, 298, 302
- Exercise ECG 29
- high blood pressure 76
- resting ECG 29
- rheumatic fever 45

Electroencephalogram (EEG) 95, 97, 106, 108, 109, 113, 114, 117, 119, 298

Emotion 95
Emotional instability 281
Emotional shock 106
Emotional stress 154
Emphysema 157
Endemic iodine deficiency goitre 221, 222
Endoscope 167
Endoscope ultrasound (EUS) 167
Enzyme linked immunosorbent assay (ELISA)
- acquired immune deficiency syndrome (AIDS) 275, 299
- tuberculosis 136, 299

Epilepsy 93-120
- antiepileptic drugs – withdrawal 116
- attacks – details 95
- cause of disturbance in the brain 98
- causes of transitory unconsciousness 105
- childhood epilepsy 102
- drop attacks 108
- first seizure 113
- general guidelines 118
- hysterical convulsions 104
- mental health 109
- pitfalls in detecting occult/hidden cases 100
- prevention 116
- refractory epilepsy 115
- status epilepticus 113
- treatment 111
- *See also* pages 8, 59, 208, 290, 298, 303

Epileptic attacks/fits 2, 8, 93, 98, 208
Epileptic convulsions 103, 104
Erythrocyte sedimentation rate (ESR) 45, 48

Escherichia coli (E. coli) 170, 183, 190 (vaccine)
Ethanol 289
Exercise
- diabetes 66, 73
- for the prevention/treatment 314-316 (appendix VIII)
- high blood pressure 77
- high blood uric acid 86
- lack of exercise – coronary artery disease (CAD) 27
- obesity 293
- regular exercises 38
- stroke 91

Exercise electrocardiogram (ECG) 29, 298
Exopthalmos 224
External cardiac massage 301 (fig.), 302
Extracorporeal shock-wave lithotripsy (ESWL) 176
Extradural haemorrhage 307
Extrapulmonary tuberculosis 137
Eyes
- high blood pressure 74
- pallor 2, 9
Eyewitness 95, 96, 102, 103, 109, 110, 111

Fall in the elderly
- causes 283
Family history
- asthma 152
- coronary artery disease (CAD) 27, 28, 29, 38
- diabetes 60, 65
- epilepsy 117
- graves' disease 224
- high blood pressure 78
- hypothyroidism 227
- prostate cancer 6
Fasting blood sugar 297
Fasting glucose test 61
Fat (low) diet 20
Feathers of birds – asthma 155
Female breast 15
- cancer 11

Index

Female hormones
- malignancy 16

Fever
- epilepsy 117
- low grade (unexplained) 2
- old age 279
- Plague epidemic (sudden high fever) 266
- poliomyelitis 122
- rheumatic 42

Fibrillation
- atrial – rheumatic heart disease (RHD) 47

Fibroid tumour of the uterus 6

Fine needle aspiration cytology (FNAC) 137, 223, 298

First-aid
- diabetic coma 303
- epilepsy 303, 111
- for prevention/immediate control of some common serious diseases 300-309 (appendix VI)
- injury to the head, spine, chest, abdomen, fractures and burn injuries 303
- heart attack 300
- rabies (urgent steps after the bite) 243
- reviving the heart 302
- technique for reviving the heart 302
- scorpion-sting (immediate local care) 248
- snake-bite (immediately after the bite) 239

First seizure 113
Fits/attacks – epileptic 2
Flashes 117
Flea-bitten kidney 192
Flickers 117
Focal convulsions 94
Focal epilepsy 94, 95, 97, 100, 103, 138
Foetal echocardiography
- prevention of CHD 59
Food-pipe 30, 222, 289
- cancer 287
- carcinoma 3

Foods
- allergy/asthma 153

Fractures 282, 303, 307
- of the skull 306

Frightened 94
Frothing 96
Functional problems of the elderly 284
Fundi examination
- high blood pressure 76
Fungal infection
- diabetes 65

Gallbladder 164, 298
- Inflamed 1, 4
- Malignancy 9
Gallstones 1, 4, 30, 164, 292
- high blood uric acid 87
Gangrene foot
- diabetes 71
Gastric/duodenal peptic ulcer 1, 3, 297
Gastric peptic ulcer 287
Gastritis 30
Gastrointestinal endoscopy 167
Generalized epileptic convulsions 93, 94, 117
Genetic counselling
- prevention of CHD 58
Genetic factors 291
- asthma 154, 156
Genetic/family history
- diabetes 65
Geriatrics 277
German measles
- prevention of congenital heart disease (CHD) 59
Ghee
- blood cholesterol 79
Giddiness 141, 283
Gland/s 128, 266
- Prostate gland 177
Glandular swellings 2, 9
- enlargement 10, 268
Glomerulonephritis (GN) 191-199
- acute GN 192

- cause 191
- chronic GN 196
- how to suspect 195
- prognosis and treatment 195
- prophylaxis of GN 198
- subacute GN (nephrotic syndrome – NS) 193
- symptoms 191

Glucocorticoids 225

Glucose test
- fasting 61
- post challenge 62
- postprandial 61

Glucose tolerance test (GTT) 62, 297

Glyceryl trinitrate 26, 40

Goitre 221
- iodine deficiency goiter 221
- investigating a case of goitre and/or solitary nodule/s 221
- prophylaxis 222
- other causes of goitre 222
- toxic goiter 223
- *See also* 5, 223

Gonorrhoea 276

Gout
- acute attack 89
- high blood uric acid 86

Grand mal epilepsy 93, 95, 97

Graves' disease 223

Gray rat (rattus noryegicus) 263, 264

Green vegetables – cooked/salad 66

Group A-beta haemolytic streptococcus (GABHS) 44, 49,191

Gum
- oozing of blood from gums 9

Gynecomastia 17

Haematamesis 207
Haematuria 5
Haemoglobin (Hb.) 208, 296
Haemoptysis 134, 279
Haemorrhage 91, 304
- chronic renal failure 207
- gastric/duodenal ulcer 279
- plague 267
- scorpion sting 250

- stroke 90
- viper's bite 237

Haemorrhagic spots 9, 267

Hair-dyes
- asthma 155

Hallucinations
- of smell or taste 94

Head injury 100, 116, 298, 304

Headache
- recurrent 8
- with or without vomiting 2, 8

Hearing 94, 141

Heart attack 25-42
- diabetes 65
- female hormone 17
- high blood uric acid 84
- old age 278, 280,281
- *See also* 199, 200, 209, 250, 297, 299

Heart enlargement
- rheumatic fever (RF)/rheumatic heart disease (RHD) 48

Heart muscle
- damage 25, 32
- stress echocardiography 35
- thallium test 33
- viability 35

Hemiplegia 90, 250

Hepatitis 9
- alcoholic 289

Hereditary disease
- diabetes 63

Heredity 100, 101
- prevention of congenital heart disease (CHD) 58

Hernia 168

Hiccoughs 207

Hidden/occult/silent/symptomless/subclinical/undetected/concealed diseases/silent human killers
- appendicitis (old age) 279
- asthma 163
- chronic renal failure 197, 203, 206, 211
- congenital heart disease (detection) 56

Index

- coronary artery disease 21, 28, 33, 37
- diabetes 73, 207
- diseases of the kidneys 169
- gallbladder diseases 164
- glomerulonephritis (GN) subacute and chronic 192
- hyperactive thyroid gland 224
- hypertension (high blood pressure) 74, 78, 207
- Hypothyroidism (subclinical) 227
- malignancy 17
- pyelonephritis 173
- respiratory infection (old age) 279
- sore throat: rheumatic fever/ rheumatic heart disease (RF/ RHD) 49
- tuberculosis 126, 131, 133
- urinary tract infection 174, 190

High blood cholesterol 79-83
- harmful effects 81
- high density lipoprotein cholesterol (HDL-cholesterol) 82
- how to bring back normal levels 81
- low density lipoprotein cholesterol (LDL-cholesterol) 83
- source of cholesterol in blood/ body 79
- *See also* 27 29, 33, 36, 91, 196, 292, 294, 297, 310, 314

High blood pressure 74 -78
- *See also* 27, 29, 33, 38, 189, 292, 310
- *See also* hypertension

High blood sugar
- *See under* diabetes
- *See also* pages 29, 32, 33

High blood uric acid 84-89
- and syndrome X 88
- as a result of various diseases/ drugs 87
- control 86
- harm 86
- normal range of blood uric acid 86
- sources of uric acid in blood 84
- *See also* pages 27, 29, 33, 36, 91, 294, 297, 310, 312
- *See also* hyperuricaemia

High density lipoprotein (HDL) cholesterol 82, 291

High fibre diet
- cancer 20
- diabetes 66
- high blood pressure 77

Hoarse voice 1
- unusual hoarseness 2

Hoarseness of voice
- thyroid gland 5

Hoffkine's vaccine 271
Holter monitoring 32, 106
Holter test 110, 298
Homocyctein (Hcy) 39
Horseshoe kidneys 172, 177
- urinary tract infection (UTI) 181

Human immunodeficiency virus (HIV) 273
Hydatiform mole 7
Hydronephrosis 179
Hydroureters 179
Hyperactive thyroid gland *See under* (hyperfunction of thyroid gland) *See also* 221
Hypercholesterolaemia (*See under* high blood cholesterol)
- *See also* 194, 287
Hyperfunction of thyroid gland (also called hyperthyroidism/thyrotoxicosis/hyperactive/over active thyroid/toxic goiter 223-226
- *See under* diseases of the thyroid gland
Hyperglycaemia (*See under* diabetes)
- *See also* 230
Hypertension – (*See under* high blood pressure)
- *See also* 56, 65, 91, 119, 173, 182, 193, 209, 214, 217, 294, 314
- pulmonary 54
Hypertensive kidney 182
Hyperthyroidism (*See under* hyperfunction of thyroid gland)
- *See also* 279

- unusual manifestations (personal experience) 232
Hyperuricaemia - See high blood uric acid
- See also 209
Hypofunction of thyroid gland 226-231 (also called hypothyroidism/ myxoedema/underactive thyroid) - See under diseases of thyroid gland - subclinical hypothyrpidism and hypothyroidism
Hypoglycaemia 117, 230
Hypoproteinaemia 193, 194
Hypotension
- postural/orthostatic 283
Hysterical convulsions 104, 114
Hysteroscopy 299

Iatrogenic cases
- acute renal failure 199
Immature cells 10
Immunization
- rabies 244
Immunological disease
- rheumatic fever 44
Immunotherapy
- asthma 162
Impaired glucose tolerance test (IGT) 68
Impaired vision 8
Impotence
- diabetes 65
- hypothyroidism 229
Incubation period
- acquired immune deficiency syndrome (AIDS) 273
- rabies 243
- Tetanus 259
Indigestion (persistent) 1, 3
Indiscriminate use of drugs 199, 209
Industrial fumes
- asthma 154
Infantile paralysis 122
Infantile syncopal attacks 104
Infection - tuberculosis 130

Inflamed gallbladder/gallstone 1, 4
Inflammation
- anterior horn cells - in cases of poliomyelitis 120
- food-pipe (oesophagus) 30, 289
- gallbladder 30
- grey matter - in cases of poliomyelitis 120
- pancreas 30
- pleura (membrane covering the lungs) 30
- stomach or duodenum 30, 289
Inhaled steroids 161
Inhalers 160
- bronchodilators 161
Injury 103, 116
- birth injury 100
- burn injuries 308
- fractures 303
- head injury/ies 100, 116, 303
- head, spine, chest, abdomen, fractures and burn injuries 303
- minor 9
- of heart muscle 25
- tongue-bite 104
Insect debris in the environment
- asthma 155
Insect repellent oils/cream 271
Instructions for diabetics 69
Insulin
- self-insulin injection 69
- sites for taking insulin injections 68
Insulin-producing cells 65
Intensive care unit (ICU) 26, 294
Intercourse
- contact bleeding 6
Intermenstrual bleeding 6
Intestinal canal 170
Intestine 120, 137, 170
- haemorrhage 207, 279
- ulceration 207
Intestine of horses and other animals 256
Intravenous pyelography 177, 181, 185, 206
Intrinsic factors - asthma 154, 156

Index

Involuntary movements 8
Iodine 220
Iodine deficiency goitre 221, 222
Iron 282 (old age)
Ischaemic heart disease (IHD)
- *See under* coronary artery disease, *and also* 298
Islets of Langerhans 65
Isolated systolic hypertension (ISH) 281
Isoniazid 141, 144
Itching 209
- diabetes 65

Jacksonian epilepsy 93
Jaundice-pallor of eyes 2, 9,141,165
Jerky movements 44, 105
Jogging 315
Joints
- high blood uric acid 84
- RF (rheumatic fever) 43
- tuberculosis 137

Kernig's sign 138
Kidneys
- carcinoma 5
- failure 65, 100,190, 191, 199, 205 (renal failure), 206
- high blood pressure 74, 78
- high blood uric acid 87
- tests 296, 297
- tuberculosis 5, 129, 137
- ultrasonography 7
- urinary tract infection (UTI) 170, 175, 178, 182
Kidney function tests 296, 297
Kraits 235, 238
Krait's bite 237

Lactic dehydrogenase (LDH) 32
Laryngeal carcinoma 299
Laryngoscopy 2, 299
Larynx
- malignancy 2
- papiloma (benign)

- tetanus 260
- tuberculosis 2, 137
Late cyanotic cases of CHD 54
Lepromin skin test 272
Leprosy 272
- lepromatous 272
- tuberculoid type 272
Lethargic 227
Leukaemias 9, 296
- acute 9
- chronic 9
- high blood uric acid 87
Libido 229
Life-style
- childhood (prevention of coronary artery disease) 42
Lipids 297
- blood 17
Lipidogram 32, 297
Lithium
- prevention of CHD 59
Lithotripsy 176
Liver
- cancer 165, 289
- cirrhosis 165
- dialysis 166
- fatty change 289
- malignancy 9
- tests 296, 297
- transplant 166
- ultrasonography 7
Liver function tests 141, 296, 297
Lockjaw 258, 259
Loss of appetite 3, 4
- unexplained 2, 11, 134
Loss of memory 8
Loss of smell 8
Loss of speech 90
Loss of sweating
- diabetes 65
Loss of vision 90
- diabetes 65
- high blood pressure 74
Loss of weight 3, 4, 134, 224
- diabetes (sudden) 65
- thyroid hyperactivity 224
- unexplained 2, 11

Low defence mechanism 280
Low-fat diet 20
  - diabetes 66
Low-grade fever 134
  - prolonged 165
  - unexplained 2, 11
Low protein diet 218
Lucid interval 305, 306
Lump
  - abdomen (carcinoma of the kidney) 5
  - breast 1, 4, 13, 17
  - testes 1, 4, 13
Lungs
  - alveoli 127
  - bronchial asthma 151
  - cancer 2, 15, 287, 296, 298, 299
  - pleurisy 136
  - pleura – its inflammation 30
  - tuberculosis 2, 128, 296
  - uraemic (lungs) 208

Madness-myxoedema 230
Magnetic resonance imaging (MRI) 8, 65, 92, 99, 111, 202, 206, 223, 298
Malaena 207
Male breasts 17
  - carcinoma 18
Malignancy
  - abdomen 15
  - bile duct 9
  - brain 99
  - cervix 14
  - diseases of old age 279
  - gallbladder 9
  - kidneys 194
  - larynx 2
  - liver 9
  - pancreas 9
  - pleura 299
  - skin/oral cavity 8
  - thyroid gland 221, 222 (cancer)
Malignancy and use of female hormones 16
Malignant
  - brain tumour 87
  - cells – sputum 296
  - Growth/lump 298
  - Hypertension 200
  - pleural effusion 299
  - Tumour 87
Mammography 13, 299
Mania
  - myxoedema 230
Mantoux skin test 132, 135, 150
Mastectomy 18
Meats – high blood uric acid 84
Mediastinal glands 137
Medicolegal cases
  - lucid interval 306
Meningitis
  - tuberculosis 100, 137
Menopause 17, 282
Menorrhagia 229
Menstrual disturbance 229
Mental health
  - epilepsy 109
Mental/psychiatric disorders 225
Mental retardation 103, 231
Microalbuminuria 206
Multi-drug resistant tuberculosis (MDRT) 147

Nasal regurgitation 8
Nasal septum (perforation)
  - leprosy 272
National tuberculosis programme (NTP) 142, 147
Neck
  - cervical spondylosis 282
  - Glandular swelling (signals of cancer) 2, 9
  - Thyroid gland 219
  - Tuberculosis
    - glands of the neck 137
Needle biopsy
  - ultrasonographically guided needle biopsy of prostate 6
Neomercazole (carbimazole) 226
Nephrotic syndrome (NS) 193
Neuritis 141
Neuropathy 208 (chronic renal failure - CRF), 290 (alcoholic)

Index

Nicotine 287
Night sweat 134
Nipple
- bleeding or discharge 1, 4, 13
Nodule
- cancer of prostate 180
- cancer warning signals 8
- parotid gland 1, 5
- testes 1, 4
- thyroid gland 1, 5
Non-invasive test
- computed tomographic (CT) coronary angiogram 34
- computed tomographic (CT) scanning 110
- magnetic resonance imaging (MRI) 111
- stress echocardiography 35
- thallium stress test 33
Non-paralytic poliomyelitis 122
Non-pharmacological measures of
- lowering of hypertension 76
Non-vegetarian food/diet 79
Nose
- bleeding 9
Nutrition (old age) 282

Obese 292
- children – urgent tests 89
Obesity 27, 292, 314
Occult blood 14
- stools 296
- urine 296
Occult cases/diseases
- *See under* hidden diseases
Occult nature of diseases
- *See under* hidden diseases
Occupational diseases 130
Oedema-feet (nephrotic syndrome) 195
Oesophagus
- cancer/ulcer 287, 298
- carcinoma 3
- goiter – press the underlying oesophagus 222
- upper gastrointestinal (GI) endoscopy 7

Oesophagogastro-duodenoscopy (OGD) 167
Oestrogen 15, 19, 63
Old age – diseases 277
Old peoples' homes 286
Old scar 2, 8
Oligomenorrhoea 230
Oozing of blood
- gum 9
Operator-dependent 165
Oral cavity
- ulceration 8
Oral contraceptives 16, 28, 29, 37, 72, 76
Oral polio vaccine (OPV) 124
Oral steroids 161
Orthrostatic hypotension 283
Osteoarthritis 282, 292
Osteoporosis 282, 299
Out growing asthma 163
Overactive thyroid gland 223
- *See* hyperfunction of thyroid gland
Overcrowding 142
Overeating 313
Overweight 29, 37, 65, 77, 91, 292

Pain
- abdomen 1, 3
- anginal 23, 25
- chest 23, 25, 30, 134, 278
- heart attack 26
- joints (fleeting pain) – rheumatic fever 43
Painless swelling anywhere 4
Pallor of eyes (jaundice) 2, 9, 141,165
Palpitation 224
Pancreas
- diabetes 65
- magnetic resonance imaging (MRI) 65
- malignancy 9
- test 298
- ultrasonographic examination 65
Pancreatitis 30, 250
- acute and chronic 289, 290

Pap smear 14, 298
Papilloma (benign)
 - larynx 2
 - pelvis of the kidney 5
 - urinary bladder 5
Papilloedema 8
Paralysis 74, 90, 122, 281, 305, 306
Paresthesias
 - diabetes 65
Parotid gland
 - cancerous growth 5
 - swelling
Passive smoking 159, 288
Patent ductus arteriosus (PDA) 54
Patient with first seizure 113
Peak expiratory flow rate (PEFR) 157
Peak flow charts 162
Peak flow meter (PFM) 161
Pelvis of the kidney
 - papilloma (benign) 5
Pentalogy of Fallot
 - early symptoms/warning signals 53
Peptic ulcer 1, 3, 30
 - duodenum 287
 - gastric 287
Pericardial effusion 45 (RF), 229 (hypothyroidism)
Pericarditis – chronic renal failure (CRF) 208
Perineal hygiene 187
Peripheral blood film (PBF) 10, 296
Peripheral neuropathy 141
Peritonitis 168
Persistent headache 138
Persistent indigestion 1, 3
Persistently troublesome cough 1, 3
Petit mal epilepsy 93, 97,105
Pharynx
 - cancer 3, 287
Photic stimulation 109
Photosensitive epilepsy 117
Plague epidemic 263-271
 - early symptoms/warning signals 265
 - forecast 265
 - management 269

 - Pneumonic plague 267
 - prediction 269
 - prevention 269
 - rats transmit the disease 264
 - septicaemia of plague 267
 - tests 268
Pleura 136
 - inflammation 30
 - Malignancy 299
Pleural biopsy 299
Pleural cavity 136
Pleural effusion 136, 299
Pleural fluid 136
 - analysis 299
Pleurisy 136, 167, 298
Pleuritis 30
Poliomyelitis 120-124
 - age of the patient 122
 - incubation period 122
 - infection 120, 121
 - paralytic stage of poliomyelitis 122
 - signs and symptoms 122
 - treatment of poliomyelitis 123
 - vaccination 123
Poliovirus 120
Pollens – asthma 155
Polyunsaturated fats 79
Polyvalent anti-snake venom (ASV) 240
Porencephaly 110
Pork tapeworm (Taenia solium) 111
Postchallenge glucose test (2-hour) 62, 297
Postcoital voiding 188
Post-epileptic oedema 110
Postmenopausal/intermenstrual bleeding through vagina 6
Postmenopausal osteoporosis 282
Postprandial glucose test (2-hour) 61, 297
Post-streptococcal glomerulo-nephritis (PSGN) 191
Post-traumatic epilepsy 305
Post-traumatic porencephaly 305
Post-traumatic scarring 110
Postural hypotension 78, 108, 283

Index 333

Potassium
- high blood pressure 77

Prediabetes
- prevention of CHD 59

Prediabetics 60

Pregnancy/pregnant mother/woman
- acquired immune deficiency syndrome (AIDS) 275
- alcohol and diseases 289
- asthma 159
- congenital heart disease 58
- foetal echocardiography 59
- high blood pressure 76
- smoking and tobacco chewing 287
- tetanus 257

Pre-natal check-up 182

Prevention/prophylaxis
- abdomen diseases 164-168
- acute renal failure 203
- acquired immune deficiency syndrome (AIDS) 273, 275
- asthma 157-160
- cancer 1, 13, 19, 164, 223
- chronic renal failure 210
- congenital heart disease 58
- coronary artery disease 37
- diabetes - complications 66
- epilepsy 116
- glomerulonephritis 198
- heart damage (heart attack) 300
- high blood cholesterol 83
- high blood pressure 74 -78
- high blood uric acid 84 – 89
- iodine deficiency goiter 222
- osteoarthritis 282
- osteoporosis 282
- plague epidemic 265, 269
- poliomyelitis (vaccination) 123
- rabies (immunization) 244
- rheumatic fever/rheumatic heart disease RF/RHD 49
- scorpion-sting 253
- sexually transmitted diseases 276
- snake-bite 241

- stroke 91
- subacute bacterial endocarditis 57
- sudden cardiac death 294 -295
- tests 89, 296
- tetanus 261
- tuberculosis 14
- urinary tract infection (UTI) 187

Primary complex 128, 143

Primary infection – tuberculosis 128

Primary prevention – coronary artery disease (CAD) 37

Proctoscopy 14, 299

Prostate 171
- bone scan
- cancer 6, 14, 284
- family history 6
- magnetic resonance imaging (MRI) 6
- prostate acid phosphatase 6
- prostate specific antigen (PSA)
- ultrasonography 298
- urine examination 296
- *See also* benign enlargement of prostate

Prostate-specific antigen (PSA) 6, 297

Prostatic acid phosphatase 6, 297

Prostatitis 178

Protective devices-radiation 19

Protein – chronic renal failure (CRF) 210

Protein diet
- chronic renal failure (CRF) 218

Proteinuria 193

Psychogenic factors-asthma 154

Psychogenic seizures 104

Psychological aspects of diabetics 72

Psychological stress 163

Psychological symptoms
- unexplained 2, 8

Puberty goitre 220

Pulmonary function tests 157

Pulmonary hypertension 54

Pulmonary stenosis (PS) 52, 56

Pulmonary tuberculosis 2
- *See also* page 125

Pulse pressure 224, 22

Pulse polio immunisation programme (PPI) 12
Pus cells
- urine 172, 296
Pyelonephritis 17
Pyrexia of uncertain origin (PUO) 165

Rabid dog 241, 246
Rabies 241-248
- care of the wound 244
- immunisation 244
- prevention 247
- schedule of vaccination 245
- symptoms and signs 243
- treatment 247
- urgent steps after the bite 244
Radiation 19, 59
Radio-iodine therapy-thyroid gland 227
Radioisotope scanning 223, 299
Rats 263, 264
- sudden death 270
- wild/urban 269
Rat fleas (Xenopsylla cheopis) 263, 264
Rectum
- blood 4
- cancer 4, 7, 14
- sigmoidoscopy 7
Recurrent headache 8
Red blood cells (RBCs)
- stools 296
- urine 29
Refractory asthma 163
Refractory epilepsy 115
Rehabilitation
- after heart attack 41
Renal biopsy 185
Renal colic 176
Renal function tests
- high blood pressure 76
Renal hypertension 182, 197
Renal insufficiency 180
Renal (kidney) failure
- acute 199
- chronic 203

Renal osteodystrophy 208
Renal transplant 203
Renovascular hypertension 75
Residual paralysis 123
Residual urine 17
Resting electrocardiogram (ECG) 29
Retinae
- high blood pressure 76
Retinal detachment
- diabetes 6
- high blood pressure 74
Retrosternal
- pain in the centre of the chest 26
Reviving the heart 302
Rheumatic activity 45, 48
Rheumatic chorea 44, 45
Rheumatic fever (RF) and rheumatic heart disease (RHD) 42
- allergic response 44
- RF 42
- cause of RF 44
- diagnosis of RF 45
- early diagnosis vital 46
- RHD 47
- prognosis 47
- treatment of acute RF/RHD 48
- treatment of chronic RHD 49
- prophylaxis of RF/RHD 49
Right ventricle hypertrophy (RVH) 53
Ringing in the ears 8
Rupture of sinus of valsalva
- case 57
Russel's viper 235, 238

Safflower oil
- blood cholesterol 79
Salad
- green vegetables-diabetes 66
Salt intake
- high blood pressure 76
Saturated fat
- blood cholesterol 79
Saw-scaled viper 235, 238
Scar
- old 2, 8

Index

Scorpion antivenin 253
Scorpion-sting 248 – 255
- caution 250
- early signs, symptoms/warning signals 251, 252
- fatal symptoms and signs 249
- local care of sting 252
- preventive measures 253
- scorpion antivenin 253
- treatment 251
- types of scorpion, dangerous 248
Seasonal allergy 152, 159
Secondary prevention of CAD 40
Self-examination of the breasts 13
Self-examination of testes 13
Self-insulin injections 69
Senile osteoporosis 282
Serum alkaline phosphatase 297
Serum bilirubin 297
Serum cholesterol 79 (blood cholesterol), 297
Serum creatinine 141, 185, 197, 200, 209, 213, 297
Serum free T_4 (thyroxine or tetra-iodothyroninc) 299
Serum glutamic oxaloacetic transaminase (SGOT) 297
Serum glutamic pyruvic transaminase (SGPT) 297
Serum hepatitis 165
Serum uric acid (fasting) 297
Sex and CAD (coronary artery disease) 40
- secondary prevention of CAD 40
Sexually-transmitted diseases 276
Shavasana 77
Sigmoidoscope 167
Sigmoidoscopy 167
Signals/early symptoms
- cancers 1
- diabetes 65
- heart attack 26
- rheumatic fever 43
Silent diseases – *See under* hidden diseases
Silent human killer
- coronary artery disease (CAD) 21

- high blood pressure 78
- *See also* under hidden diseases
Skin tests - asthma 152, 157
Skull injury 116
Sleep apnea 292
Sleep deprivation electroencephalogram 109
Smell 8, 94
Smoke
- asthma 154
Smoking 19, 29, 63, 76, 78, 91, 222, 287, 294
- passive 288
Smoking and tobacco chewing-related diseases 287
Snake-bite 235-41
- anti-snake venom (ASV) and other measures 240
- ASV vaccine 241
- common poisonous snakes 235
- general preventive measures 241
- how is ASV prepared ? 240
- symptoms of snake-bite 23
- what should be done immediately after snake-bite? 239
Social stigma 98
Sonography
- transvaginal 14
Sore throat
- glomerulonephritis 198
- rheumatic fever/rheumatic heart disease 44, 45, 47
Soybean oil
- blood cholesterol 7
Spacehalers 160
Space-occupying lesions 100
Speech
- difficulty 8
- loss 90
Spino-cerebellar degeneration 233
Spleen
- enlargement 10
Sputum culture
- tubercle bacilli 135
Sputum examination
- for malignant cells 296

- for tubercle bacilli 296
Sputum laden with tubercle bacilli 126, 127
Sputum smears 139
Status asthmaticus 151, 161
Sterility 229
Sternal tenderness 10
Steroids- inhaled 161
Stokes-Adams attack 106
Stomach
- cancer/ulcer 298
- carcinoma/peptic ulcer 3
- haemorrhage 279
- ulceration 30, 207
- upper gastrointestinal (Gl) endoscopy 7
Stone
- calcium oxalate 176
- calcium phosphate 176
- gallbladder 30
- high blood uric acid 87
- urinary 176, 296
Stone analysis
- urinary stones 177
Stool
- blood 1,4
Stool examination
- for red blood cells (RBC)/occult blood 14, 296
Streptococcal infection-throat 44
Streptococcal vaccine
- rheumatic fever (RF)/rheumatic heart disease (RHD) 51
Stress
- echocardiography 35
- diabetes 72
- glucose tolerance test 62
- treadmill stress test (TMT) 33
Strip test
- Troponin I (TnI) 32
- Troponin T (TnT) 32
- testing of sugar in urine 62
Stroke 17, 65, 66, 74, 84, 90-93, 281, 284, 287, 290, 292, 298, 314
Subacute bacterial endocarditis 50
- prevention 57
Subacute glomerulonephritis 192

Subclinical hypothyroidism 227
- treatment 228
Sudden cardiac death (SCD) 294
Sudden fall
- epilepsy 104
- in cardiac output (syncope) 106
- in blood pressure (syncope) 106
Sugar
- urine (fasting and/or postprandial) 296
Sunlight 20
Surgery
- congenital heart disease (CHD) 56
- coronary artery disease (CAD) 25
- rheumatic heart disease (RHD) 49
- thyroid gland 227
Swallowing
- difficulty 3, 8, 259
Sweetener (artificial)
- diabetes 66
Swelling 110
- face 192
- feet 193
- glandular 2, 9
- joints 42, 45
- painless 4
- parotid gland 5
- testes 1, 4
- thyroid gland 5
Syncopal attacks 105
- infantile paralysis 104
Syncope 27, 105, 107, 108, 280, 283, 290
Syndrome X 88
Syphilis 276
Systolic hypertension 281

Takayasu arteritis 75
Tea 310
- high blood uric acid 84, 88
Teratogenic effect
- antiepileptic drugs (prevention of CHD – congenital heart disease) 59

Index

- on the foetus 113
- thalidomide 59

Testes
- cancer 4
- change in size 1, 4, 13
- gynecomastia 18
- lump/nodule 1, 4, 13
- self examination 13
- swelling or feeling of heaviness/ discomfort 1, 4
- ultrasonography 7
- undescended testes 4

Tests
- acute renal failure 202
- asthma 157
- bone densitometry (old age) 283
- for the detection of various common serious diseases 296
- hyperactive thyroid gland 225
- in elderly persons 285
- plague epidemic 268
- prevention of cancer 19
- Troponin I (TnI) 32, 299
- Troponin T (TnT) 32, 299
- urgent tests for the detection of common serious diseases 296
- urinary tract infection 183
- Viral markers for hepatitis ABCDE 166

Tetanus 255-262
- hospitalisation 260
- infection 256
- other clinical manifestations 259
- preventive measures 261
- tetanus breaks in wards 257
- tetanus spores 255
- types of wounds responsible

Tetanus toxoid 304
Tetraiodothyronine -T_4 220, 299
Tetralogy/pentalogy of Fallot 53
- early symptoms/warning signals 53

Thalidomide
- teratogenic effect (prevention of CHD) 59

Thallium stress test 33, 298

Thirst
- excessive-diabetes 65

Thrombosis 90-stroke
- coronary artery 25

Thyroid cancer
- test for detection 223
- prophylaxis 223

Thyroid function tests 225, 226
Thyroid gland 219-234
- cancer 222
- crisis 5
- hyperactive 223
- hyperfunction 223
- hypothyroidism 226
- overactive 223
- radio-iodine therapy 227
- surgery 227
- swelling/nodules 1, 5
- toxic goiter 223
- underactive 226

Thyroid stimulating hormone (TSH) 227, 299
Thyrotoxic crisis 225
Thyrotoxic myopathy 225
Thyrotoxicosis 223
Thyroxine 299
- tetraiodothyronine (T4) 220

Tinnitus 8
Tobacco-chewing 287, 294
Tongue-bite (epilepsy) 9
Tooth extraction
- bleeding 9

Tophi (uric acid) 86
Total leucocyte count (TLC) 296
Toxic goitre 223
Toxic thyroid 5
Tourniquet 308
- complications 239
- release 239
- snake-bite 239

Transitory fall in blood pressure 105
Transitory generalised convulsions 103
Transitory jerky movement 97, 103
Transient ischaemic attack (TIA) 91, 108
Transient spells of TIA 91

Transitory unconsciousness 27, 97, 104, 105, 108
Trans-rectal prostate sonography 180
Transurethral resection of the prostate (TURP) 181
Transvaginal sonography 14, 15
Traumatic epilepsy 116
Treadmill stress test (TMT) 33, 298
Tremors 8, 208, 224, 290
Tricuspid strenosis/regurgitation (TS/TR) 56
Triglycerides 83
Triiodothyronine – T3 220, 299
Tropical diseases 235
- Plague epidemic 263
- rabies 241
- scorpion-sting 248
- snake-bite 235
- tetanus 255
Troponin I (TnI) 32, 299
Troponin T (TnT) 32, 299
Tubercle bacilli 126, 128, 129, 135
Tuberculins 133
- test surveys 143
Tuberculin skin test 132
Tubercular lesion 132
Tuberculoma 100, 110
Tuberculosis 125-150
- acid-fast bacillus (AFB) 126
- antituberculosis treatment 139
- chest X-ray 135
- common drugs for tuberculosis 140
- defence mechanism of the body 129
- diagnosis 135
- dormant tubercle bacilli 129
- drug toxicity 141
- early symptoms 134
- efficacy of treatment 140
- ELISA test for tuberculosis 136
- extrapulmonary tuberculosis 137
- infection and clinical manifestations 130
- pleurisy 136
- prevention 142
- primary complex 128
- site of infection 129
- sputum examination for tubercle bacilli 135
- sputum culture for tubercle bacilli 135
- treatment 140
- tubercle bacilli 126
- tuberculin skin test 132
- tuberculin/Mantoux test 135
- tuberculous meningitis 137
- warning signals 134
- *See also* 2, 5, 9, 100, 110, 279, 296, 299
Tuberculous meningitis 100, 137
Tuberculous pleural effusion 299 (see Pleurisy) 136
Tumour
- brain 2, 7, 100
- uterus-fibroid 6
Twitchings 102, 105

Ulcer/ulceration
- food-pipe, stomach-ulceration 289
- gastric/duodenal-peptic ulcer 1, 3
- gastric/duodenal ulcer 279
- mouth - ulceration 207
- peptic ulcer 207
- skin ulcers - diabetes 65
- skin/mouth ulcers 2
- skin/oral cavity ulceration 8
- stomach or duodenum ulceration 30
- stomach ulceration 207
Ultrasonography/ultrasonographic examination
- abdomen 15
- acute renal failure (ARF) 202
- adrenal glands, urinary tract in high blood pressure cases 76
- cancers of kidneys, urinary bladder, uterus (most important being cervix), testes, liver, prostate, gall bladder 7
- chronic renal failure (CRF) 206

Index

- detection of subclinical disease of the abdomen 15, 164
- high blood pressure 76
- in various disorders 298
- operator dependent 165
- other predisposing/obstructive factors of urinary tract infection (UTI) 181
- pancreas-diabetes 65
- pleural effusion 136
- prevention of congenital heart disease (CHD) 58
- prostate 15, 179
- residual urine – benign enlargement of prostate (BEP) 179
- urinary stones 177
- urinary tract infection (UTI) 185
- uterus 17

Ultrasonographically guided needle biopsy
- prostate 6

Ultrasonologist 165

Unconsciousness
- diabetes 65
- epilepsy 97
- head injury 304
- stroke 90
- syncope 105
- transitory 27
- vaso-vagal syncope 105

Unexpected bleeding 2, 9

Unexplained
- loss of appetite 3, 11
- low-grade fever 2, 11
- loss of weight 2, 11
- psychological symptoms 2, 8

Unilateral deafness 8

Unstable angina 29

Unusually hoarse voice (hoarseness) 1

Upper gastrointestinal (GI) endoscopy 7, 298

Uraemia 208

Uraemic lung 208

Urethritis 178, 276

Urgent dietary measures for the prevention of common serious diseases 310-313

Urgent tests for the detection of various common serious diseases 296-299

Urgent tests
- in childhood 89

Urgent tips : first-aid for prevention/immediate control of some common serious diseases 300-309
- diabetic comma 303
- epilepsy 303
- heart attack 300
- injury to head, spine, chest, abdomen, fractures and burn injuries 303
- reviving the heart 302
- technique of reviving the heart 302

Uric acid-blood
- See high blood uric acid

Uric acid-stone 176

Urinary incontinence 284 (old age)

Urinary stones 176, 296

Urinary tract
- cancer 14

Urinary tract infection 170, 284, 296

Urinary tract infection (UTI) and catheter 189

Urinary tract infection (UTI) vaccine 190/191

Urine
- albumin- chronic renal failure (CRF) 206
- blood/RBC 1, 5, 14
- examination 296
- high blood pressure 76
- urinary tract infection 171

Urine culture 184

Uterus
- cancer/malignancy 6, 14
- fibroid tumour 6

Vaccine
- acquired immune deficiency syndrome (AIDS) 276
- anti-snake venom (ASV) 240, 241
- E.coli 190/191
- Haffkine's 271
- plague 271

- streptococcal- RF/RHD 51
- urinary tract infection (UTI) 190
Vaccination
- BCG 144
- hepatitis-B 166
- poliomyelitis 124
- rabies 245
- tetanus 261
Vaginal
- bleeding or discharge 2, 6
Vague aches/pains
- high blood uric acid 86
Vascular diseases
- stroke 28, 90
Vaso-vagal syncope 105
Vegetarian diet
- high blood uric acid
Ventricle septal defect (VSD) 52
Vertebro-basilar artery insufficiency 108
Vertigo 27, 91, 141, 280
Viral hepatitis 165
Viral markers for hepatitis ABCDE 166
Viper's bite 237
Vision
- double 8
- impaired 8
Visual-field defects 8
Voice
- unusual (hoarseness) 1, 2
Vomiting
- brain tumours 2, 7

Wall of the heart
- blood supply 24
Warning signals
- asthma 151
- cancers 1
- diabetes 65
- epilepsy 117
- heart attack 27
- hyperactive thyroid gland 224
- plague epidemic 265

- pneumonic plague 268
- rheumatic fever 43, 51
- scorpion-sting 252
- stroke 91
- tetanus 258, 262
- tetralogy/pentalogy of Fallot 53
- tuberculosis 134, 146
Wart 2, 8
Weakness
- in one of the limbs or of the limbs of the same side 8
Weather
- CAD 38
Weight
- body weight 17
- increase in weight of the body 28
Western blot test 275, 299
Wheat (whole)
- diabetes 66
Wheezing sound 151
Wild/urban rats 264, 269
- population 269
- trapped and killed 270
Wine
- high blood uric acid 84, 88
Withdrawal of alcohol 113
Withdrawal of antiepileptic drugs 116
Withdrawal of drug 113
World health organization (WHO) 139, 166
Worms infestations 120
Wound 304, 307
- responsible for causing tetanus 256

X-ray/s 15, 19, 32, 34, 59, 111, 131, 136, 143, 150, 157, 176, 185, 267, 279, 298
X-ray radiation 132

Yersinia pestis 263

Zyloric 89